Teen Health Series

Genetic Disorders
SOURCEBOOK

Fourth Edition

Health Reference Series

Fourth Edition

Genetic Disorders SOURCEBOOK

Basic Consumer Health Information about Heritable Disorders, Including Disorders Resulting from Abnormalities in Specific Genes, Such as Hemophilia, Sickle Cell Disease, and Cystic Fibrosis, Chromosomal Disorders, Such as Down Syndrome, Fragile X Syndrome, and Klinefelter Syndrome, and Complex Disorders with Environmental and Genetic Components, Such as Alzheimer Disease, Cancer, Heart Disease, and Obesity

Along with Information about the Human Genome Project, Genetic Testing and Privacy Concerns, the Special Needs of Children with Genetic Disorders, Current Research Initiatives, a Glossary of Terms, and a Directory of Resources for Further Help and Information

Edited by
Sandra J. Judd

Omnigraphics

P.O. Box 31-1640, Detroit, MI 48231

Bibliographic Note

Because this page cannot legibly accommodate all the copyright notices, the Bibliographic Note portion of the Preface constitutes an extension of the copyright notice.

Edited by Sandra J. Judd

Health Reference Series

Karen Bellenir, *Managing Editor*
David A. Cooke, MD, FACP, *Medical Consultant*
Elizabeth Collins, *Research and Permissions Coordinator*
Cherry Edwards, *Permissions Assistant*
EdIndex, Services for Publishers, *Indexers*

* * *

Omnigraphics, Inc.

Matthew P. Barbour, *Senior Vice President*
Kevin M. Hayes, *Operations Manager*

* * *

Peter E. Ruffner, *Publisher*

Copyright © 2010 Omnigraphics, Inc.

ISBN 978-0-7808-1076-1

Library of Congress Cataloging-in-Publication Data

Genetic disorders sourcebook : basic consumer health information about heritable disorders, including disorders resulting from abnormalities in specific genes ... / edited by Sandra J. Judd. -- 4th ed.
    p. cm. -- (Health reference series)
    Summary: "Provides basic consumer health information about disorders caused by gene and chromosome abnormalities and those with genetic and environmental components, genetic testing, treatment research, and guidance for parents of children with special needs. Includes index, glossary of related terms, and other resources"--Provided by publisher.
    Includes bibliographical references and index.
    ISBN 978-0-7808-1076-1 (hardcover : alk. paper) 1. Human chromosome abnormalities--Popular works. I. Judd, Sandra J.
    RB155.5.G455 2009
    616'.042--dc22

                                                                2009039792

∞

Printed in the United States

Table of Contents

Visit www.healthreferenceseries.com to view *A Contents Guide to the Health Reference Series*, a listing of more than 15,000 topics and the volumes in which they are covered.

Part III: Chromosome Abnormalities

Part IV: Complex Disorders with Genetic and Environmental Components

Part V: Genetic Research

Part VI: Information for Parents of Children with Genetic Disorders

Part VII: Additional Help and Information

Preface

About This Book

Genes provide the information that directs the human body's basic cellular activities. Research on the human genome has shown that the DNA sequences of any two individuals are 99.9 percent identical. That 0.1 percent variation, however, is profoundly important. It contributes to visible differences, like height and hair color, and also to invisible differences, such as increased risk for—or protection from—a myriad of diseases and disorders.

As medical researchers unlock the secrets of the human genome, they are learning that nearly all diseases have a genetic component. Some are caused by a mutation in a gene or group of genes. Such mutations can occur randomly or due to an environmental exposure. Other disorders are hereditary. These can be passed down from generation to generation within a family. Finally, many—perhaps most—genetic disorders are caused by a combination of small variations in genes operating in concert with environmental factors.

Genetic Disorders Sourcebook, Fourth Edition offers information on how genes work, and it and provides facts about the most common genetic disorders, including those that arise from mutations in specific genes—for example, muscular dystrophy, sickle cell anemia, and cystic fibrosis—as well as those arising from chromosomal abnormalities—such as Down syndrome and fragile X syndrome. A section on disorders with genetic and environmental components explains the hereditary components of such disorders as cancer, diabetes, mental illness, obesity, and addiction. Reports on current research initiatives provide detailed information on the newest breakthroughs in the causes and treatments of genetic disorders. The research also looks at strategies, like gene therapy and pharmacogenetics, that could radically change how we treat these disorders in the future. A section for parents of children with genetic disorders offers information about assistive technologies, educational options, transition to adulthood, and estate planning. Information about genetic counseling, prenatal testing, newborn screening, and preventing genetic discrimination is also provided. The book concludes with a glossary of genetic terms and a list of resources for additional help and information.

How to Use This Book

This book is divided into parts and chapters. Parts focus on broad areas of interest. Chapters are devoted to single topics within a part.

Part I: Introduction to Genetics provides basic information about how genes work, how they are inherited, and how changes in genes can affect health. It also includes information about genetic counseling, prenatal testing, and newborn screening, as well as a discussion of concerns regarding genetic discrimination.

Part II: Disorders Resulting from Abnormalities in Specific Genes describes disorders associated with the mutation or malfunction of a single gene or genes, including albinism, hemophilia and other blood clotting disorders, sickle cell anemia, dwarfism and other growth disorders, hereditary deafness, and muscular dystrophy. Information about the known causes of these disorders is provided, and treatment strategies are discussed.

Part III: Chromosome Abnormalities provides information about disorders caused by changes in the number or form of the chromosomes. These include Angelman syndrome, Down Syndrome and other trisomy disorders, Fragile X syndrome, and Klinefelter syndrome. Methods of diagnosis, treatment options, and strategies for living with the disorder are included for each.

Part IV: Complex Disorders with Genetic and Environmental Components describes the hereditary components of such disorders as Alzheimer disease, cancer, diabetes, mental illness, obesity, and heart disease. Reports on current research initiatives detail the latest breakthroughs in the research into the causes and treatment of these disorders and the potential for future preventative strategies.

Part V: Genetic Research details current insights into the human genome, and it provides information on how researchers hope to use those insights to prevent or treat genetic disorders in the future. Chapters on pharmacogenetics and nutrigenomics describe efforts to tailor medicine and diet to the individual. A chapter on gene therapy describes current efforts to develop a method of correcting defective genes.

Part VI: Information for Parents of Children with Genetic Disorders offers information about early intervention, assistive technology, and educational options to help parents meet the challenge of parenting a child with an inherited disability. Information on transition to adulthood and estate planning is also included.

Part VII: Additional Help and Information includes a glossary of terms related to genetics and a directory of resources offering additional help and support.

Bibliographic Note

This volume contains documents and excerpts from publications issued by the following U.S. government agencies: Centers for Disease Control and Prevention (CDC); Federal Trade Commission; Genetics Home Reference; Human Genome Project Information; National Cancer Institute (NCI); National Dissemination Center for Children with Disabilities (NICHCY); National Heart, Lung, and Blood Institute (NHLBI); National Human Genome Research Institute (NHGRI); National Institute of Arthritis and Musculoskeletal and Skin Diseases (NIAMS); National Institute of Child Health and Human Development (NICHD); National Institute of Diabetes and Digestive and Kidney Diseases (NIDDK); National Institute of General Medical Sciences (NIGMS); National Institute of Neurological Disorders and Stroke (NINDS); National Institute on Aging; National Institute on Alcohol Abuse and Alcoholism (NIAAA); National Institute on Deafness and other Communication Disorders (NIDCD); National Institute on Drug Abuse (NIDA); National Institutes of Health; National Women's Health Information Center (NWHIC); NIH Clinical Center; and the U.S. Department of Education.

In addition, this volume contains copyrighted documents from the following organizations and individuals: A.D.A.M., Inc.; American Liver Foundation; American Optometric Association; Cincinnati Children's

Hospital Medical Center; Columbia University Department of Surgery; Emory University School of Medicine/Department of Human Genetics; EP Global Communications; Genetic Science Learning Center; HealthDay/ScoutNews LLC; Howard Hughes Medical Institute; Johns Hopkins University Genetics and Public Policy Center; Mary Ann Liebert Publishers; Madisons Foundation; MAGIC Foundation; March of Dimes; Masonic Medical Research Laboratory; Jeffrey H. Minde; Michigan State University News; Missouri Department of Health and Senior Services; National Center on Secondary Education and Transition; National Craniofacial Association (FACES); National Marfan Foundation; National Urea Cycle Disorders Foundation; Nemours Foundation; New Zealand Dermatological Society; PACER Center; Prader-Willi Syndrome Association; PsychCentral; Simon Fraser University Public Affairs; Spastic Paraplegia Foundation; United Mitochondrial Disease Foundation; University of Iowa News Services; University of Maryland School of Medicine Office of Public Affairs; University of Michigan Health System; University of Virginia Inside UVA; Washington State Department of Health—Newborn Screening Program; and Wrightslaw.com.

Acknowledgements

Thanks go to the many organizations, agencies, and individuals who have contributed materials for this *Sourcebook* and to medical consultant Dr. David Cooke and document engineer Bruce Bellenir. Special thanks go to managing editor Karen Bellenir and permissions coordinator Liz Collins for their help and support.

About the Health Reference Series

The *Health Reference Series* is designed to provide basic medical information for patients, families, caregivers, and the general public. Each volume takes a particular topic and provides comprehensive coverage. This is especially important for people who may be dealing with a newly diagnosed disease or a chronic disorder in themselves or in a family member. People looking for preventive guidance, information about disease warning signs, medical statistics, and risk factors for health problems will also find answers to their questions in the *Health Reference Series*. The *Series*, however, is not intended to serve as a tool for diagnosing illness, in prescribing treatments, or as a substitute for the physician/patient relationship. All people concerned about medical symptoms or the possibility of disease are encouraged to seek professional care from an appropriate healthcare provider.

A Note about Spelling and Style

Health Reference Series editors use *Stedman's Medical Dictionary* as an authority for questions related to the spelling of medical terms and the *Chicago Manual of Style* for questions related to grammatical structures, punctuation, and other editorial concerns. Consistent adherence is not always possible, however, because the individual volumes within the *Series* include many documents from a wide variety of different producers and copyright holders, and the editor's primary goal is to present material from each source as accurately as is possible following the terms specified by each document's producer. This sometimes means that information in different chapters or sections may follow other guidelines and alternate spelling authorities. For example, occasionally a copyright holder may require that eponymous terms be shown in possessive forms (Crohn's disease *vs.* Crohn disease) or that British spelling norms be retained (leukaemia *vs.* leukemia).

Locating Information within the Health Reference Series

The *Health Reference Series* contains a wealth of information about a wide variety of medical topics. Ensuring easy access to all the fact sheets, research reports, in-depth discussions, and other material contained within the individual books of the series remains one of our highest priorities. As the *Series* continues to grow in size and scope, however, locating the precise information needed by a reader may become more challenging.

A Contents Guide to the Health Reference Series was developed to direct readers to the specific volumes that address their concerns. It presents an extensive list of diseases, treatments, and other topics of general interest compiled from the Tables of Contents and major index headings. To access *A Contents Guide to the Health Reference Series*, visit www.healthreferenceseries.com.

Medical Consultant

Medical consultation services are provided to the *Health Reference Series* editors by David A. Cooke, MD, FACP. Dr. Cooke is a graduate of Brandeis University, and he received his M.D. degree from the University of Michigan. He completed residency training at the University of Wisconsin Hospital and Clinics. He is board-certified in Internal Medicine. Dr. Cooke currently works as part of the University of Michigan

Health System and practices in Ann Arbor, MI. In his free time, he enjoys writing, science fiction, and spending time with his family.

Our Advisory Board

We would like to thank the following board members for providing guidance to the development of this series:

Dr. Lynda Baker, Associate Professor of Library and Information Science, Wayne State University, Detroit, MI

Nancy Bulgarelli, William Beaumont Hospital Library, Royal Oak, MI

Karen Imarisio, Bloomfield Township Public Library, Bloomfield Township, MI

Karen Morgan, Mardigian Library, University of Michigan-Dearborn, Dearborn, MI

Rosemary Orlando, St. Clair Shores Public Library, St. Clair Shores, MI

Health Reference Series *Update Policy*

The inaugural book in the *Health Reference Series* was the first edition of *Cancer Sourcebook* published in 1989. Since then, the *Series* has been enthusiastically received by librarians and in the medical community. In order to maintain the standard of providing high-quality health information for the layperson the editorial staff at Omnigraphics felt it was necessary to implement a policy of updating volumes when warranted.

Medical researchers have been making tremendous strides, and it is the purpose of the *Health Reference Series* to stay current with the most recent advances. Each decision to update a volume is made on an individual basis. Some of the considerations include how much new information is available and the feedback we receive from people who use the books. If there is a topic you would like to see added to the update list, or an area of medical concern you feel has not been adequately addressed, please write to:

Editor, *Health Reference Series*
Omnigraphics, Inc.
P.O. Box 31-1640
Detroit, MI 48231
E-mail: editorial@omnigraphics.com

Part One

Introduction to Genetics

Chapter 1

Genes and How They Work

Cells and DNA

What is a cell?

Cells are the basic building blocks of all living things. The human body is composed of trillions of cells. They provide structure for the body, take in nutrients from food, convert those nutrients into energy, and carry out specialized functions. Cells also contain the body's hereditary material and can make copies of themselves.

Cells have many parts, each with a different function. Some of these parts, called organelles, are specialized structures that perform certain tasks within the cell.

What is DNA?

DNA, or deoxyribonucleic acid, is the hereditary material in humans and almost all other organisms. Nearly every cell in a person's body has the same DNA. Most DNA is located in the cell nucleus (where it is called nuclear DNA), but a small amount of DNA can also be found in the mitochondria (where it is called mitochondrial DNA or mtDNA).

The information in DNA is stored as a code made up of four chemical bases: adenine (A), guanine (G), cytosine (C), and thymine (T). Human DNA consists of about three billion bases, and more than 99

Excerpted from "Cells and DNA" and "How Genes Work," *Genetics Home Reference*, a service of the U.S. National Library of Medicine, January 2, 2009 percent of those bases are the same in all people. The order, or sequence, of these bases determines the information available for building and maintaining an organism, similar to the way in which letters of the alphabet appear in a certain order to form words and sentences.

DNA bases pair up with each other, A with T and C with G, to form units called base pairs. Each base is also attached to a sugar molecule and a phosphate molecule. Together, a base, sugar, and phosphate are called a nucleotide. Nucleotides are arranged in two long strands that form a spiral called a double helix. The structure of the double helix is somewhat like a ladder, with the base pairs forming the ladder's rungs and the sugar and phosphate molecules forming the vertical sidepieces of the ladder.

An important property of DNA is that it can replicate, or make copies of itself. Each strand of DNA in the double helix can serve as a pattern for duplicating the sequence of bases. This is critical when cells divide because each new cell needs to have an exact copy of the DNA present in the old cell.

What is mitochondrial DNA?

Although most DNA is packaged in chromosomes within the nucleus, mitochondria also have a small amount of their own DNA. This genetic material is known as mitochondrial DNA or mtDNA.

Mitochondria are structures within cells that convert the energy from food into a form that cells can use. Each cell contains hundreds to thousands of mitochondria, which are located in the fluid that surrounds the nucleus (the cytoplasm).

Mitochondria produce energy through a process called oxidative phosphorylation. This process uses oxygen and simple sugars to create adenosine triphosphate (ATP), the cell's main energy source. A set of enzyme complexes, designated as complexes I–V, carry out oxidative phosphorylation within mitochondria.

In addition to energy production, mitochondria play a role in several other cellular activities. For example, mitochondria help regulate the self-destruction of cells (apoptosis). They are also necessary for the production of substances such as cholesterol and heme (a component of hemoglobin, the molecule that carries oxygen in the blood).

Mitochondrial DNA contains thirty-seven genes, all of which are essential for normal mitochondrial function. Thirteen of these genes provide instructions for making enzymes involved in oxidative phosphorylation. The remaining genes provide instructions for making molecules called transfer RNAs (tRNAs) and ribosomal RNAs (rRNAs), which are chemical cousins of DNA. These types of RNA help assemble protein building blocks (amino acids) into functioning proteins.

What is a gene?

A gene is the basic physical and functional unit of heredity. Genes, which are made up of DNA, act as instructions to make molecules called proteins. In humans, genes vary in size from a few hundred DNA bases to more than two million bases. The Human Genome Project has estimated that humans have between twenty thousand and twenty-five thousand genes.

Every person has two copies of each gene, one inherited from each parent. Most genes are the same in all people, but a small number of genes (less than 1 percent of the total) are slightly different between people. Alleles are forms of the same gene with small differences in their sequence of DNA bases. These small differences contribute to each person's unique physical features.

What is a chromosome?

In the nucleus of each cell, the DNA molecule is packaged into thread-like structures called chromosomes. Each chromosome is made up of DNA tightly coiled many times around proteins called histones that support its structure.

Chromosomes are not visible in the cell's nucleus—not even under a microscope—when the cell is not dividing. However, the DNA that makes up chromosomes becomes more tightly packed during cell division and is then visible under a microscope. Most of what researchers know about chromosomes was learned by observing chromosomes during cell division.

Each chromosome has a constriction point called the centromere, which divides the chromosome into two sections, or "arms." The short arm of the chromosome is labeled the "p arm." The long arm of the chromosome is labeled the "q arm." The location of the centromere on each chromosome gives the chromosome its characteristic shape, and can be used to help describe the location of specific genes.

How many chromosomes do people have?

In humans, each cell normally contains twenty-three pairs of chromosomes, for a total of forty-six. Twenty-two of these pairs, called autosomes, look the same in both males and females. The 23rd pair, the sex chromosomes, differs between males and females. Females

5

have two copies of the X chromosome, while males have one X and one Y chromosome.

How Genes Work

What are proteins and what do they do?

Proteins are large, complex molecules that play many critical roles in the body. They do most of the work in cells and are required for the structure, function, and regulation of the body's tissues and organs.

Proteins are made up of hundreds or thousands of smaller units called amino acids, which are attached to one another in long chains. There are twenty different types of amino acids that can be combined to make a protein. The sequence of amino acids determines each protein's unique three-dimensional structure and its specific function.

Proteins can be described according to their large range of functions in the body:

- **Antibody:** Antibodies bind to specific foreign particles, such as viruses and bacteria, to help protect the body.

- **Enzyme:** Enzymes carry out almost all of the thousands of chemical reactions that take place in cells. They also assist with the formation of new molecules by reading the genetic information stored in DNA.

- **Messenger:** Messenger proteins, such as some types of hormones, transmit signals to coordinate biological processes between different cells, tissues, and organs.

- **Structural component:** These proteins provide structure and support for cells. On a larger scale, they also allow the body to move.

- **Transport/storage:** These proteins bind and carry atoms and small molecules within cells and throughout the body.

How do genes direct the production of proteins?

Most genes contain the information needed to make functional molecules called proteins. (A few genes produce other molecules that help the cell assemble proteins.) The journey from gene to protein is complex and tightly controlled within each cell. It consists of two major

6

steps: transcription and translation. Together, transcription and translation are known as gene expression.

During the process of transcription, the information stored in a gene's DNA is transferred to a similar molecule called RNA (ribonucleic acid) in the cell nucleus. Both RNA and DNA are made up of a chain of nucleotide bases, but they have slightly different chemical properties. The type of RNA that contains the information for making a protein is called messenger RNA (mRNA) because it carries the information, or message, from the DNA out of the nucleus into the cytoplasm.

Translation, the second step in getting from a gene to a protein, takes place in the cytoplasm. The mRNA interacts with a specialized complex called a ribosome, which "reads" the sequence of mRNA bases. Each sequence of three bases, called a codon, usually codes for one particular amino acid. (Amino acids are the building blocks of proteins.) A type of RNA called transfer RNA (tRNA) assembles the protein, one amino acid at a time. Protein assembly continues until the ribosome encounters a "stop" codon (a sequence of three bases that does not code for an amino acid).

The flow of information from DNA to RNA to proteins is one of the fundamental principles of molecular biology. It is so important that it is sometimes called the "central dogma."

Can genes be turned on and off in cells?

Each cell expresses, or turns on, only a fraction of its genes. The rest of the genes are repressed, or turned off. The process of turning genes on and off is known as gene regulation. Gene regulation is an important part of normal development. Genes are turned on and off in different patterns during development to make a brain cell look and act different from a liver cell or a muscle cell, for example. Gene regulation also allows cells to react quickly to changes in their environments. Although we know that the regulation of genes is critical for life, this complex process is not yet fully understood.

Gene regulation can occur at any point during gene expression, but most commonly occurs at the level of transcription (when the information in a gene's DNA is transferred to mRNA). Signals from the environment or from other cells activate proteins called transcription factors. These proteins bind to regulatory regions of a gene and increase or decrease the level of transcription. By controlling the level of transcription, this process can determine the amount of protein product that is made by a gene at any given time.

How do cells divide?

There are two types of cell division: mitosis and meiosis. Most of the time when people refer to "cell division," they mean mitosis, the process of making new body cells. Meiosis is the type of cell division that creates egg and sperm cells.

Mitosis is a fundamental process for life. During mitosis, a cell duplicates all of its contents, including its chromosomes, and splits to form two identical daughter cells. Because this process is so critical, the steps of mitosis are carefully controlled by a number of genes. When mitosis is not regulated correctly, health problems such as cancer can result.

The other type of cell division, meiosis, ensures that humans have the same number of chromosomes in each generation. It is a two-step process that reduces the chromosome number by half—from forty-six to twenty-three—to form sperm and egg cells. When the sperm and egg cells unite at conception, each contributes twenty-three chromosomes so the resulting embryo will have the usual forty-six. Meiosis also allows genetic variation through a process of DNA shuffling while the cells are dividing.

How do genes control the growth and division of cells?

A variety of genes are involved in the control of cell growth and division. The cell cycle is the cell's way of replicating itself in an organized, step-by-step fashion. Tight regulation of this process ensures that a dividing cell's DNA is copied properly, any errors in the DNA are repaired, and each daughter cell receives a full set of chromosomes. The cycle has checkpoints (also called restriction points), which allow certain genes to check for mistakes and halt the cycle for repairs if something goes wrong.

If a cell has an error in its DNA that cannot be repaired, it may undergo programmed cell death (apoptosis). Apoptosis is a common process throughout life that helps the body get rid of cells it doesn't need. Cells that undergo apoptosis break apart and are recycled by a type of white blood cell called a macrophage. Apoptosis protects the body by removing genetically damaged cells that could lead to cancer, and it plays an important role in the development of the embryo and the maintenance of adult tissues.

Cancer results from a disruption of the normal regulation of the cell cycle. When the cycle proceeds without control, cells can divide without order and accumulate genetic defects that can lead to a cancerous tumor.

What are gene families?

A gene family is a group of genes that share important characteristics. In many cases, genes in a family share a similar sequence of DNA building blocks (nucleotides). These genes provide instructions for making products (such as proteins) that have a similar structure or function. In other cases, dissimilar genes are grouped together in a family because proteins produced from these genes work together as a unit or participate in the same process.

Classifying individual genes into families helps researchers describe how genes are related to each other. Researchers can use gene families to predict the function of newly identified genes based on their similarity to known genes. Similarities among genes in a family can also be used to predict where and when a specific gene is active (expressed). Additionally, gene families may provide clues for identifying genes that are involved in particular diseases.

Sometimes not enough is known about a gene to assign it to an established family. In other cases, genes may fit into more than one family. No formal guidelines define the criteria for grouping genes together. Classification systems for genes continue to evolve as scientists learn more about the structure and function of genes and the relationships between them.

Chapter 2

Genetic Mutations and Health

What is a gene mutation and how do mutations occur?

A gene mutation is a permanent change in the deoxyribonucleic acid (DNA) sequence that makes up a gene. Mutations range in size from a single DNA building block (DNA base) to a large segment of a chromosome.

Gene mutations occur in two ways: they can be inherited from a parent or acquired during a person's lifetime. Mutations that are passed from parent to child are called hereditary mutations or germline mutations (because they are present in the egg and sperm cells, which are also called germ cells). This type of mutation is present throughout a person's life in virtually every cell in the body.

Mutations that occur only in an egg or sperm cell, or those that occur just after fertilization, are called new (de novo) mutations. De novo mutations may explain genetic disorders in which an affected child has a mutation in every cell, but has no family history of the disorder.

Acquired (or somatic) mutations occur in the DNA of individual cells at some time during a person's life. These changes can be caused by environmental factors such as ultraviolet radiation from the sun, or can occur if a mistake is made as DNA copies itself during cell division. Acquired mutations in somatic cells (cells other than sperm and egg cells) cannot be passed on to the next generation.

Excerpted from "Mutations and Health," *Genetics Home Reference*, a service of the U.S. National Library of Medicine, January 2, 2009.

11

Mutations may also occur in a single cell within an early embryo. As all the cells divide during growth and development, the individual will have some cells with the mutation and some cells without the genetic change. This situation is called mosaicism.

Some genetic changes are very rare; others are common in the population. Genetic changes that occur in more than 1 percent of the population are called polymorphisms. They are common enough to be considered a normal variation in the DNA. Polymorphisms are responsible for many of the normal differences between people such as eye color, hair color, and blood type. Although many polymorphisms have no negative effects on a person's health, some of these variations may influence the risk of developing certain disorders.

How can gene mutations affect health and development?

To function correctly, each cell depends on thousands of proteins to do their jobs in the right places at the right times. Sometimes, gene mutations prevent one or more of these proteins from working properly. By changing a gene's instructions for making a protein, a mutation can cause the protein to malfunction or to be missing entirely. When a mutation alters a protein that plays a critical role in the body, it can disrupt normal development or cause a medical condition. A condition caused by mutations in one or more genes is called a genetic disorder.

In some cases, gene mutations are so severe that they prevent an embryo from surviving until birth. These changes occur in genes that are essential for development, and often disrupt the development of an embryo in its earliest stages. Because these mutations have very serious effects, they are incompatible with life.

It is important to note that genes themselves do not cause disease— genetic disorders are caused by mutations that make a gene function improperly. For example, when people say that someone has "the cystic fibrosis gene," they are usually referring to a mutated version of the CFTR gene, which causes the disease. All people, including those without cystic fibrosis, have a version of the CFTR gene.

Do all gene mutations affect health and development?

No; only a small percentage of mutations cause genetic disorders— most have no impact on health or development. For example, some mutations alter a gene's DNA base sequence but do not change the function of the protein made by the gene.

Often, gene mutations that could cause a genetic disorder are repaired by certain enzymes before the gene is expressed (makes a protein). Each cell has a number of pathways through which enzymes recognize and repair mistakes in DNA. Because DNA can be damaged or mutated in many ways, DNA repair is an important process by which the body protects itself from disease.

A very small percentage of all mutations actually have a positive effect. These mutations lead to new versions of proteins that help an organism and its future generations better adapt to changes in their environment. For example, a beneficial mutation could result in a protein that protects the organism from a new strain of bacteria.

What kinds of gene mutations are possible?

The DNA sequence of a gene can be altered in a number of ways. Gene mutations have varying effects on health, depending on where they occur and whether they alter the function of essential proteins. The types of mutations include:

- **Missense mutation:** This type of mutation is a change in one DNA base pair that results in the substitution of one amino acid for another in the protein made by a gene.

- **Nonsense mutation:** A nonsense mutation is also a change in one DNA base pair. Instead of substituting one amino acid for another, however, the altered DNA sequence prematurely signals the cell to stop building a protein. This type of mutation results in a shortened protein that may function improperly or not at all.

- **Insertion:** An insertion changes the number of DNA bases in a gene by adding a piece of DNA. As a result, the protein made by the gene may not function properly.

- **Deletion:** A deletion changes the number of DNA bases by removing a piece of DNA. Small deletions may remove one or a few base pairs within a gene, while larger deletions can remove an entire gene or several neighboring genes. The deleted DNA may alter the function of the resulting protein(s).

- **Duplication:** A duplication consists of a piece of DNA that is abnormally copied one or more times. This type of mutation may alter the function of the resulting protein.

- **Frameshift mutation:** This type of mutation occurs when the addition or loss of DNA bases changes a gene's reading frame. A reading frame consists of groups of three bases that each code for one amino acid. A frameshift mutation shifts the grouping of these bases and changes the code for amino acids. The resulting protein is usually nonfunctional. Insertions, deletions, and duplications can all be frameshift mutations.

- **Repeat expansion:** Nucleotide repeats are short DNA sequences that are repeated a number of times in a row. For example, a trinucleotide repeat is made up of three-base-pair sequences, and a tetranucleotide repeat is made up of four-base-pair sequences. A repeat expansion is a mutation that increases the number of times that the short DNA sequence is repeated. This type of mutation can cause the resulting protein to function improperly.

Can a change in the number of genes affect health and development?

People have two copies of most genes, one copy inherited from each parent. In some cases, however, the number of copies varies—meaning that a person can be born with one, three, or more copies of particular genes. Less commonly, one or more genes may be entirely missing. This type of genetic difference is known as copy number variation (CNV).

Copy number variation results from insertions, deletions, and duplications of large segments of DNA. These segments are big enough to include whole genes. Variation in gene copy number can influence the activity of genes and ultimately affect many body functions.

Researchers were surprised to learn that copy number variation accounts for a significant amount of genetic difference between people. More than 10 percent of human DNA appears to contain these differences in gene copy number. While much of this variation does not affect health or development, some differences likely influence a person's risk of disease and response to certain drugs. Future research will focus on the consequences of copy number variation in different parts of the genome and study the contribution of these variations to many types of disease.

Can changes in the number of chromosomes affect health and development?

Human cells normally contain twenty-three pairs of chromosomes, for a total of forty-six chromosomes in each cell. A change in the number of chromosomes can cause problems with growth, development, and function of the body's systems. These changes can occur during the formation of reproductive cells (eggs and sperm), in early fetal development, or in any cell after birth. A gain or loss of chromosomes from the normal forty-six is called aneuploidy.

A common form of aneuploidy is trisomy, or the presence of an extra chromosome in cells. "Tri-" is Greek for "three"; people with trisomy have three copies of a particular chromosome in cells instead of the normal two copies. Down syndrome is an example of a condition caused by trisomy. People with Down syndrome typically have three copies of chromosome 21 in each cell, for a total of forty-seven chromosomes per cell.

Monosomy, or the loss of one chromosome in cells, is another kind of aneuploidy. "Mono-" is Greek for "one"; people with monosomy have one copy of a particular chromosome in cells instead of the normal two copies. Turner syndrome is a condition caused by monosomy. Women with Turner syndrome usually have only one copy of the X chromosome in every cell, for a total of forty-five chromosomes per cell.

Rarely, some cells end up with complete extra sets of chromosomes. Cells with one additional set of chromosomes, for a total of sixty-nine chromosomes, are called triploid. Cells with two additional sets of chromosomes, for a total of ninety-two chromosomes, are called tetraploid. A condition in which every cell in the body has an extra set of chromosomes is not compatible with life.

In some cases, a change in the number of chromosomes occurs only in certain cells. When an individual has two or more cell populations with a different chromosomal makeup, this situation is called chromosomal mosaicism. Chromosomal mosaicism occurs from an error in cell division in cells other than eggs and sperm. Most commonly, some cells end up with one extra or missing chromosome (for a total of forty-five or forty-seven chromosomes per cell), while other cells have the usual forty-six chromosomes. Mosaic Turner syndrome is one example of chromosomal mosaicism. In females with this condition, some cells have forty-five chromosomes because they are missing one copy of the X chromosome, while other cells have the usual number of chromosomes.

Many cancer cells also have changes in their number of chromosomes. These changes are not inherited; they occur in somatic cells (cells other than eggs or sperm) during the formation or progression of a cancerous tumor.

Can changes in the structure of chromosomes affect health and development?

Changes that affect the structure of chromosomes can cause problems with growth, development, and function of the body's systems.

These changes can affect many genes along the chromosome and disrupt the proteins made from those genes.

Structural changes can occur during the formation of egg or sperm cells, in early fetal development, or in any cell after birth. Pieces of DNA can be rearranged within one chromosome or transferred between two or more chromosomes. The effects of structural changes depend on their size and location, and whether any genetic material is gained or lost. Some changes cause medical problems, while others may have no effect on a person's health.

Changes in chromosome structure include the following:

- **Translocations:** A translocation occurs when a piece of one chromosome breaks off and attaches to another chromosome. This type of rearrangement is described as balanced if no genetic material is gained or lost in the cell. If there is a gain or loss of genetic material, the translocation is described as unbalanced.

- **Deletions:** Deletions occur when a chromosome breaks and some genetic material is lost. Deletions can be large or small, and can occur anywhere along a chromosome.

- **Duplications:** Duplications occur when part of a chromosome is copied (duplicated) too many times. This type of chromosomal change results in extra copies of genetic material from the duplicated segment.

- **Inversions:** An inversion involves the breakage of a chromosome in two places; the resulting piece of DNA is reversed and reinserted into the chromosome. Genetic material may or may not be lost as a result of the chromosome breaks. An inversion that involves the chromosome's constriction point (centromere) is called a pericentric inversion. An inversion that occurs in the long (q) arm or short (p) arm and does not involve the centromere is called a paracentric inversion.

- **Isochromosomes:** An isochromosome is a chromosome with two identical arms. Instead of one long (q) arm and one short (p) arm, an isochromosome has two long arms or two short arms. As a result, these abnormal chromosomes have an extra copy of some genes and are missing copies of other genes.

- **Dicentric chromosomes:** Unlike normal chromosomes, which have a single constriction point (centromere), a dicentric chromosome contains two centromeres. Dicentric chromosomes result from the abnormal fusion of two chromosome pieces, each of which includes a centromere. These structures are unstable and often involve a loss of some genetic material.

- **Ring chromosomes:** Ring chromosomes usually occur when a chromosome breaks in two places and the ends of the chromosome arms fuse together to form a circular structure. The ring may or may not include the chromosome's constriction point (centromere). In many cases, genetic material near the ends of the chromosome is lost.

Additionally, as was noted earlier, changes in chromosome structure also occur in many types of cancer cells. These changes happen when a cancerous tumor is formed or as it grows. Cancerous changes differ from inherited changes.

Can changes in mitochondrial DNA affect health and development?

Mitochondria are structures within cells that convert the energy from food into a form that cells can use. Although most DNA is packaged in chromosomes within the nucleus, mitochondria also have a small amount of their own DNA (known as mitochondrial DNA or mtDNA). In some cases, inherited changes in mitochondrial DNA can cause problems with growth, development, and function of the body's systems. These mutations disrupt the mitochondria's ability to generate energy efficiently for the cell.

Conditions caused by mutations in mitochondrial DNA often involve multiple organ systems. The effects of these conditions are most pronounced in organs and tissues that require a lot of energy (such as the heart, brain, and muscles). Although the health consequences of inherited mitochondrial DNA mutations vary widely, frequently observed features include muscle weakness and wasting, problems with movement, diabetes, kidney failure, heart disease, loss of intellectual functions (dementia), hearing loss, and abnormalities involving the eyes and vision.

Mitochondrial DNA is also prone to noninherited (somatic) mutations. Somatic mutations occur in the DNA of certain cells during a person's lifetime, and typically are not passed to future generations. Because mitochondrial DNA has a limited ability to repair itself when it is damaged, these mutations tend to build up over time. A buildup of somatic mutations in mitochondrial DNA has been associated with some forms of cancer and an increased risk of certain age-related disorders such as heart disease, Alzheimer disease, and Parkinson disease.

Additionally, research suggests that the progressive accumulation of these mutations over a person's lifetime may play a role in the normal process of aging.

What are complex or multifactorial disorders?

Researchers are learning that nearly all conditions and diseases have a genetic component. Some disorders, such as sickle cell anemia and cystic fibrosis, are caused by mutations in a single gene. The causes of many other disorders, however, are much more complex. Common medical problems such as heart disease, diabetes, and obesity do not have a single genetic cause—they are likely associated with the effects of multiple genes in combination with lifestyle and environmental factors. Conditions caused by many contributing factors are called complex or multifactorial disorders.

Although complex disorders often cluster in families, they do not have a clear-cut pattern of inheritance. This makes it difficult to determine a person's risk of inheriting or passing on these disorders. Complex disorders are also difficult to study and treat because the specific factors that cause most of these disorders have not yet been identified. By 2010, however, researchers predict they will have found the major contributing genes for many common complex disorders.

What information about a genetic condition can statistics provide?

Statistical data can provide general information about how common a condition is, how many people have the condition, or how likely it is that a person will develop the condition. Statistics are not personalized, however—they offer estimates based on groups of people. By taking into account a person's family history, medical history, and other factors, a genetics professional can help interpret what statistics mean for a particular patient.

Chapter 3

Genetic Inheritance

What does it mean if a disorder seems to run in my family?

A particular disorder might be described as "running in a family" if more than one person in the family has the condition. Some disorders that affect multiple family members are caused by gene mutations, which can be inherited (passed down from parent to child). Other conditions that appear to run in families are not caused by mutations in single genes. Instead, environmental factors such as dietary habits or a combination of genetic and environmental factors are responsible for these disorders.

It is not always easy to determine whether a condition in a family is inherited. A genetics professional can use a person's family history (a record of health information about a person's immediate and extended family) to help determine whether a disorder has a genetic component. He or she will ask about the health of people from several generations of the family, usually first-, second-, and third-degree relatives:

- **First-degree relatives:** Parents, children, brothers, and sisters
- **Second-degree relatives:** Grandparents, aunts and uncles, nieces and nephews, and grandchildren
- **Third-degree relatives:** First cousins

Excerpted from "Inheriting Genetic Conditions," *Genetics Home Reference*, a service of the U.S. National Library of Medicine, January 12, 2009.

Why is it important to know my family medical history?

A family medical history is a record of health information about a person and his or her close relatives. A complete record includes information from three generations of relatives, including children, brothers and sisters, parents, aunts and uncles, nieces and nephews, grandparents, and cousins.

Families have many factors in common, including their genes, environment, and lifestyle. Together, these factors can give clues to medical conditions that may run in a family. By noticing patterns of disorders among relatives, healthcare professionals can determine whether an individual, other family members, or future generations may be at an increased risk of developing a particular condition.

A family medical history can identify people with a higher-than-usual chance of having common disorders, such as heart disease, high blood pressure, stroke, certain cancers, and diabetes. These complex disorders are influenced by a combination of genetic factors, environmental conditions, and lifestyle choices. A family history also can provide information about the risk of rarer conditions caused by mutations in a single gene, such as cystic fibrosis and sickle cell anemia.

While a family medical history provides information about the risk of specific health concerns, having relatives with a medical condition does not mean that an individual will definitely develop that condition. On the other hand, a person with no family history of a disorder may still be at risk of developing that disorder.

Knowing one's family medical history allows a person to take steps to reduce his or her risk. For people at an increased risk of certain cancers, healthcare professionals may recommend more frequent screening (such as mammography or colonoscopy) starting at an earlier age. Healthcare providers may also encourage regular checkups or testing for people with a medical condition that runs in their family. Additionally, lifestyle changes such as adopting a healthier diet, getting regular exercise, and quitting smoking help many people lower their chances of developing heart disease and other common illnesses.

The easiest way to get information about family medical history is to talk to relatives about their health. Have they had any medical problems, and when did they occur? A family gathering could be a good time to discuss these issues. Additionally, obtaining medical records and other documents (such as obituaries and death certificates) can help complete a family medical history. It is important to keep this information up-to-date and to share it with a healthcare professional regularly.

What are the different ways in which a genetic condition can be inherited?

Some genetic conditions are caused by mutations in a single gene. These conditions are usually inherited in one of several straightforward patterns, depending on the gene involved:

- **Autosomal dominant:** One mutated copy of the gene in each cell is sufficient for a person to be affected by an autosomal dominant disorder. Each affected person usually has one affected parent. Autosomal dominant disorders tend to occur in every generation of an affected family.

- **Autosomal recessive:** Two mutated copies of the gene are present in each cell when a person has an autosomal recessive disorder. An affected person usually has unaffected parents who each carry a single copy of the mutated gene (and are referred to as carriers). Autosomal recessive disorders are typically not seen in every generation of an affected family.

- **X-linked dominant:** X-linked dominant disorders are caused by mutations in genes on the X chromosome. Females are more frequently affected than males, and the chance of passing on an X-linked dominant disorder differs between men and women. Families with an X-linked dominant disorder often have both affected males and affected females in each generation. A striking characteristic of X-linked inheritance is that fathers cannot pass X-linked traits to their sons (no male-to-male transmission).

- **X-linked recessive:** X-linked recessive disorders are also caused by mutations in genes on the X chromosome. Males are more frequently affected than females, and the chance of passing on the disorder differs between men and women. Families with an X-linked recessive disorder often have affected males, but rarely affected females, in each generation. A striking characteristic of X-linked inheritance is that fathers cannot pass X-linked traits to their sons (no male-to-male transmission).

- **Codominant:** In codominant inheritance, two different versions (alleles) of a gene can be expressed, and each version makes a slightly different protein. Both alleles influence the genetic trait or determine the characteristics of the genetic condition.

- **Mitochondrial:** This type of inheritance, also known as maternal inheritance, applies to genes in mitochondrial DNA. Mitochondria, which are structures in each cell that convert molecules into energy, each contain a small amount of DNA. Because only egg cells contribute mitochondria to the developing embryo, only females can pass on mitochondrial conditions to their children. Mitochondrial disorders can appear in every generation of a family and can affect both males and females, but fathers do not pass mitochondrial traits to their children.

Many other disorders are caused by a combination of the effects of multiple genes or by interactions between genes and the environment. Such disorders are more difficult to analyze because their genetic causes are often unclear, and they do not follow the patterns of inheritance described above. Examples of conditions caused by multiple genes or gene/environment interactions include heart disease, diabetes, schizophrenia, and certain types of cancer.

If a genetic disorder runs in my family, what are the chances that my children will have the condition?

When a genetic disorder is diagnosed in a family, family members often want to know the likelihood that they or their children will develop the condition. This can be difficult to predict in some cases because many factors influence a person's chances of developing a genetic condition. One important factor is how the condition is inherited. For example:

- **Autosomal dominant inheritance:** A person affected by an autosomal dominant disorder has a 50 percent chance of passing the mutated gene to each child. The chance that a child will not inherit the mutated gene is also 50 percent.

- **Autosomal recessive inheritance:** Two unaffected people who each carry one copy of the mutated gene for an autosomal recessive disorder (carriers) have a 25 percent chance with each pregnancy of having a child affected by the disorder. The chance with each pregnancy of having an unaffected child who is a carrier of the disorder is 50 percent, and the chance that a child will not have the disorder and will not be a carrier is 25 percent.

- **X-linked dominant inheritance:** The chance of passing on an X-linked dominant condition differs between men and women because men have one X chromosome and one Y chromosome, while women have two X chromosomes. A man passes on his Y chromosome to all of his sons and his X chromosome to all of his daughters. Therefore, the sons of a man with an X-linked dominant disorder will not be affected, but all of his daughters will inherit the condition. A woman passes on one or the other of her X chromosomes to each child. Therefore, a woman with an X-linked dominant disorder has a 50 percent chance of having an affected daughter or son with each pregnancy.

- **X-linked recessive inheritance:** Because of the difference in sex chromosomes, the probability of passing on an X-linked recessive disorder also differs between men and women. The sons of a man with an X-linked recessive disorder will not be affected, and his daughters will carry one copy of the mutated gene. With each pregnancy, a woman who carries an X-linked recessive disorder has a 50 percent chance of having sons who are affected and a 50 percent chance of having daughters who carry one copy of the mutated gene.

- **Codominant inheritance:** In codominant inheritance, each parent contributes a different version of a particular gene, and both versions influence the resulting genetic trait. The chance of developing a genetic condition with codominant inheritance, and the characteristic features of that condition, depend on which versions of the gene are passed from parents to their child.

- **Mitochondrial inheritance:** Mitochondria, which are the energy-producing centers inside cells, each contain a small amount of DNA. Disorders with mitochondrial inheritance result from mutations in mitochondrial DNA. Although mitochondrial disorders can affect both males and females, only females can pass mutations in mitochondrial DNA to their children. A woman with a disorder caused by changes in mitochondrial DNA will pass the mutation to all of her daughters and sons, but the children of a man with such a disorder will not inherit the mutation.

It is important to note that the chance of passing on a genetic condition applies equally to each pregnancy. For example, if a couple has a child with an autosomal recessive disorder, the chance of having another child with the disorder is still 25 percent (or 1 in 4). Having one child with a disorder does not "protect" future children from inheriting the condition. Conversely, having a child without the condition does not mean that future children will definitely be affected.

Although the chances of inheriting a genetic condition appear straightforward, factors such as a person's family history and the results of genetic testing can sometimes modify those chances. In addition, some people with a disease-causing mutation never develop any health problems or may experience only mild symptoms of the disorder. If a disease that runs in a family does not have a clear-cut inheritance pattern, predicting the likelihood that a person will develop the condition can be particularly difficult.

Estimating the chance of developing or passing on a genetic disorder can be complex. Genetics professionals can help people understand these chances and help them make informed decisions about their health.

What are reduced penetrance and variable expressivity?

Reduced penetrance and variable expressivity are factors that influence the effects of particular genetic changes. These factors usually affect disorders that have an autosomal dominant pattern of inheritance, although they are occasionally seen in disorders with an autosomal recessive inheritance pattern.

Reduced penetrance: Penetrance refers to the proportion of people with a particular genetic change (such as a mutation in a specific gene) who exhibit signs and symptoms of a genetic disorder. If some people with the mutation do not develop features of the disorder, the condition is said to have reduced (or incomplete) penetrance. Reduced penetrance often occurs with familial cancer syndromes. For example, many people with a mutation in the BRCA1 or BRCA2 gene will develop cancer during their lifetime, but some people will not. Doctors cannot predict which people with these mutations will develop cancer or when the tumors will develop.

Reduced penetrance probably results from a combination of genetic, environmental, and lifestyle factors, many of which are unknown. This phenomenon can make it challenging for genetics professionals to interpret a person's family medical history and predict the risk of passing a genetic condition to future generations.

Variable expressivity: Although some genetic disorders exhibit little variation, most have signs and symptoms that differ among affected individuals. Variable expressivity refers to the range of signs and symptoms that can occur in different people with the same genetic condition. For example, the features of Marfan syndrome vary widely—some people have only mild symptoms (such as being tall and thin with long, slender fingers), while others also experience life-threatening complications involving the heart and blood vessels. Although the features are highly variable, most people with this disorder have a mutation in the same gene (FBN1).

As with reduced penetrance, variable expressivity is probably caused by a combination of genetic, environmental, and lifestyle factors, most of which have not been identified. If a genetic condition has highly variable signs and symptoms, it may be challenging to diagnose.

What do geneticists mean by anticipation?

The signs and symptoms of some genetic conditions tend to become more severe and appear at an earlier age as the disorder is passed from one generation to the next. This phenomenon is called anticipation. Anticipation is most often seen with certain genetic disorders of the nervous system, such as Huntington disease, myotonic dystrophy, and fragile X syndrome.

Anticipation typically occurs with disorders that are caused by an unusual type of mutation called a trinucleotide repeat expansion. A trinucleotide repeat is a sequence of three DNA building blocks (nucleotides) that is repeated a number of times in a row. DNA segments with an abnormal number of these repeats are unstable and prone to errors during cell division. The number of repeats can change as the gene is passed from parent to child. If the number of repeats increases, it is known as a trinucleotide repeat expansion. In some cases, the trinucleotide repeat may expand until the gene stops functioning normally. This expansion causes the features of some disorders to become more severe with each successive generation.

Most genetic disorders have signs and symptoms that differ among affected individuals, including affected people in the same family. Not all of these differences can be explained by anticipation. A combination of genetic, environmental, and lifestyle factors is probably responsible for the variability, although many of these factors have not been identified. Researchers study multiple generations of affected family members and consider the genetic cause of a disorder before determining that it shows anticipation.

What are genomic imprinting and uniparental disomy?

Genomic imprinting and uniparental disomy are factors that influence how some genetic conditions are inherited.

Genomic imprinting: People inherit two copies of their genes—one from their mother and one from their father. Usually both copies of each gene are active, or "turned on," in cells. In some cases, however, only one of the two copies is normally turned on. Which copy is active depends on the parent of origin: some genes are normally active only when they are inherited from a person's father; others are active only when inherited from a person's mother. This phenomenon is known as genomic imprinting.

In genes that undergo genomic imprinting, the parent of origin is often marked, or "stamped," on the gene during the formation of egg and sperm cells. This stamping process, called methylation, is a chemical reaction that attaches small molecules called methyl groups to certain segments of DNA. These molecules identify which copy of a gene was inherited from the mother and which was inherited from the father. The addition and removal of methyl groups can be used to control the activity of genes.

Only a small percentage of all human genes undergo genomic imprinting. Researchers are not yet certain why some genes are imprinted and others are not. They do know that imprinted genes tend to cluster together in the same regions of chromosomes. Two major clusters of imprinted genes have been identified in humans, one on the short (p) arm of chromosome 11 (at position 11p15) and another on the long (q) arm of chromosome 15 (in the region 15q11 to 15q13).

Uniparental disomy: Uniparental disomy (UPD) occurs when a person receives two copies of a chromosome, or part of a chromosome, from one parent and no copies from the other parent. UPD can occur as a random event during the formation of egg or sperm cells or may happen in early fetal development.

In many cases, UPD likely has no effect on health or development. Because most genes are not imprinted, it doesn't matter if a person inherits both copies from one parent instead of one copy from each parent. In some cases, however, it does make a difference whether a gene is inherited from a person's mother or father. A person with UPD may lack any active copies of essential genes that undergo genomic imprinting. This loss of gene function can lead to delayed development, mental retardation, or other medical problems.

Several genetic disorders can result from UPD or a disruption of normal genomic imprinting. The most well-known conditions include Prader-Willi syndrome, which is characterized by uncontrolled eating and obesity, and Angelman syndrome, which causes mental retardation and impaired speech. Both of these disorders can be caused by UPD or other errors in imprinting involving genes on the long arm of chromosome 15. Other conditions, such as Beckwith-Wiedemann syndrome (a disorder characterized by accelerated growth and an increased risk of cancerous tumors), are associated with abnormalities of imprinted genes on the short arm of chromosome 11.

Are chromosomal disorders inherited?

Although it is possible to inherit some types of chromosomal abnormalities, most chromosomal disorders (such as Down syndrome and Turner syndrome) are not passed from one generation to the next.

Some chromosomal conditions are caused by changes in the number of chromosomes. These changes are not inherited, but occur as random events during the formation of reproductive cells (eggs and sperm). An error in cell division called nondisjunction results in reproductive cells with an abnormal number of chromosomes. For example, a reproductive cell may accidentally gain or lose one copy of a chromosome. If one of these atypical reproductive cells contributes to the genetic makeup of a child, the child will have an extra or missing chromosome in each of the body's cells.

Changes in chromosome structure can also cause chromosomal disorders. Some changes in chromosome structure can be inherited, while others occur as random accidents during the formation of reproductive cells or in early fetal development. Because the inheritance of these changes can be complex, people concerned about this type of chromosomal abnormality may want to talk with a genetics professional.

Some cancer cells also have changes in the number or structure of their chromosomes. Because these changes occur in somatic cells (cells other than eggs and sperm), they cannot be passed from one generation to the next.

Why are some genetic conditions more common in particular ethnic groups?

Some genetic disorders are more likely to occur among people who trace their ancestry to a particular geographic area. People in an ethnic group often share certain versions of their genes, which have been passed down from common ancestors. If one of these shared genes contains a disease-causing mutation, a particular genetic disorder may be more frequently seen in the group.

Examples of genetic conditions that are more common in particular ethnic groups are sickle cell anemia, which is more common in people of African, African-American, or Mediterranean heritage; and Tay-Sachs disease, which is more likely to occur among people of

Ashkenazi (eastern and central European) Jewish or French Canadian ancestry. It is important to note, however, that these disorders can occur in any ethnic group.

Chapter 4

Genetic Counseling

What is a genetic consultation?

A genetic consultation is a health service that provides information and support to people who have, or may be at risk for, genetic disorders. During a consultation, a genetics professional meets with an individual or family to discuss genetic risks or to diagnose, confirm, or rule out a genetic condition.

Genetics professionals include medical geneticists (doctors who specialize in genetics) and genetic counselors (certified healthcare workers with experience in medical genetics and counseling). Other healthcare professionals such as nurses, psychologists, and social workers trained in genetics can also provide genetic consultations.

Consultations usually take place in a doctor's office, hospital, genetics center, or other type of medical center. These meetings are most often in-person visits with individuals or families, but they are occasionally conducted in a group or over the telephone.

Why might someone have a genetic consultation?

Individuals or families who are concerned about an inherited condition may benefit from a genetic consultation. The reasons that a person might be referred to a genetic counselor, medical geneticist, or other genetics professional include the following:

Excerpted from "Genetic Consultation," *Genetics Home Reference*, a service of the U.S. National Library of Medicine, January 12, 2009.

- A personal or family history of a genetic condition, birth defect, chromosomal disorder, or hereditary cancer

- Two or more pregnancy losses (miscarriages), a stillbirth, or a baby who died

- A child with a known inherited disorder, a birth defect, mental retardation, or developmental delay

- A woman who is pregnant or plans to become pregnant at or after age 35 (some chromosomal disorders occur more frequently in children born to older women)

- Abnormal test results that suggest a genetic or chromosomal condition

- An increased risk of developing or passing on a particular genetic disorder on the basis of a person's ethnic background

- People related by blood (for example, cousins) who plan to have children together (a child whose parents are related may be at an increased risk of inheriting certain genetic disorders)

A genetic consultation is also an important part of the decision-making process for genetic testing. A visit with a genetics professional may be helpful even if testing is not available for a specific condition, however.

What happens during a genetic consultation?

A genetic consultation provides information, offers support, and addresses a patient's specific questions and concerns. To help determine whether a condition has a genetic component, a genetics professional asks about a person's medical history and takes a detailed family history (a record of health information about a person's immediate and extended family). The genetics professional may also perform a physical examination and recommend appropriate tests.

If a person is diagnosed with a genetic condition, the genetics professional provides information about the diagnosis, how the condition is inherited, the chance of passing the condition to future generations, and the options for testing and treatment.

During a consultation, a genetics professional will do the following things:

- Interpret and communicate complex medical information

- Help each person make informed, independent decisions about their health care and reproductive options

- Respect each person's individual beliefs, traditions, and feelings

A genetics professional will not do the following things:

- Tell a person which decision to make

- Advise a couple not to have children

- Recommend that a woman continue or end a pregnancy

- Tell someone whether to undergo testing for a genetic disorder

How can I find a genetics professional in my area?

To find a genetics professional in your community, you may wish to ask your doctor for a referral. If you have health insurance, you can also contact your insurance company to find a medical geneticist or genetic counselor in your area who participates in your plan.

Chapter 5

Genetic Testing

Chapter Contents

Section 5.1

An Overview of Genetic Testing

Excerpted from "Genetic Testing," *Genetics Home Reference*,
a service of the U.S. National Library of Medicine, June 26, 2009

What is genetic testing?

Genetic testing is a type of medical test that identifies changes in chromosomes, genes, or proteins. Most of the time, testing is used to find changes that are associated with inherited disorders. The results of a genetic test can confirm or rule out a suspected genetic condition or help determine a person's chance of developing or passing on a genetic disorder. Several hundred genetic tests are currently in use, and more are being developed.

Genetic testing is voluntary. Because testing has both benefits and limitations, the decision about whether to be tested is a personal and complex one. A genetic counselor can help by providing information about the pros and cons of the test and discussing the social and emotional aspects of testing.

What are the types of genetic tests?

Genetic testing can provide information about a person's genes and chromosomes. Available types of testing include the following:

- **Newborn screening:** Newborn screening is used just after birth to identify genetic disorders that can be treated early in life. Millions of babies are tested each year in the United States. All states currently test infants for phenylketonuria (a genetic disorder that causes mental retardation if left untreated) and congenital hypothyroidism (a disorder of the thyroid gland). Most states also test for other genetic disorders.

- **Diagnostic testing:** Diagnostic testing is used to identify or rule out a specific genetic or chromosomal condition. In many cases, genetic testing is used to confirm a diagnosis when a particular condition is suspected based on physical signs and symptoms. Diagnostic testing can be performed before birth or at any time during a person's life, but is not available for all genes or all genetic conditions. The results of a diagnostic test can influence a person's choices about health care and the management of the disorder.

- **Carrier testing:** Carrier testing is used to identify people who carry one copy of a gene mutation that, when present in two copies, causes a genetic disorder. This type of testing is offered to individuals who have a family history of a genetic disorder and to people in certain ethnic groups with an increased risk of specific genetic conditions. If both parents are tested, the test can provide information about a couple's risk of having a child with a genetic condition.

- **Prenatal testing:** Prenatal testing is used to detect changes in a fetus's genes or chromosomes before birth. This type of testing is offered during pregnancy if there is an increased risk that the baby will have a genetic or chromosomal disorder. In some cases, prenatal testing can lessen a couple's uncertainty or help them make decisions about a pregnancy. It cannot identify all possible inherited disorders and birth defects, however.

- **Preimplantation testing:** Preimplantation testing, also called preimplantation genetic diagnosis (PGD), is a specialized technique that can reduce the risk of having a child with a particular genetic or chromosomal disorder. It is used to detect genetic changes in embryos that were created using assisted reproductive techniques such as in-vitro fertilization. In-vitro fertilization involves removing egg cells from a woman's ovaries and fertilizing them with sperm cells outside the body. To perform preimplantation testing, a small number of cells are taken from these embryos and tested for certain genetic changes. Only embryos without these changes are implanted in the uterus to initiate a pregnancy.

- **Predictive and presymptomatic testing:** Predictive and presymptomatic types of testing are used to detect gene mutations associated with disorders that appear after birth, often later in life. These tests can be helpful to people who have a family member with a genetic disorder, but who have no features of the disorder themselves at the time of testing. Predictive testing can identify mutations that increase a person's risk of developing disorders with a genetic basis, such as certain types of cancer.

Presymptomatic testing can determine whether a person will develop a genetic disorder, such as hemochromatosis (an iron overload disorder), before any signs or symptoms appear. The results of predictive and presymptomatic testing can provide information about a person's risk of developing a specific disorder and help with making decisions about medical care.

- **Forensic testing:** Forensic testing uses deoxyribonucleic acid (DNA) sequences to identify an individual for legal purposes. Unlike the tests described above, forensic testing is not used to detect gene mutations associated with disease. This type of testing can identify crime or catastrophe victims, rule out or implicate a crime suspect, or establish biological relationships between people (for example, paternity).

How is genetic testing done?

Once a person decides to proceed with genetic testing, a medical geneticist, primary care doctor, specialist, or nurse practitioner can order the test. Genetic testing is often done as part of a genetic consultation.

Genetic tests are performed on a sample of blood, hair, skin, amniotic fluid (the fluid that surrounds a fetus during pregnancy), or other tissue. For example, a procedure called a buccal smear uses a small brush or cotton swab to collect a sample of cells from the inside surface of the cheek. The sample is sent to a laboratory where technicians look for specific changes in chromosomes, DNA, or proteins, depending on the suspected disorder. The laboratory reports the test results in writing to a person's doctor or genetic counselor.

Newborn screening tests are done on a small blood sample, which is taken by pricking the baby's heel. Unlike other types of genetic testing, a parent will usually receive the result only if it is positive. If the test result is positive, additional testing is needed to determine whether the baby has a genetic disorder.

Before a person has a genetic test, it is important that he or she understands the testing procedure, the benefits and limitations of the test, and the possible consequences of the test results. The process of educating a person about the test and obtaining permission is called informed consent.

What is direct-to-consumer genetic testing?

Traditionally, genetic tests have been available only through healthcare providers such as physicians, nurse practitioners, and genetic counselors. Healthcare providers order the appropriate test from a laboratory, collect and send the samples, and interpret the test results. Direct-to-consumer genetic testing refers to genetic tests that are marketed directly to consumers via television, print advertisements, or the internet. This form of testing, which is also known as at-home genetic testing, provides access to a person's genetic information without necessarily involving a doctor or insurance company in the process.

If a consumer chooses to purchase a genetic test directly, the test kit is mailed to the consumer instead of being ordered through a doctor's office. The test typically involves collecting a DNA sample at home, often by swabbing the inside of the cheek, and mailing the sample back to the laboratory. In some cases, the person must visit a health clinic to have blood drawn. Consumers are notified of their results by mail or over the telephone, or the results are posted online. In some cases, a genetic counselor or other healthcare provider is available to explain the results and answer questions. The price for this type of at-home genetic testing ranges from several hundred dollars to more than a thousand dollars.

The growing market for direct-to-consumer genetic testing may promote awareness of genetic diseases, allow consumers to take a more proactive role in their health care, and offer a means for people to learn about their ancestral origins. At-home genetic tests, however, have significant risks and limitations. Consumers are vulnerable to being misled by the results of unproven or invalid tests. Without guidance from a healthcare provider, they may make important decisions about treatment or prevention based on inaccurate, incomplete, or misunderstood information about their health. Consumers may also experience an invasion of genetic privacy if testing companies use their genetic information in an unauthorized way.

Genetic testing provides only one piece of information about a person's health—other genetic and environmental factors, lifestyle choices, and family medical history also affect a person's risk of developing many disorders. These factors are discussed during a consultation with a doctor or genetic counselor, but in many cases are not addressed by at-home genetic tests. More research is needed to fully understand the benefits and limitations of direct-to-consumer genetic testing.

How can consumers be sure a genetic test is valid and useful?

Before undergoing genetic testing, it is important to be sure that the test is valid and useful. A genetic test is valid if it provides an accurate result. Two main measures of accuracy apply to genetic tests: analytical validity and clinical validity. Another measure of the quality of a genetic test is its usefulness, or clinical utility.

Analytical validity refers to how well the test predicts the presence or absence of a particular gene or genetic change. In other words, can the test accurately detect whether a specific genetic variant is present or absent?

Clinical validity refers to how well the genetic variant being analyzed is related to the presence, absence, or risk of a specific disease.

Clinical utility refers to whether the test can provide information about diagnosis, treatment, management, or prevention of a disease that will be helpful to a consumer.

All laboratories that perform health-related testing, including genetic testing, are subject to federal regulatory standards called the Clinical Laboratory Improvement Amendments (CLIA) or even stricter state requirements. CLIA standards cover how tests are performed, the qualifications of laboratory personnel, and quality control and testing procedures for each laboratory. By controlling the quality of laboratory practices, CLIA standards are designed to ensure the analytical validity of genetic tests.

CLIA standards do not address the clinical validity or clinical utility of genetic tests. The Food and Drug Administration (FDA) requires information about clinical validity for some genetic tests. Additionally, the state of New York requires information on clinical validity for all laboratory tests performed for people living in that state. Consumers, health providers, and health insurance companies are often the ones who determine the clinical utility of a genetic test.

It can be difficult to determine the quality of a genetic test sold directly to the public. Some providers of direct-to-consumer genetic tests are not CLIA-certified, so it can be difficult to tell whether their tests are valid. If providers of direct-to-consumer genetic tests offer easy-to-understand information about the scientific basis of their tests, it can help consumers make more informed decisions. It may also be helpful to discuss any concerns with a health professional before ordering a direct-to-consumer genetic test.

What do the results of genetic tests mean?

The results of genetic tests are not always straightforward, which often makes them challenging to interpret and explain. Therefore, it is important for patients and their families to ask questions about the potential meaning of genetic test results both before and after the test is performed. When interpreting test results, healthcare professionals consider a person's medical history, family history, and the type of genetic test that was done.

A positive test result means that the laboratory found a change in a particular gene, chromosome, or protein of interest. Depending on the purpose of the test, this result may confirm a diagnosis, indicate that a person is a carrier of a particular genetic mutation, identify an increased risk of developing a disease (such as cancer) in the future, or suggest a need for further testing. Because family members have some genetic material in common, a positive test result may also have implications for certain blood relatives of the person undergoing testing. It is important to note that a positive result of a predictive or presymptomatic genetic test usually cannot establish the exact risk of developing a disorder. Also, health professionals typically cannot use a positive test result to predict the course or severity of a condition.

A negative test result means that the laboratory did not find a change in the gene, chromosome, or protein under consideration. This result can indicate that a person is not affected by a particular disorder, is not a carrier of a specific genetic mutation, or does not have an increased risk of developing a certain disease. It is possible, however, that the test missed a disease-causing genetic alteration because many tests cannot detect all genetic changes that can cause a particular disorder. Further testing may be required to confirm a negative result.

In some cases, a negative result might not give any useful information. This type of result is called uninformative, indeterminate, inconclusive, or ambiguous. Uninformative test results sometimes occur because everyone has common, natural variations in their DNA, called polymorphisms, that do not affect health. If a genetic test finds a change in DNA that has not been associated with a disorder in other people, it can be difficult to tell whether it is a natural polymorphism or a disease-causing mutation. An uninformative result cannot confirm or rule out a specific diagnosis, and it cannot indicate whether a person has an increased risk of developing a disorder. In some cases, testing other affected and unaffected family members can help clarify this type of result.

What is the cost of genetic testing, and how long does it take to get the results?

The cost of genetic testing can range from under $100 to more than $2,000, depending on the nature and complexity of the test. The cost increases if more than one test is necessary or if multiple family members must be tested to obtain a meaningful result. For newborn screening, costs vary by state. Some states cover part of the total cost, but most charge a fee of $15 to $60 per infant.

From the date that a sample is taken, it may take a few weeks to several months to receive the test results. Results for prenatal testing are usually available more quickly because time is an important consideration in making decisions about a pregnancy. The doctor or genetic counselor who orders a particular test can provide specific information about the cost and time frame associated with that test.

Will health insurance cover the costs of genetic testing?

In many cases, health insurance plans will cover the costs of genetic testing when it is recommended by a person's doctor. Health insurance providers have different policies about which tests are covered, however. A person interested in submitting the costs of testing may wish to contact his or her insurance company beforehand to ask about coverage.

Some people may choose not to use their insurance to pay for testing because the results of a genetic test can affect a person's health insurance coverage. Instead, they may opt to pay out-of-pocket for the test. People considering genetic testing may want to find out more about their state's privacy protection laws before they ask their insurance company to cover the costs.

What are the benefits of genetic testing?

Genetic testing has potential benefits whether the results are positive or negative for a gene mutation. Test results can provide a sense of relief from uncertainty and help people make informed decisions about managing their health care. For example, a negative result can eliminate the need for unnecessary checkups and screening tests in some cases. A positive result can direct a person toward available prevention, monitoring, and treatment options. Some test results can also help people make decisions about having children. Newborn screening can identify genetic disorders early in life so treatment can be started as early as possible.

What are the risks and limitations of genetic testing?

The physical risks associated with most genetic tests are very small, particularly for those tests that require only a blood sample or buccal smear (a procedure that samples cells from the inside surface of the cheek). The procedures used for prenatal testing carry a small but real risk of losing the pregnancy (miscarriage) because they require a sample of amniotic fluid or tissue from around the fetus.

Many of the risks associated with genetic testing involve the emotional, social, or financial consequences of the test results. People may feel angry, depressed, anxious, or guilty about their results. In some cases, genetic testing creates tension within a family because the results can reveal information about other family members in addition to the person who is tested. The possibility of genetic discrimination in employment or insurance is also a concern.

Genetic testing can provide only limited information about an inherited condition. The test often can't determine if a person will show symptoms of a disorder, how severe the symptoms will be, or whether the disorder will progress over time. Another major limitation is the lack of treatment strategies for many genetic disorders once they are diagnosed.

A genetics professional can explain in detail the benefits, risks, and limitations of a particular test. It is important that any person who is considering genetic testing understand and weigh these factors before making a decision.

What is genetic discrimination?

Genetic discrimination occurs when people are treated differently by their employer or insurance company because they have a gene mutation that causes or increases the risk of an inherited disorder. People who undergo genetic testing may be at risk for genetic discrimination.

The results of a genetic test are normally included in a person's medical records. When a person applies for life, disability, or health insurance, the insurance company may ask to look at these records before making a decision about coverage. An employer may also have the right to look at an employee's medical records. As a result, genetic test results could affect a person's insurance coverage or employment. People making decisions about genetic testing should be aware that when test results are placed in their medical records, the results might not be kept private.

Fear of discrimination is a common concern among people considering genetic testing. Several laws at the federal and state levels help protect people against genetic discrimination; however, genetic testing is a fast-growing field and these laws don't cover every situation.

How does genetic testing in a research setting differ from clinical genetic testing?

The main differences between clinical genetic testing and research testing are the purpose of the test and who receives the results. The goals of research testing include finding unknown genes, learning how genes work, and advancing our understanding of genetic conditions. The results of testing done as part of a research study are usually not available to patients or their healthcare providers. Clinical testing, on the other hand, is done to find out about an inherited disorder in an individual patient or family. People receive the results of a clinical test and can use them to help them make decisions about medical care or reproductive issues.

It is important for people considering genetic testing to know whether the test is available on a clinical or research basis. Clinical and research testing both involve a process of informed consent in which patients learn about the testing procedure, the risks and benefits of the test, and the potential consequences of testing.

Section 5.2

Prenatal Testing

The terms prenatal screening and prenatal diagnosis refer broadly to a number of different techniques and procedures that can be performed during a pregnancy to provide information about the health of a developing fetus. Screening tests indicate whether the fetus has an average, greater than average, or below average risk of being affected by a particular genetic condition or birth defect. When the result of a screening shows increased risk, the pregnant patient may be offered other diagnostic tests to confirm whether the fetus is, in fact, affected. Diagnostic tests may also be offered directly to women whose pregnancies are considered high risk because of age, family history, or other factors.

It is important to note that a normal result on either a diagnostic or screening test does not guarantee the birth of a normal baby. These tests are designed to look for specific conditions, but not all conditions can be detected and no test is 100 percent accurate.

Decisions about Prenatal Diagnosis

The decision to undergo a prenatal screening or diagnostic test should be carefully considered. Genetic counseling is often recommended prior to screening or to chorionic villi sampling (CVS) or amniocentesis. After reviewing medical and family histories, a genetic counselor assesses the specific genetic risks to a pregnancy and helps the patient decide whether or not to undergo prenatal screening or testing based on the parent's own values and beliefs.

If an abnormality is detected, the options for the family will be specific to what is found and what treatment is available. The courses of action—including continuing or terminating the pregnancy—are determined solely by the parents-to-be in consultation with their primary care provider and other resources that they may choose to consult.

Prenatal Screening

Ultrasound is a noninvasive procedure that may be performed at any stage of a pregnancy. The procedure uses high-frequency sound waves to produce an image of the fetus inside the uterus. When an abdominal ultrasound is performed, a gel that acts as a sound wave conductor is placed on the mother's abdomen. The doctor or technician who is performing the ultrasound moves a small instrument, called a transducer, back and forth over the abdomen, directing sound waves into the uterus. The sound waves reflect off bones and tissue and are converted into black and white images to produce a picture of the fetus. Ultrasounds can also be done vaginally by introducing the transducer into the mother's vagina to allow a closer examination of the fetus.

Ultrasound is used to determine the age of a fetus based on fetal measurements, to monitor fetal growth, to determine why bleeding is occurring in a pregnancy, to check the baby's position in the uterus, to detect multiple births (e.g., twins), and to evaluate the general development of the fetus. Ultrasound may also provide the first indication of a problem with the fetus by revealing major fetal structural abnormalities or abnormalities of function in certain fetal organs. The procedure is also used as a guide to visualize the fetus when invasive prenatal diagnostic procedures, such as amniocentesis and chorionic villi sampling (CVS), are performed. Accurate ultrasound requires technically proficient physicians and technicians.

Nuchal fold translucency (NT) is an ultrasound performed by a specially trained ultrasonographer at approximately eleven to thirteen weeks of pregnancy. The ultrasonographer measures the size of the fluid-filled sack at the back of the fetal neck, called the nuchal fold. An increase in the size of the nuchal fold may indicate the presence of a number of conditions, including a chromosome abnormality such as Down syndrome or other abnormalities such as a heart defect. An NT measurement is often done in conjunction with a first trimester maternal serum screen (see below).

Maternal serum marker screening is a blood test that is offered to pregnant women during the first (eleven to thirteen weeks) or second trimester (fifteen to eighteen weeks of pregnancy) to screen for two chromosome disorders, Down syndrome and trisomy 18, in the first trimester; and for Down syndrome, trisomy 18, and neural tube defects in the second trimester.

Second trimester maternal serum marker screening measures the concentration of proteins (alpha-fetoprotein, unconjugated estriol, and human chorionic gonadotropin in the "triple screen," and these three proteins plus inhibin A in the "quad screen") that are made by the fetus during pregnancy, and that circulate in the blood of a pregnant woman. The normal levels of these proteins depend on a number of factors, including the gestational age of the fetus, the number of fetuses, maternal weight and race, and the presence of maternal diabetes.

To calculate risk for Down syndrome, the results of the maternal serum screen are used to adjust a woman's age-related risk for Down syndrome up or down. If her adjusted risk equals that of a thirty-five-year-old (who would generally be offered amniocentesis based on age alone), additional follow-up, possibly including diagnostic testing, is offered. A woman who is at risk because of age who would prefer not to go directly to an invasive procedure may use maternal serum screening to adjust her age-related risk. If her risk goes down based on the results of the serum screen, she may choose not to pursue additional diagnostic testing.

Maternal serum screening will not detect every baby with Down syndrome, trisomy 18, or a neural tube defect. Seventy percent of pregnancies in which the baby has Down syndrome can be detected with the triple screen and 80 percent with the quad screen. The alpha-fetoprotein analysis detects about 90 percent of babies with open structural defects of the fetal abdominal wall or the neural tube (open spina bifida and anencephaly).

In addition, screening tests may yield what are called false positives. The false-positive rate is the chance that a test is abnormal, or "positive," even though the condition being tested for is not present. The goal of any screening program is to balance the possible benefits of detecting an abnormality with the risks of subjecting women to the anxieties of a positive result or the risks of invasive diagnostic testing.

First trimester maternal serum marker screening is becoming more available as an alternative or adjunct to second trimester screening. Two proteins are measured in the maternal serum, free beta human chorionic gonadotropin and pregnancy-associated plasma protein A (PAPP-A). The results of the blood test are often combined with the results of an NT measurement that is done at the same time to adjust the woman's age-related risk for Down syndrome up or down. When a first trimester serum screen is combined with an NT measurement, 80 to 85 percent of Down syndrome cases will be detected.

There are a number of ways that first trimester screening may be offered, either as a stand-alone test or in combination with a second trimester screen. When both first and second trimester screens are done, however, they should not be reported out independently as the false-positive rates (the chance that someone has a positive result, but the fetus is chromosomally normal) are additive, leading to more unnecessary invasive testing. Some of the approaches that physicians and patients may consider include:

- **Integrated screening:** In integrated screening, first and second trimester screening is done but only one final result is reported after the second screen. This has the highest detection rate of all the approaches.

- **Stepwise sequential screening:** In stepwise sequential screening, a woman has a first trimester serum screen, with or without an NT measurement. If she is found to have an increased risk, she is referred for follow-up counseling and possible diagnostic testing. If she is not at an increased risk based on the first screen, she is given the option of a second screen in the second trimester and given a final risk that incorporates the result of both tests.

- **Contingent sequential screening:** In a variation on the above, a woman has a first trimester screen and if she is has an increased risk, she is referred for follow-up counseling and possible diagnostic testing just like in the stepwise sequential screen. However, if her risk is not significantly increased, what happens next depends on her result. If her risk is adjusted to a very low risk, no further screening is offered. If she has an intermediate risk, she is offered a second trimester screen to clarify that risk further.

Which approach is appropriate for any one woman or obstetrician's office will depend on many factors: a woman's gestational age at the time the pregnancy is diagnosed and her access to care in the first trimester, the availability of trained ultrasonographers to do NT measurement, the availability of first trimester diagnostic testing (CVS) if there is a positive first trimester screen, the presence of multiple fetuses, and personal preference, among others.

Prenatal Diagnostic Tests

Amniocentesis is among the most commonly performed prenatal diagnostic procedures, and is used to detect chromosomal abnormalities as well as other specific genetic diseases.

Amniocentesis is usually performed in the second trimester of pregnancy, at approximately fifteen to twenty weeks from the first day of the last menstrual period. During the procedure a thin needle is inserted through the abdomen to allow for the withdrawal of a small quantity (usually one to two tablespoons) of amniotic fluid from the sac that holds the developing fetus. The fetal cells found in the amniotic fluid are grown in a cell culture and studied to detect chromosome abnormalities. Specific enzyme or deoxyribonucleic acid (DNA) analyses, which may be indicated based on family or medical history, can also be performed on the fetal cells derived from amniotic fluid.

Amniocentesis is a relatively simple and safe procedure when performed by an experienced physician, but there is some risk for miscarriage. That risk has been quoted at being about 1 in 200. However, recent data suggests that in experienced hands, the risk may be much lower. Infection is another rare complication of amniocentesis. There is also a small increased risk of clubfoot when amniocentesis is performed before thirteen weeks of pregnancy.

The results from amniocentesis are highly accurate. The complete chromosome analysis is usually completed one to two weeks after the procedure is performed. Additional testing such as biochemical (enzyme) analyses and DNA testing usually take an additional two to four weeks, while the amniotic fluid alpha-fetoprotein analysis takes only a few days.

Amniocentesis is commonly recommended for a variety of reasons:

- Increased risk for fetal chromosome abnormalities:
  - Maternal age (thirty-five or greater at delivery)
  - Having a previous child with a chromosome problem, such as Down syndrome
  - Increased risk of Down syndrome or trisomy 18 based on maternal serum markers
  - One of the parents has a balanced chromosome rearrangement
- Increased risk for open neural tube defects or fetal abdominal wall defect:
  - One of the parents or a previous child has had a neural tube defect
  - Elevated AFP (alpha-fetoprotein) concentration in the second trimester screening
- Increased risk for a specific genetic condition:
  - A previous child or relative has had birth defects or a metabolic or other known genetic condition
  - Both parents are known to carry genes for an inherited disorder, such as Tay-Sachs, sickle cell anemia, thalassemia, or cystic fibrosis
  - The mother's male relatives (brothers, sons, uncles, fathers) have inherited conditions such as muscular dystrophy or hemophilia

If amniocentesis results indicate that the fetus is affected with a particular condition, further counseling is usually recommended.

Chorionic villi sampling (CVS) is a test performed to detect specific genetic abnormalities early in pregnancy. By performing a biopsy of the cells that will become the placenta (villi), fetal cells are obtained and genetic analyses can be performed. CVS is performed by inserting either a catheter through the vagina and cervix, or a needle through the abdomen, into the villi. CVS is generally done at ten to thirteen weeks from the first day of the pregnant woman's last menstrual period, significantly earlier than amniocentesis is usually performed. The greatest success exists when the physician performing the procedure is experienced at performing both the transcervical and transabdominal techniques because the location of the placenta and uterine anatomy will often dictate the best or easiest approach to obtaining villi.

Preliminary CVS results (which are not always accurate) can be available within two to four days after the procedure is performed; final results are available in about seven to ten days. Many biochemical and molecular (DNA) analyses can be accurately performed using chorionic villi.

CVS can be used to determine virtually all disorders that can be diagnosed by amniocentesis except the presence of neural tube defects (spina bifida).

CVS carries a slightly higher increased risk of miscarriage (still less than 1 percent) than amniocentesis. Other complications, such as vaginal bleeding (spotting) or cramping, and maternal infection, occur more frequently after CVS than after amniocentesis. There is concern about the risks of CVS performed before ten weeks gestation because of reports of a higher risk of limb anomalies with this very early procedure.

Discovering a problem in the first trimester has several benefits. These include peace of mind for the family when no abnormality is detected, or earlier fetal treatment with surgery or medication if the condition detected is amenable to treatment. The option of a first trimester termination, which is safer and easier than a second trimester procedure, also makes CVS appealing to some individuals or couples whose pregnancy is at high risk.

Future Directions

New noninvasive techniques being developed focus on ensuring diagnostic accuracy while eliminating the risks associated with invasive procedures such as amniocentesis and CVS. Studies are underway to determine how to best obtain and concentrate fetal cells or fetal DNA that normally circulate in maternal blood during pregnancy so that chromosome, biochemical, and DNA analyses can be performed using those cells.

Ultrasound imaging techniques, such as three-dimensional and color imaging, continue to improve to allow better visualization of fetal anomalies.

Section 5.3

Newborn Screening

Newborn screening is the practice of testing every newborn for certain harmful or potentially fatal disorders that aren't otherwise apparent at birth. Many of these are metabolic disorders, often called "inborn errors of metabolism," which interfere with the body's use of nutrients to maintain healthy tissues and produce energy. Other disorders that may be detected through screening include problems with hormones) or the blood.

In general, metabolic and other inherited disorders can hinder an infant's normal physical and mental development in a variety of ways. And parents can pass along the gene for a certain disorder without even knowing that they're carriers.

With a simple blood test, doctors can often tell whether newborns have certain conditions that could eventually cause problems. Even though these conditions are considered rare and most babies are given a clean bill of health, early diagnosis and proper treatment can make the difference between lifelong impairment and healthy development.

Newborn Screening: Past, Present, and Future

In the early 1960s, scientist Robert Guthrie, Ph.D., developed a blood test that could determine whether newborn babies had a metabolic disorder known as phenylketonuria (PKU). People with PKU lack an enzyme needed to process the amino acid phenylalanine. This amino acid is necessary for normal growth in infants and children and for normal protein use throughout life. However, if too much of it builds up, it damages the brain tissue and can eventually cause mental retardation.

When babies with PKU are put on a special diet right away, they can often avoid the mental retardation that children with PKU experienced in the past. By following certain dietary restrictions, these children can lead normal lives.

Since the development of the PKU test, researchers have developed additional blood tests that can screen newborns for other disorders that, unless detected and treated early, can cause physical problems, mental retardation, and in some cases, death.

Most states, the District of Columbia, Puerto Rico, and the U.S. Virgin Islands now have their own mandatory newborn screening programs (in some states, such as Wyoming and Maryland, the screening is not mandatory). Because the federal government has set no national standard, screening requirements vary from state to state, as determined by individual state public health departments.

Consequently, the comprehensiveness of these programs varies, with states routinely screening for anywhere from four to thirty disorders. The average state program tests from four to ten disorders.

State requirements tend to change periodically as well. In fact, the pace of change is speeding up, thanks to the development of a new screening technique known as tandem mass spectrometry (often abbreviated as MS/MS). This technology can detect the blood components that are elevated in certain disorders, and is capable of screening for more than twenty inherited metabolic disorders with a single test.

About half of the states are offering expanded screening with tandem mass spectrometry on every baby. However, there's some controversy over whether the new technology has been tested adequately. Also, some experts want more evidence that early detection of every disease tested for will actually offer babies some long-term benefit. Equally important, parents may not want to know ahead of time that their child will develop a serious condition when there are no medical treatments or dietary changes that can improve the outcome. And some questions about who will pay (states, insurance companies, or parents) for the newer technology have yet to be resolved.

The American Academy of Pediatrics (AAP) and the federal government's Health Resources and Services Administration convened a task force of experts to grapple with these issues and recommend next steps. Their report identified some flaws and inconsistencies in the current state-driven screening system and proposed the following:

- All state screening programs should reflect current technology.
- All states should test for the same disorders.

- Parents should be informed about screening procedures and have the right to refuse screening, as well as the right to keep the results private and confidential.

- Parents should be informed about the benefits and risks associated with newborn screening.

All of this can be a little confusing (and anxiety-provoking) for a new parent. The inconsistencies among state requirements mean that there's no clear consensus on what's really necessary. On the one hand, it's important to keep in mind that the disorders being screened for are rare. On the other hand, no parent wants to take any unnecessary chances with the quality of his or her child's life—no matter how small the risk.

How Do States and Hospitals Determine Which Tests They Offer?

Traditionally, state decisions about what to screen for have been based on weighing the costs against the benefits. "Cost" considerations include:

- the risk of false positive results (and the unnecessary anxiety they cause);

- the availability of treatments proven to help the condition;

- financial costs.

And states often face conflicting priorities when determining their budgets. For instance, a state may face a choice between expanding newborn screening and ensuring that all expectant mothers get sufficient prenatal care. Of course, this offers little comfort to parents whose children have a disorder that could have been found through a screening test but wasn't.

So what can you do? Your best strategy is to stay informed. Discuss this issue with both your obstetrician or health care provider and your future baby's doctor before you give birth. Know what tests are routinely done in your state and in the hospital where you'll deliver (some hospitals go beyond what's required by state law).

If your state isn't offering screening for the expanded panel of disorders, you may want to ask your doctors about supplemental screening. Keep in mind, though, that you'll probably have to pay for the additional tests out of your own pocket.

If you're the parent of an infant and are concerned about whether your child was screened for certain conditions, ask your child's doctor for information about which tests were performed and whether further tests are recommended.

What Disorders Will Be Screened for in My Newborn?

Newborn screening varies by state and is subject to change, especially given advancements in technology. However, the disorders listed here are the ones typically included in newborn screening programs and are listed in order from the most common (all states screen for the first two) to least common (ranging from three-fourths or one-half of states to just a few). Incidence figures included in this list are according to a 1996 AAP policy statement.

PKU: When this disorder is detected early, feeding an infant a special formula low in phenylalanine can prevent mental retardation. A low-phenylalanine diet will need to be followed throughout childhood and adolescence and perhaps into adult life. This diet cuts out all high-protein foods, so people with PKU often need to take a special artificial formula as a nutritional substitute. Incidence: 1 in 10,000 to 25,000.

Congenital hypothyroidism: This is the disorder most commonly identified by routine screening. Affected babies don't have enough thyroid hormone and so develop retarded growth and brain development. (The thyroid, a gland at the front of the neck, releases chemical substances that control metabolism and growth.) If the disorder is detected early, a baby can be treated with oral doses of thyroid hormone to permit normal development. Incidence: 1 in 4,000.

Galactosemia: Babies with galactosemia lack the enzyme that converts galactose (one of two sugars found in lactose) into glucose, a sugar the body is able to use. As a result, milk (including breast milk) and other dairy products must be eliminated from the diet. Otherwise, galactose can build up in the system and damage the body's cells and organs, leading to blindness, severe mental retardation, growth deficiency, and even death. Incidence: 1 in 60,000 to 80,000. There are several less severe forms of galactosemia that may be detected by newborn screening. These may not require any intervention.

Sickle cell disease: Sickle cell disease is an inherited blood disease in which red blood cells stretch into abnormal "sickle" shapes and can cause episodes of pain, damage to vital organs such as the lungs and kidneys, and even death. Young children with sickle cell disease are especially prone to certain dangerous bacterial infections, such as pneumonia (inflammation of the lungs) and meningitis (inflammation of the brain and spinal cord). Studies suggest that newborn screening can alert doctors to begin antibiotic treatment before infections occur and to monitor symptoms of possible worsening more closely. The screening test can also detect other disorders affecting hemoglobin (the oxygen-carrying substance in the blood). Incidence: about 1 in every 500 African-American births and 1 in every 1,000 to 1,400 Hispanic-American births; also occurs with some frequency among people of Hispanic, Mediterranean, Middle Eastern, and South Asian descent.

Biotinidase deficiency: Babies with this condition don't have enough biotinidase, an enzyme that recycles biotin (one of the B vitamins) in the body. The deficiency may cause seizures, poor muscle control, immune system impairment, hearing loss, mental retardation, coma, and even death. If the deficiency is detected in time, however, problems can be prevented by giving the baby extra biotin. Incidence: 1 in 72,000 to 126,000.

Congenital adrenal hyperplasia: This is actually a group of disorders involving a deficiency of certain hormones produced by the adrenal gland. It can affect the development of the genitals and may cause death due to loss of salt from the kidneys. Lifelong treatment through supplementation of the missing hormones manages the condition. Incidence: 1 in 12,000.

Maple syrup urine disease (MSUD): Babies with MSUD are missing an enzyme needed to process three amino acids that are essential for the body's normal growth. When these are not processed properly, they can build up in the body, causing urine to smell like maple syrup or sweet, burnt sugar. These babies usually have little appetite and are extremely irritable. If not detected and treated early, MSUD can cause mental retardation, physical disability, and even death. A carefully controlled diet that cuts out certain high-protein foods containing those amino acids can prevent these outcomes. Like people with PKU, those with MSUD are often given a formula that supplies the necessary nutrients missed in the special diet they must follow. Incidence: 1 in 250,000.

Homocystinuria: This metabolic disorder results from a deficiency of one of several enzymes for normal development. If untreated, it can lead to dislocated lenses of the eyes, mental retardation, skeletal abnormalities, and abnormal blood clotting. However, a special diet combined with dietary supplements may help prevent most of these problems. Incidence: 1 in 50,000 to 150,000.

Tyrosinemia: Babies with this disorder have trouble processing the amino acid tyrosine. If it accumulates in the body, it can cause mild retardation, language skill difficulties, liver problems, and even death from liver failure. A special diet and sometimes a liver transplant are needed to treat the condition. Early diagnosis and treatment seem to offset long-term problems, although more information is needed. Incidence: not yet determined. Some babies have a mild self-limited form of tyrosinemia cystic fibrosis. Cystic fibrosis is an inherited disorder expressed in the various organs that causes cells to release a thick mucus, which can lead to chronic respiratory disease, problems with digestion, and poor growth. There is no known cure—treatment involves trying to prevent the serious lung infections associated with it and providing adequate nutrition. Some infections may be prevented with antibiotics. Detecting the disease early may help doctors reduce the lung and nutritional problems associated with cystic fibrosis, but the real impact of newborn screening is yet to be determined. Incidence: 1 in 2,000 Caucasian babies; less common in African-Americans, Hispanics, and Asians.

Toxoplasmosis: Toxoplasmosis is a parasitic infection that can be transmitted through the mother's placenta to an unborn child. The disease-causing organism, which is found in uncooked or undercooked meat, can invade the brain, eye, and muscle, possibly resulting in blindness and mental retardation. The benefit of early detection and treatment is uncertain. Incidence: 1 in 1,000. But only one or two states screen for toxoplasmosis.

These aren't the only disorders that can be detected through newborn screening. Certain other rare disorders of body chemistry can also be detected. Other conditions that are candidates for newborn screening include:

- Duchenne muscular dystrophy, a childhood form of muscular dystrophy that can be detected through a blood test;
- human immunodeficiency virus (HIV);
- neuroblastoma, a type of cancer that can be detected with a urine test.

Hearing Screening

Most, but not all states require newborns' hearing to be screened before they are discharged from the hospital. If your infant isn't examined at that time, it's important to make sure that he or she does get screened within the first three weeks of life. A child develops critical speaking and language skills in the first few years of life, and if a hearing loss is caught early, doctors can treat it so that it doesn't interfere with that development.

Should I Request Additional Tests?

If you answer "yes" to any of the questions below, talk to your child's future doctor and perhaps a genetic counselor about requesting additional tests.

- Do you have a positive family history of an inherited disorder?
- Have you previously given birth to a child who's affected by a disorder?
- Did an infant in your family die because of a suspected metabolic disorder?
- Do you have another reason to believe that your child may be at risk for a certain condition?

If your hospital can't or won't make expanded screening available to you, and your doctors believe additional testing would be worthwhile, you may want to contact outside laboratory services that provide supplemental testing for more than thirty metabolic disorders through a mail-order service available anywhere in the United States. The labs send out kits that are used to collect additional blood at the time of your baby's regular screening, and this sample is then mailed back for analysis. The cost ranges from $25 to $50.

How Is Newborn Screening Performed?

Within the first two or three days of life, your baby's heel will be pricked and a small sample of her blood will then be applied to a filter paper. Most states have identified a state or regional laboratory to which hospitals should send the samples for analysis. (If your hospital offers expanded screening that uses the new technology, your baby's sample may be sent to a private laboratory. Some states use a private lab for all of their studies.)

It's generally recommended that the sample be taken after the first twenty-four hours of life. Some tests, such as the one for PKU, may not be as sensitive if they're done too soon after birth. However, because mothers and newborns are often discharged within a day, some babies may be tested within the first twenty-four hours. If this happens, the AAP recommends that a repeat sample be taken no more than one to two weeks later. It's especially important that the PKU screening test be run again for accurate results. Some states routinely do two tests on all infants.

Getting the Results

Different labs have different procedures for notifying families and pediatricians of the results. Some may send them to the hospital where your child was born and not directly to your child's doctor, which may mean a delay in getting the results to you. And although some states have a system that allows doctors to access the results via phone or computer, others may not. Ask your child's doctor how you will get the results and when you should expect them.

If a test result should come back abnormal, try not to panic. This does not necessarily mean that your child has the disorder in question. A screening test is not the same as diagnostic test. The initial screening provides only preliminary information that must be followed up with more specific diagnostic testing.

If testing confirms that your child does have a disorder, your child's doctor may refer you to a specialist for further evaluation and treatment. Keep in mind that dietary restrictions and supplements, along with proper medical supervision, can often avert most of the serious physical and mental problems that were associated with metabolic disorders in the past.

You may also wonder whether the disorder can be passed on to any future children. This is a matter you'll want to discuss with your child's doctor and perhaps a genetic counselor. Also, if you have other children who weren't screened for the disorder, you may want to have this done. Again, talk this over with your children's doctor.

Know Your Options

Because state programs are subject to change, you'll want to find up-to-date information about your state's (and individual hospital's) program. Talk to your child's doctor or contact your state's department of health for more information.

Section 5.4

Preventing Genetic Discrimination

Reprinted from "Genetic Information Nondiscrimination Act of 2008," National Human Genome Research Institute, December 18, 2008.

What's genetic discrimination?

Genetic discrimination occurs if people are treated unfairly because of differences in their deoxyribonucleic acid (DNA) that increase their chances of getting a certain disease. For example, a health insurer might refuse to give coverage to a woman who has a DNA difference that raises her odds of getting breast cancer. Employers also could use DNA information to decide whether to hire or fire workers.

Who needs protection from genetic discrimination?

Everyone should care about the potential for genetic discrimination. Every person has dozens of DNA differences that could increase or decrease his or her chance of getting a disease such as diabetes, heart disease, cancer, or Alzheimer disease. It's important to remember that these DNA differences don't always mean someone will develop a disease, just that the risk to get the disease may be greater.

More and more tests are being developed to find DNA differences that affect our health. Called genetic tests, these tests will become a routine part of health care in the future. Health care providers will use information about each person's DNA to develop more individualized ways of detecting, treating, and preventing disease. But unless this DNA information is protected, it could be used to discriminate against people.

What's the Genetic Information Nondiscrimination Act (GINA)?

The Genetic Information Nondiscrimination Act of 2008, also referred to as GINA, is a new federal law that protects Americans from being treated unfairly because of differences in their DNA that may

57

affect their health. The new law prevents discrimination from health insurers and employers. The president signed the act into federal law on May 21, 2008. The parts of the law relating to health insurers will take effect by May 2009, and those relating to employers will take effect by November 2009.

Why was the law needed?

The law was needed to help ease concerns about discrimination that might keep some people from getting genetic tests that could benefit their health. The law also enables people to take part in research studies without fear that their DNA information might be used against them in health insurance or the workplace.

What's included in the law?

The law protects people from discrimination by health insurers and employers on the basis of DNA information.

What's not included?

The law does not cover life insurance, disability insurance, and long-term care insurance.

How does the federal law affect state laws?

Before the federal law was passed, many states had passed laws against genetic discrimination. The degree of protection from these laws varies widely among the different states. The federal law sets a minimum standard of protection that must be met in all states. It does not weaken the protections provided by any state law.

Part Two

Disorders Resulting from Abnormalitites in Specific Genes

Chapter 6

Albinism

What Is Albinism?

Albinism is a condition in which people have little or no melanin pigment (compound that creates color) in their eyes, skin, or hair. Because of this people with albinism look a little different from other members of their family without albinism. They have very fair skin which is prone to sunburn, their hair is white or a very light color, and they may squint a lot as their eyes are sensitive to sunlight.

Classification of Albinism

There are two main categories of albinism.

Oculocutaneous

- Involves dilution of the color of the hair, skin, and eyes
- Most common form of albinism

Ocular

- Melanin pigment mainly missing from the eyes while the skin and hair appear normal or only slightly lighter

This information is reprinted with permission from DermNet, the website of the New Zealand Dermatological Society. Visit www.dermnetnz.org for patient information on numerous skin conditions and their treatment. © 2009 New Zealand Dermatological Society.

- Accounts for 10 to 15 percent of all albinism cases

Oculocutaneous albinism (OCA) makes up a group of different types of albinism based on the specific albinism gene involved. Oculocutaneous albinism type 1 and type 2 are the most common types of oculocutaneous albinism.

Types of Oculocutaneous Albinism

Type 1 (Tyrosinase-Related Albinism)

- Sub-groups include OCA1, OCA1A, and OCA1B
- Very little or no pigmentation
- Genetic defect of the tyrosinase enzyme that helps the body to change the amino acid tyrosine into melanin pigment

Type 2 (P-Gene Related Albinism)

- Slight pigmentation
- Genetic defect of the P gene on chromosome 15

Hermansky-Pudlak Syndrome

- Variable pigmentation
- Genetic defect of the P gene on chromosome 10
- Also associated with abnormal platelets leading to bleeding, lung fibrosis, and gastrointestinal problems

Other Less Common OCA Types

- Chédiak-Higashi syndrome
- Prader-Willi and Angelman syndrome
- TRP1-related OCA

How Do You Get Albinism?

Albinism is mostly a recessively inherited disease, which means that you have inherited two albinism genes (one from each parent). If your parents are only carriers of albinism (each having one albinism gene and one normal gene) they will have enough genetic information to make normal pigment and will not show any signs of albinism.

Who Is at Risk of Albinism?

Albinism occurs worldwide and affects people of all races. Males and females alike can have the condition although ocular albinism occurs primarily in males.

About 1 in 70 people have a gene for albinism. Couples who are each carriers of the recessive albinism gene have a 1 in 4 chance of producing a child with albinism.

What Are the Problems Associated with Albinism?

The main problems of albinism are caused by the inability of the body to produce melanin pigment (whose major role in the skin is to absorb ultraviolet [UV] light from the sun so skin is not sun-damaged). It also has a role in the development of normal vision of the eye. Having white or light-colored hair due to lack of melanin is no cause for concern, however, lack of melanin in the skin and eyes can cause the following problems:

- Skin problems:

  - Easily sunburn

  - Increased chance of getting skin cancers

- Eye problems:

  - **Impaired vision:** Although not "blind," vision is impaired and may not be fully corrected with glasses. Varying degrees of nearsightedness or farsightedness exist.

  - **Photophobia:** Sensitivity to light or glare.

  - **Nystagmus:** Involuntary movement of the eyes back and forth.

  - **Strabismus:** Eyes do not fixate and track together.

  - **Retinal involvement:** This is an important area of the eye as it is responsible for sending signals to the brain. Impaired transmission of signals causes various vision disorders.

Other less common types of albinism may also involve problems with blood clotting, immune deficiency, or problems with hearing.

One concern that should not be overlooked is the risk of isolation in people with albinism. People with albinism, especially children, need to be treated normally and included in all activities. They develop normally and have normal intelligence. It is a myth that people with albinism are mentally impaired or intellectually challenged.

What Treatment or Precautions Can Be Taken?

It is important for people with albinism to protect themselves from UV exposure and thus prevent the damaging effects it can have on the skin.

Sun avoidance methods:

- Wear protective clothing (long sleeves and pants, shirts with collars, tightly woven fabrics that don't let light through), hats (wide-brimmed), and eyewear (specifically made to protect from UV rays).

- Use broad-spectrum sunscreens with SPF of 15 or greater: apply to all exposed areas.

Undergo frequent skin examinations by someone who has been taught to recognize signs of skin cancer.

Because the patient has no, or little, pigmentation, skin cancers will often have no or little pigmentation. Report to your doctor any suspicious spots or growths immediately.

Specialist eye doctors cannot cure eye problems but can help with various optical aids to improve vision for people with albinism.

Chapter 7

Alpha-1 Antitrypsin Deficiency

What is alpha-1 antitrypsin deficiency?

Alpha-1 antitrypsin deficiency (AATD) is an inherited condition that causes low levels of, or no, alpha-1 antitrypsin (AAT) in the blood. AATD occurs in approximately 1 in 2,500 individuals. This condition is found in all ethnic groups; however, it occurs most often in whites of European ancestry.

Alpha-1 antitrypsin (AAT) is a protein that is made in the liver. The liver releases this protein into the bloodstream. AAT protects the lungs so they can work normally. Without enough AAT, the lungs can be damaged, and this damage may make breathing difficult.

Everyone has two copies of the gene for AAT and receives one copy of the gene from each parent. Most people have two normal copies of the alpha-1 antitrypsin gene. Individuals with AATD have one normal copy and one damaged copy, or they have two damaged copies. Most individuals who have one normal gene can produce enough alpha-1 antitrypsin to live healthy lives, especially if they do not smoke.

People who have two damaged copies of the gene are not able to produce enough alpha-1 antitrypsin, which leads them to have more severe symptoms.

Reprinted from "Learning about Alpha-1 Antitrypsin Deficiency (AATD)," National Human Genome Research Institute, National Institutes of Health, March 10, 2008.

What are the symptoms of alpha-1 antitrypsin deficiency (AATD)?

AATD can present as lung disease in adults and can be associated with liver disease in a small portion of affected children. In affected adults, the first symptoms of AATD are shortness of breath with mild activity, reduced ability to exercise, and wheezing. These symptoms usually appear between the ages of twenty and forty. Other signs and symptoms can include repeated respiratory infections, fatigue, rapid heartbeat upon standing, vision problems, and unintentional weight loss.

Some individuals with AATD have emphysema, in which the small air sacs (alveoli) in the lungs are damaged. Symptoms of emphysema include difficulty breathing, a hacking cough, and a barrel-shaped chest. Smoking or exposure to tobacco smoke increases the appearance of symptoms and damage to the lungs. Other common diagnoses include chronic obstructive pulmonary disease (COPD), asthma, chronic bronchitis, and bronchiectasis—a chronic inflammatory or degenerative condition of one or more bronchi or bronchioles.

Liver disease, called cirrhosis of the liver, is another symptom of AATD. It can be present in some affected children, about 10 percent, and has also been reported in 15 percent of adults with AATD. In its late stages signs and symptoms of liver disease can include a swollen abdomen, coughing up blood, swollen feet or legs, and yellowing of the skin and the whites of the eyes (jaundice).

Rarely, AATD can cause a skin condition known as panniculitis, which is characterized by hardened skin with painful lumps or patches. Panniculitis varies in severity and can occur at any age.

How is alpha-1 antitrypsin deficiency diagnosed?

Alpha-1 antitrypsin deficiency (AATD) is diagnosed through testing of a blood sample, when a person is suspected of having AATD. For example, AATD may be suspected when a physical examination reveals a barrel-shaped chest, or, when listening to the chest with a stethoscope, wheezing, crackles or decreased breath sounds are heard.

Testing for AATD, using a blood sample from the individual, is simple, quick, and highly accurate. Three types of tests are usually done on the blood sample:

- Alpha-1 genotyping, which examines a person's genes and determines their genotype

- Alpha-1 antitrypsin PI type of phenotype test, which determines the type of AAT protein that a person has

- Alpha-1 antitrypsin level test, which determines the amount of AAT in a person's blood

Individuals who have symptoms that suggest AATD or who have a family history of AATD should consider being tested.

What is the treatment for alpha-1 antitrypsin deficiency?

Treatment of alpha-1 antitrypsin deficiency (AATD) is based on a person's symptoms. There is currently no cure. The major goal of AATD management is preventing or slowing the progression of lung disease.

Treatments include bronchodilators and prompt treatment with antibiotics for upper respiratory tract infections. Lung transplantation may be an option for those who develop end-stage lung disease. Quitting smoking, if a person with AATD smokes, is essential.

Replacement (augmentation) therapy with the missing AAT protein is available, although it is used only under special circumstances. It is not known how effective this is once disease has developed or which people would benefit most.

Is alpha-1 antitrypsin deficiency inherited?

Alpha-1 antitrypsin deficiency is inherited in families in an autosomal codominant pattern. Codominant inheritance means that two different variants of the gene (alleles) may be expressed, and both versions contribute to the genetic trait.

The M gene is the most common allele of the alpha-1 gene. It produces normal levels of the alpha-1 antitrypsin protein.

The Z gene is the most common variant of the gene. It causes alpha-1 antitrypsin deficiency. The S allele is another, less common variant that causes ATTD.

If a person inherits one M gene and one Z gene or one S gene ("type PiMZ" or "type PiMS"), that person is a carrier of the disorder. While such a person may not have normal levels of alpha-1 antitrypsin, there should be enough to protect the lungs. However, carriers with the MZ alleles have an increased risk for lung disease, particularly if they smoke.

A person who inherits the Z gene from each parent is called "type PiZZ." This person has very low alpha-1 antitrypsin levels, allowing elastase—an enzyme especially of pancreatic juice that digests elastin—

to damage the lungs. A person who inherits an altered version called S and Z is also likely to develop AATD.

Chapter 8

Blood Clotting Deficiency Disorders

Chapter Contents

Section 8.1

Factor V Leiden Thrombophilia

Reprinted from "Learning about Factor V Leiden Thrombophilia,"
National Human Genome Research Institute, National Institutes of
Health, September 14, 2007.

What is factor V Leiden thrombophilia?

Factor V Leiden thrombophilia is an inherited disorder of blood clotting. Factor V Leiden is the name of a specific mutation (genetic alteration) that results in thrombophilia, or an increased tendency to form abnormal blood clots in blood vessels. People who have the factor V Leiden mutation are at somewhat higher than average risk for a type of clot that forms in large veins in the legs (deep venous thrombosis, or DVT) or a clot that travels through the bloodstream and lodges in the lungs (pulmonary embolism, or PE).

Factor V Leiden is the most common inherited form of thrombophilia. Between 3 and 8 percent of the Caucasian (white) U.S. and European populations carry one copy of the factor V Leiden mutation, and about 1 in 5,000 people have two copies of the mutation. The mutation is less common in other populations.

A mutation in the factor V gene (F5) increases the risk of developing factor V Leiden thrombophilia. The protein made by F5 called factor V plays a critical role in the formation of blood clots in response to injury. The factor V protein is involved in a series of chemical reactions that hold blood clots together. A molecule called activated protein C (APC) prevents blood clots from growing too large by inactivating factor V. In people with the factor V Leiden mutation, APC is unable to inactivate factor V normally. As a result, the clotting process continues longer than usual, increasing the chance of developing abnormal blood clots.

What are the symptoms of factor V Leiden thrombophilia?

The symptoms of factor V Leiden vary among individuals. There are some individuals who have the F5 gene and who never develop thrombosis, while others have recurring thrombosis before the age of thirty years. This variability is influenced by the number of F5 gene mutation a person has, the presence of other gene alterations related to blood clotting, and circumstantial risk factors, such as surgery, use of oral contraceptives, and pregnancy.

Symptoms of factor V Leiden include the following:

- Having a first DVT or PE before fifty years of age

- Having recurring DVT or PE

- Having venous thrombosis in unusual sites in the body such as the brain or the liver

- Having a DVT or PE during or right after pregnancy

- Having a history of unexplained pregnancy loss in the second or third trimester

- Having a DVT or PE and a strong family history of venous thromboembolism

The use of hormones, such as oral contraceptive pills (OCPs) and hormone replacement therapy (HRT), including estrogen and estrogen-like drugs taken after menopause, increases the risk of developing DVT and PE. Healthy women taking OCPs have a three- to four-fold increased risk of developing a DVT or PE compared with women who do not take OCP. Women with factor V Leiden who take OCPs have about a thirty-five–fold increased risk of developing a DVT or PE compared with women without factor V Leiden and those who do not take OCPs. Likewise, postmenopausal women taking HRT have a two- to three-fold higher risk of developing a DVT or PE than women who do not take HRT, and women with factor V Leiden who take HRT have a fifteen-fold higher risk. Women with heterozygous factor V Leiden who are making decisions about OCP or HRT use should take these statistics into consideration when weighing the risks and benefits of treatment.

How is factor V Leiden thrombophilia diagnosed?

Your doctor would suspect a diagnosis of thrombophilia if you have a history of venous thrombosis and/or a family history of venous thrombosis. The diagnosis is made using a screening test called a coagulation screening test or by genetic testing (deoxyribonucleic acid [DNA] analysis) of the F5 gene.

How is factor V Leiden thrombophilia treated?

The management of individuals with factor V Leiden depends on the clinical circumstances. People with factor V Leiden who have had a DVT or PE are usually treated with blood thinners, or anticoagulants. Anticoagulants such as heparin are given for varying amounts of time depending on the person's situation. It is not usually recommended that people with factor V Leiden be treated lifelong with anticoagulants if they have had only one DVT or PE, unless there are additional risk factors present. Having had a DVT or PE in the past increases a person's risk for developing another one in the future, but having factor V Leiden does not seem to add to the risk of having a second clot. In general, individuals who have factor V Leiden but have never had a blood clot are not routinely treated with an anticoagulant. Rather, these individuals are counseled about reducing or eliminating other factors that may add to one's risk of developing a clot in the future. In addition, these individuals may require temporary treatment with an anticoagulant during periods of particularly high risk, such as major surgery.

Factor V Leiden increases the risk of developing a DVT during pregnancy by about seven-fold. Women with factor V Leiden who are planning pregnancy should discuss this with their obstetrician and/or hematologist. Most women with factor V Leiden have normal pregnancies and require close follow-up only during pregnancy. For those with a history of DVT or PE, treatment with an anticoagulant during a subsequent pregnancy can prevent recurrent problems.

What do we know about heredity and factor V Leiden thrombophilia?

Factor V Leiden is the most common inherited form of thrombophilia. The risk of developing a clot in a blood vessel depends on whether a person inherits one or two copies of the factor V Leiden mutation. Inheriting one copy of the mutation from a parent increases by four-fold to eight-fold the chance of developing a clot. People who inherit two copies of the mutation, one from each parent, may have up to eighty times the usual risk of developing this type of blood clot. Considering that the risk of developing an abnormal blood clot averages about 1 in 1,000 per year in the general population, the presence of one copy of the factor V Leiden mutation increases that risk to 1 in 125 to 1 in 250. Having two copies of the mutation may raise the risk as high as 1 in 12.

Section 8.2

Hemophilia

Reprinted from "Learning about Hemophilia," National
Human Genome Research Institute, National Institutes of Health,
August 15, 2008.

What is hemophilia?

Hemophilia is a bleeding disorder that slows down the blood clotting process. People who have hemophilia often have longer bleeding after an injury or surgery. People who have severe hemophilia have spontaneous bleeding into the joints and muscles. Hemophilia occurs more commonly in males than in females.

The two most common types of hemophilia are hemophilia A (also known as classic hemophilia) and hemophilia B (also known as Christmas disease). People who have hemophilia A have low levels of a blood-clotting factor called factor eight (FVIII). People who have hemophilia B have low levels of factor nine (FIX).

The two types of hemophilia are caused by permanent gene changes (mutations) in different genes. Mutations in the FVIII gene cause hemophilia A. Mutations in the FIX gene cause hemophilia B. Proteins made by these genes have an important role in the blood clotting process. Mutations in either gene keep clots from forming when there is an injury, causing too much bleeding that can be difficult to stop.

Hemophilia A is the most common type of this condition. One in 5,000 to 10,000 males worldwide have hemophilia A. Hemophilia B is less common, and it affects 1 in 20,000 to 34,500 males worldwide.

What are the symptoms of hemophilia?

Symptoms of hemophilia include prolonged oozing after injuries, tooth extractions, or surgery; renewed bleeding after initial bleeding has stopped; easy or spontaneous bruising; and prolonged bleeding.

In both severe hemophilia A and severe hemophilia B, the most frequent symptom is spontaneous joint bleeding. Other serious sites

73

of bleeding include the bowel, the brain, and soft tissues. These types of bleeding can lead to throwing up blood or passing blood in the stool, stroke, and sudden severe pain in the joints or limbs. Painful bleeding into the soft tissues of the arms and legs can lead to nerve damage.

Individuals who have severe hemophilia are usually diagnosed within the first year of life. People who have moderate hemophilia do not usually have spontaneous bleeding, but they do have longer bleeding and oozing after small injuries. They are usually diagnosed before they reach five or six years of age.

Individuals who have mild hemophilia do not have spontaneous bleeding. If they are not treated they may have longer bleeding when they have surgery, teeth removed, or major injuries. Individuals with mild hemophilia may not be diagnosed until later in life.

How is hemophilia diagnosed?

Hemophilia A and B are diagnosed by measuring factor clotting activity. Individuals who have hemophilia A have low factor VIII clotting activity. Individuals who have hemophilia B have low factor IX clotting activity.

Genetic testing is also available for the factor VIII gene and the factor IX gene. Genetic testing of the FVIII gene finds a disease-causing mutation in up to 98 percent of individuals who have hemophilia A. Genetic testing of the FIX gene finds disease-causing mutations in more than 99 percent of individuals who have hemophilia B.

Genetic testing is usually used to identify women who are carriers of a FVIII or FIX gene mutation, and to diagnose hemophilia in a fetus during a pregnancy (prenatal diagnosis). It is sometimes used to diagnose individuals who have mild symptoms of hemophilia A or B.

What is the treatment for hemophilia?

There is currently no cure for hemophilia. Treatment depends on the severity of hemophilia.

Treatment may involve slow injection of a medicine called desmopressin (DDAVP) by the doctor into one of the veins. DDAVP helps to release more clotting factor to stop the bleeding. Sometimes, DDAVP is given as a medication that can be breathed in through the nose (nasal spray).

People who have moderate to severe hemophilia A or B may need to have an infusion of clotting factor taken from donated human blood or from genetically engineered products called recombinant clotting factors to stop the bleeding. If the potential for bleeding is serious, a doctor may give infusions of clotting factor to avoid bleeding (preventive infusions) before the bleeding begins. Repeated infusions may be necessary if the internal bleeding is serious.

When bleeding has damaged joints, physical therapy is used to help them function better. Physical therapy helps to keep the joints moving and prevents the joints from becoming frozen or badly deformed. Sometimes the bleeding into joints damages them or destroys them. In this situation, the individual may be given an artificial joint.

When a person who has hemophilia has a small cut or scrape, using pressure and a bandage will take care of the wound. An ice pack can be used when there are small areas of bleeding under the skin.

Researchers have been working to develop a gene replacement treatment (gene therapy) for hemophilia A. Research of gene therapy for hemophilia A is now taking place. The results are encouraging. Researchers continue to evaluate the long-term safety of gene therapies. The hope is that there will be a genetic cure for hemophilia in the future.

Individuals who have hemophilia A and B are living much longer and with less disability than they did thirty years ago. This is because of the use of the intravenous infusion of factor VIII concentrate, home infusion programs, prophylactic treatment, and improved patient education.

Is hemophilia inherited?

Hemophilia is inherited in an X-linked recessive pattern. A condition is considered X-linked when the gene mutation that causes it is located on the X chromosome, one of the two sex chromosomes. In males (who have only one X chromosome), one altered copy of the gene in each cell is enough to cause the condition. Since females have two X chromosomes, a mutation must be present in both copies of the gene to cause the hemophilia. Males are affected by X-linked recessive disorders much more frequently than females. A major characteristic of X-linked inheritance is that fathers cannot pass X-linked traits to their sons.

A female who is a carrier has a 1 in 2 (50 percent) chance to pass on her X chromosome with the gene mutation for hemophilia A or B to a boy who will be affected. She has a 1 in 2 (50 percent) chance to pass on her X chromosome with the normally functioning gene to a boy who will not have hemophilia.

Section 8.3

Von Willebrand Disease

Reprinted from "Von Willebrand Disease," National Heart Lung
and Blood Institute, National Institutes of Health, November 2008.

What Is Von Willebrand Disease?

Von Willebrand disease (VWD) is an inherited bleeding disorder.
It affects your blood's ability to clot. If your blood doesn't clot, you can
have heavy, hard-to-stop bleeding after an injury. The bleeding can
damage your internal organs or even be life threatening, although this
is rare.

In VWD, you either have low levels of a certain protein in your
blood, or the protein doesn't work the way it should. The protein is
called von Willebrand factor, and it helps the blood clot.

Normally, when one of your blood vessels is injured, you start to
bleed. Small blood cells called platelets clump together to plug the hole
in the blood vessel and stop the bleeding. Von Willebrand factor acts
like glue to help the platelets stick together and form a blood clot.

Von Willebrand factor also carries clotting factor VIII (8), another
important protein that helps your blood clot. Factor VIII is the protein that's inactive or missing in hemophilia, another clotting disorder.

VWD is more common and usually milder than hemophilia. In fact,
VWD is the most common of all the inherited bleeding disorders. It
occurs in about 1 out of every 100 to 1,000 people. VWD affects both
males and females, while hemophilia mainly affects males.

Types of Von Willebrand Disease

There are three major types of VWD.

Type 1: In type 1 VWD, you have a low level of the von Willebrand
factor, and you may have lower levels of factor VIII than normal. This
is the mildest and most common form of the disease. About three out
of four people who have VWD have type 1.

Type 2: In type 2 VWD, the von Willebrand factor doesn't work the way it's supposed to. Type 2 is divided into subtypes: 2A, 2B, 2M, and 2N. Different gene mutations cause each type, and each is treated differently. This makes knowing the exact type of VWD that you have very important.

Type 3: In type 3 VWD, you usually have no von Willebrand factor and low levels of factor VIII. Type 3 is the most serious form of VWD, but it's very rare.

Overview

Most people with VWD have type 1, a mild form. This type usually doesn't cause life-threatening bleeding, and you may need treatment only if you have surgery, tooth extraction, or trauma. If you need treatment, medicines and medical therapies are used.

Some people with severe forms of VWD need to seek emergency treatment to stop bleeding before it becomes life threatening.

Early diagnosis is important. With the right treatment plan, even people with type 3 VWD can be helped to live normal, active lives.

What Causes Von Willebrand Disease?

Von Willebrand disease (VWD) is almost always inherited. Your parents pass the gene for the disease on to you. You can inherit type 1 or type 2 VWD when only one of your parents passes the gene on to you. You usually inherit type 3 VWD only if both of your parents pass the gene on to you. Your symptoms may be different from your parents' symptoms.

Some people carry the genes for the disease but don't have symptoms. They still can pass the disease on to their children.

Some people develop a form of VWD later in life as a result of other medical conditions. This form of VWD is called acquired von Willebrand syndrome.

What Are the Signs and Symptoms of Von Willebrand Disease?

The signs and symptoms of von Willebrand disease (VWD) depend on the type and severity of the disease. Many people have such mild symptoms that they don't know they have the disorder.

If you have type 1 or type 2 VWD, you may have the following mild-to-moderate bleeding symptoms:

- Frequent large bruises from minor bumps or injuries
- Frequent or hard to stop nosebleeds
- Extended bleeding from the gums after a dental procedure
- Heavy or extended menstrual bleeding in women
- Blood in your stools from bleeding in your intestines or stomach
- Blood in your urine from bleeding in your kidneys or bladder
- Heavy bleeding after a cut or other accident
- Heavy bleeding after surgery

People with type 3 VWD may have all of the symptoms listed above, as well as severe bleeding episodes for no reason. These bleeding episodes can be life threatening if not treated right away. They also may have bleeding into soft tissues or joints, causing severe pain and swelling.

Heavy menstrual bleeding is often the main symptom of VWD for women. Doctors call this menorrhagia. They define it as follows:

- Bleeding with clots larger than about one inch in diameter
- Anemia or low blood iron
- The need to change pads or tampons more than every hour

However, just because a woman has heavy menstrual bleeding doesn't mean she has VWD.

How Is Von Willebrand Disease Diagnosed?

Early diagnosis of von Willebrand disease (VWD) is important to make sure that you're treated and can live a normal, active life.

VWD is sometimes difficult to diagnose. People with type 1 or type 2 VWD may not have major bleeding problems. As a result, they may not be diagnosed until they have heavy bleeding after surgery or some other trauma.

On the other hand, type 3 VWD can cause major bleeding problems during infancy and childhood. As a result, children with type 3 VWD are usually diagnosed during their first year of life.

To find out if you have VWD, your doctor will review your medical history and the results from a physical exam and tests.

Medical History

Your doctor will likely ask questions about your medical history and your family's medical history. He or she may ask about the following:

- Any bleeding from a small wound that lasted more than fifteen minutes or started up again within the first seven days following the injury.

- Any extended, heavy, or repeated bleeding that required medical attention after surgery or dental extractions.

- Any bruising with little or no apparent trauma, especially if you could feel a lump under the bruise.

- Any nosebleeds that occurred for no apparent reason and lasted more than ten minutes despite pressure on the nose, or any nosebleeds that needed medical attention.

- Any blood in your stools for no apparent reason.

- Any heavy menstrual bleeding (for women). This bleeding usually involves clots or lasts longer than seven to ten days.

- Any history of muscle or joint bleeding.

- Any medicines you've taken that might cause bleeding or increase the risk of bleeding. For example, aspirin and other non-steroidal anti-inflammatory drugs (NSAIDs), clopidogrel (Plavix®), warfarin, or heparin.

- Any history of liver or kidney disease, blood or bone marrow disease, or high or low blood platelet counts.

Physical Exam

The doctor also will do a physical exam to look for unusual bruising or other signs of recent bleeding. He or she also will look for evidence of liver disease or anemia.

Diagnostic Tests

No single test can diagnose VWD. Your doctor will order a combination of blood tests to diagnose the disease. These tests may include the following:

- **Von Willebrand factor antigen:** This test measures the amount of von Willebrand factor in your blood.

- **Von Willebrand factor ristocetin cofactor activity:** This test shows how well the von Willebrand factor works.

- **Factor VIII clotting activity:** Some people with VWD have low levels of factor VIII activity, while others have normal levels.

- **Von Willebrand factor multimers:** This test is done if one or more of the first three tests are abnormal. It shows the makeup or structure of the von Willebrand factor. It helps your doctor diagnose what type of VWD you have.

- **Platelet function test:** This test measures how well your platelets are working.

Your doctor may order these tests more than once to confirm the diagnosis. He or she may also refer you to a hematologist (a doctor who specializes in treating blood diseases) to confirm the diagnosis and for follow-up care.

How Is Von Willebrand Disease Treated?

Your doctor will decide what treatment you need based on the type of von Willebrand disease (VWD) you have and how severe it is. Most cases of VWD are mild, and you may need treatment only if you have surgery, tooth extraction, or an accident.

Medicines are used to do the following:

- Increase the release of von Willebrand factor and factor VIII into the bloodstream

- Replace von Willebrand factor

- Prevent the breakdown of clots

- Control heavy menstrual bleeding in women

Specific Treatments

Desmopressin (DDAVP) is a synthetic hormone that you usually take by injection or nasal spray. It makes your body release more von Willebrand factor and factor VIII into your bloodstream. DDAVP works for most patients who have type 1 VWD and for some who have type 2 VWD.

Von Willebrand factor replacement therapy is an infusion of a concentrate of von Willebrand factor and factor VIII into a vein in your arm. This treatment can be used if any of the following are true:

- You can't take DDAVP or need extended treatment
- You have type 1 VWD that doesn't respond to DDAVP
- You have type 2 or type 3 VWD

Antifibrinolytic drugs help prevent the breakdown of blood clots. They're mostly used to stop bleeding after minor surgery, tooth extraction, or an injury. They may be used alone or together with DDAVP and replacement therapy.

Fibrin glue is medicine that's placed directly on a wound to stop the bleeding.

Treatments for Women

Treatments for women who have VWD with heavy menstrual bleeding include the following:

- **Combined oral contraceptives (birth control pills):** The hormones in these pills can increase the amount of von Willebrand factor and factor VIII in your bloodstream and reduce menstrual blood loss. They're the most recommended birth control method for women with VWD.

- **A levonorgestrel intrauterine device:** This is a contraceptive device that contains progestin. It's placed in the uterus (womb).

- **Aminocaproic acid or tranexamic acid:** These antifibrinolytic drugs can reduce bleeding by slowing the breakdown of blood clots.

- **DDAVP**

For some women who are done having children or don't want children, endometrial ablation is performed. This procedure destroys the lining of the uterus. It has been shown to reduce menstrual blood loss in women with VWD.

If you need a hysterectomy (surgical removal of the uterus) for another reason, this procedure will stop menstrual bleeding and possibly improve your quality of life. However, hysterectomy carries its own risk of bleeding complications.

Living with Von Willebrand Disease

Preventing bleeding and staying healthy are important if you have von Willebrand disease (VWD). You should do the following things:

- Avoid over-the-counter medicines that can affect blood clotting, including aspirin, ibuprofen, and other nonsteroidal anti-inflammatory drugs (NSAIDs).

- Always check with your doctor before taking any medicines.

- Tell your doctor, dentist, and pharmacist if you have VWD. Your dentist can talk to your doctor about whether you need medicine before dental work to reduce bleeding. You also should tell people like your employee health nurse, gym trainer, and sports coach about your condition.

- Consider wearing a medical identification bracelet or necklace if you have a serious form of VWD (for example, type 3). In case of a serious accident or injury, the health care team treating you will know that you have VWD.

- Exercise regularly and maintain a healthy weight. Exercise helps keep muscles flexible. It also helps prevent damage to muscles and joints. Always stretch before exercising.

Some safe exercises or activities are swimming, biking, and walking. Football, hockey, wrestling, and lifting heavy weights are not safe activities if you have bleeding problems. Always check with your doctor before starting any exercise program.

Since your parents, brothers and sisters, and children may also have von Willebrand disease, you should consider telling them about your diagnosis and suggesting that they get tested.

Pregnancy and Von Willebrand Disease

Pregnancy can be a challenge for women who have VWD. Although blood levels of von Willebrand factor and factor VIII tend to increase during pregnancy, women with VWD can have bleeding complications during delivery. They also are likely to have heavy bleeding for an extended period after delivery.

However, there are things you can do to reduce the chances of complications during pregnancy. Consult a hematologist and an obstetrician who specialize in high-risk pregnancies before you become pregnant.

Consider using a center that specializes in high-risk obstetrics and has a hematologist on the staff for prenatal care and delivery.

Before you have any invasive procedure, such as amniocentesis, ask your doctor whether anything needs to be done to prevent serious blood loss.

During your third trimester, you should have blood tests to measure von Willebrand factor and factor VIII to help plan for delivery.

You also should meet with an anesthesiologist to review your choices for anesthesia and to discuss taking medicine to reduce your bleeding risk.

With these precautions, most women with VWD can have successful pregnancies.

Children and Von Willebrand Disease

If your child has von Willebrand disease that's severe enough to pose a significant risk of bleeding, anyone who is responsible for him or her should be told about the condition.

For example, the school nurse, teacher, daycare provider, coach, or any leader of after school activities should know, particularly if your child has one of the more severe forms of VWD. This information will help them handle the situation if your child has an injury.

Chapter 9

Blood Disorders (Hemoglobinopathies)

Chapter Contents

Section 9.1

Fanconi Anemia

What is Fanconi anemia?

Fanconi anemia (FA) is a rare inherited anemia that over time leads to bone marrow failure, or aplastic anemia. It occurs when both parents carry a mutation, or defect, in one of several FA genes, and their child inherits the defective gene from both parents.

Approximately ten to twenty children are born with FA each year in the United States. Sometimes, FA may be suspected at birth by one or more of the following physical traits:

- Skin discolorations
- Hand, arm, and other skeletal anomalies
- Kidney problems
- Small head or eyes
- Low birth weight
- Gastrointestinal problems (bowel)
- Small reproductive organs in males
- Heart defects

Since these physical characteristics can be indicative of other conditions, and since some patients may have no obvious physical traits of FA, the condition may not be diagnosed at birth. In fact, children with FA are most often diagnosed between the ages of six and eight when they may exhibit symptoms such as:

- unexplained fatigue;
- recurrent colds or viral infections;

- recurrent nosebleeds;

- easy bruising;

- blood in the stool or urine;

- shortness of breath;

- poor growth/short stature.

In rare cases, symptoms do not occur until early adulthood.

How is Fanconi anemia diagnosed?

Anyone who has displayed the physical characteristics and symptoms of FA or who develops aplastic anemia should be tested for FA. Initially, blood tests will be done to check for low white blood cell, red blood cell, and platelet counts and other abnormalities.

In addition to a complete medical history and thorough physical exam, a chromosome breakage test is used to observe how blood cells respond to chemically induced damage. This test is used to confirm a diagnosis of FA.

Upon diagnosis, patients will be referred to a multidisciplinary team of specialists, including a hematologist and other specialists with expertise in Fanconi anemia, who can treat both FA and the complications of the condition. Families will also learn about treatment options and meet with the bone marrow transplant team. Routine testing on vital organs may also be conducted to check for any abnormalities.

How is Fanconi anemia treated?

The progression of the disease varies in patients and requires regular, lifelong monitoring. Treatment strategies depend on the stage of the condition and the extent of physical traits and complications that result from the condition.

Current therapies for Fanconi anemia include:

- the use of hormones to stimulate red blood cell production;

- the use of growth factors to stimulate white blood cell production;

- bone marrow transplantation (BMT) when the condition becomes severe or if patients are not candidates for hormones or growth factors (BMT can be a cure for the blood problems associated with FA);

- other novel and investigational therapies, including stem cell collection, gene transfer, and Enbrel® (etanercept) drug therapy.

Specialized therapies and surgeries can be used to treat and correct symptoms and complications of FA, such as:

- heart surgery to correct heart defects;
- orthopedic surgery to correct anomalies of the hands, fingers, and skeletal system;
- therapies for gastrointestinal (GI), kidney, or other problems associated with the condition;
- hormonal therapy to treat growth deficiency, thyroid conditions. and diabetes.

Because this condition is rare, it is important to seek out FA treatment specialists.

What is the prognosis for Fanconi anemia?

There are therapies available to treat FA at different stages of the condition. Bone marrow transplantation (BMT) is essential as FA becomes severe and can be a cure for blood problems associated with FA. Even after successful BMT, patients with FA are still at increased risk of developing gynecological and gastrointestinal (GI) cancers and should be monitored regularly.

However, quality, comprehensive care is available. Since FA research is ongoing, clinical trials and emerging therapies offer greater hope to patients and their families. Genetic counseling and educational and emotional support from the treatment team also help patients and families understand and cope with the condition.

Section 9.2

Hemochromatosis

Hereditary hemochromatosis is a genetic disease that causes the body to absorb and store too much iron. The condition gets its name from "hemo" for blood and "chroma" for color, referring to the characteristic bronze skin tone that iron overload can cause. Someone with hereditary hemochromatosis who has never taken an iron supplement could find out in later years that iron overload is causing serious health problems.

Iron is a trace mineral that plays a vital role in the body. Every red blood cell contains iron in its hemoglobin, the pigment that carries oxygen from the lungs to the tissues. We get iron from our diet, and normally the body absorbs approximately 10 percent of the iron found in foods. People with hemochromatosis absorb double that amount.

Once absorbed, the excess iron doesn't leave the body. Instead, it's stored in synovium (joints) and major organs such as the liver, heart, brain, pancreas, and lungs. Over many years, iron accumulates to toxic levels that can damage or even destroy an organ. The iron overload can cause many health problems, most frequently a form of diabetes that's often resistant to insulin treatment. Because of this, hereditary hemochromatosis is sometimes called "bronze diabetes."

Some people with the disease develop symptoms by age twenty, although signs of the condition usually appear between ages forty and sixty, when iron in the body has reached damaging levels. Women are less likely to develop symptoms of iron buildup than men, probably due to normal iron loss during menstruation.

However, hereditary hemochromatosis should not be considered a disease of older people or men. Iron buildup is often present and silently causing problems long before symptoms occur—in men, women, adolescents, and in rare cases, children.

Causes of Hereditary Hemochromatosis

Although many people have never heard of the condition, hereditary hemochromatosis actually isn't rare at all. The condition affects as many as one in every two hundred people in the United States, according to the Centers for Disease Control and Prevention (CDC).

Hereditary hemochromatosis is a genetic disorder caused by a mutation on a gene that regulates iron absorption—one in every eight to ten people in the United States carries a single copy of this defective gene, called HFE. Carriers don't necessarily have the condition themselves, but can pass the mutated gene on to their children.

Hereditary hemochromatosis is an autosomal recessive condition, which means that in order to get it, a child must inherit two mutated HFE genes—one from each parent. If a child inherits just one mutated HFE gene, the normal gene essentially balances out the defective HFE gene.

Even with two mutated genes, not everyone becomes ill. Although a majority of those with two mutated genes will eventually develop some type of iron overload, far fewer of these people will absorb enough iron to develop serious problems.

In some cases, inheriting only one mutated gene may still eventually lead to iron overload, possibly affecting the heart, according to the Iron Disorders Institute. In these people, the iron overload may be triggered by a precipitating factor, such as hepatitis (inflammation of the liver) or alcohol abuse. Individuals with one mutated gene who become ill may also have mutations in other genes, yet to be discovered, that increase iron absorption.

Signs and Symptoms

Some people who test positive for hereditary hemochromatosis remain symptom-free for life. Kids who test positive rarely have any symptoms because iron takes years to accumulate.

Patients who do have symptoms may experience:

- muscle aches and joint pain, primarily in the fingers, knees, hips, and ankles (one of the earliest symptoms is arthritis of the knuckles of the first and second fingers);
- chronic fatigue;

- depression, disorientation, or memory problems;

- stomach swelling, abdominal pain, diarrhea, or nausea;

- loss of body hair, other than that on the scalp;

- premature menopause;

- gray or bronze skin similar to a suntan;

- heart problems;

- diabetes;

- enlarged liver;

- increased susceptibility to bacterial infections.

With such a wide range of possible symptoms, the disease can be extremely difficult to diagnose. As symptoms progress, it's frequently misdiagnosed as chronic hepatitis, other forms of diabetes, Alzheimer disease, iron deficiency, gallbladder illness, menstrual problems, thyroid conditions, or polycythemia (an increase in the number of red blood cells).

It's important to understand that someone with hereditary hemochromatosis can have some symptoms without having all of them (i.e., heart problems without skin color changes, diabetes, or liver problems).

Diagnosis and Screening

Luckily, the damage from hereditary hemochromatosis is completely preventable if the condition is diagnosed and treated early. Doctors may use several blood tests to measure the amount of iron in the blood and diagnose iron overload:

- Serum ferritin measures the blood level of the protein that stores iron many places in the body.

- Serum iron measures iron concentrations in the blood.

- Total iron-binding capacity (TIBC) measures the amount of iron that can be carried in the blood.

- With these results, a transferrin saturation percentage (transferrin is a protein that carries iron in the blood) is calculated by dividing the TIBC into the serum iron. An elevated transferrin saturation percentage or serum ferritin level points to iron overload.

Several gene mutations can cause hemochromatosis. A genetic test is available for the most common type of hemochromatosis, which accounts for about 85 percent of cases in the United States. However, only some of those who test positive will actually develop serious illness. The other 15 percent of individuals with symptomatic hemochromatosis will have mutations not in the HFE gene, but in other genes, which may be unknown or for which gene testing isn't routinely available.

Therefore, in cases in which high transferrin saturation and high serum ferritin are found but gene testing doesn't confirm hemochromatosis, a liver biopsy may be needed to determine whether symptomatic hemochromatosis exists or is likely to develop.

Also, the doctor may recommend a deoxyribonucleic acid (DNA) test to confirm hereditary hemochromatosis when a spouse or first-degree relative (parent, child, or sibling) has been diagnosed with the disease.

Given the prevalence of the condition, some specialists suggest screening to detect hereditary hemochromatosis before it causes problems. The following approaches to screening have been suggested:

- The College of American Pathologists recommends transferrin saturation testing on all adults at age twenty, and every five years thereafter for anyone who has a family history of the condition.

- The American Hemochromatosis Society proposes genetic screening for newborns to potentially benefit both the child and the rest of the family.

- All children have routine iron testing at age four and that those who have a genetic risk, but remain symptom-free, be tested every five years on a lifetime basis.

If you have a family history of hereditary hemochromatosis and are concerned about your child, talk to your doctor about screening tests.

Treatment

Besides specific treatment for complications of the condition—such as insulin for diabetes—most individuals with hereditary hemochromatosis are treated by regularly drawing blood, a process called phlebotomy that's similar to making a blood donation.

Initially, blood may be drawn once or twice weekly during the "de-ironing" phase until the level of iron in the body has dropped to normal.

In many cases, it requires two or three years of periodic phlebotomy to reach the desired level.

After the de-ironing phase, when the serum ferritin level has fallen into the normal range, the patient usually remains on a maintenance schedule of three to four phlebotomy sessions a year. Doctors check ferritin levels annually to monitor iron accumulation. For most people, this treatment will continue for life.

Complications

When detected and treated early, any and all symptoms of hereditary hemochromatosis can be prevented, and the person can live a normal life. If left untreated, however, hereditary hemochromatosis can lead to damaging or even fatal iron overload.

Complications of untreated iron overload include: diabetes, arthritis, depression, impotence, hypogonadism (deficient production of sex hormones by the testicle or ovary), gallbladder disease, cirrhosis (disease and scarring of the liver), heart attack, cancer, and failure of other organs.

Caring for Your Child

Treatment for kids typically isn't as aggressive as for adults, and implementing some minor dietary changes can help slow iron accumulation.

Talk to your doctor about taking preventive measures to delay or reduce iron overload. You might:

- Limit red meat in your child's diet. Iron-rich vegetables are fine because the body doesn't absorb iron from plant sources very well.

- Include moderate amounts of black, green, or oolong tea in your child's diet. The tannin from tea helps minimize iron absorption (herbal tea doesn't contain tannin).

- Avoid breakfast cereals, breads, and snacks that are enriched with iron.

- Ensure your child is immunized against hepatitis A and B.

- Limit vitamin C supplements to less than 100 milligrams per day, because vitamin C enhances iron absorption.

- Use a children's multivitamin that doesn't contain iron.

- Avoid raw shellfish, which occasionally can be contaminated with bacteria that might be harmful to someone with an iron overload.

These simple steps can help ensure that your child will remain free of symptoms of the disease.

Section 9.3

Sickle Cell Disease

Reprinted from "Learning about Sickle Cell Disease," National Human Genome Research Institute, National Institutes of Health, May 30, 2008.

What Do We Know about Heredity and Sickle Cell Disease?

Sickle cell disease is the most common inherited blood disorder in the United States. Approximately eighty thousand Americans have the disease.

In the United States, sickle cell disease is most prevalent among African Americans. About one in twelve African Americans and about one in one hundred Hispanic Americans carry the sickle cell trait, which means they are carriers of the disease.

Sickle cell disease is caused by a mutation in the hemoglobin-Beta gene found on chromosome 11. Hemoglobin transports oxygen from the lungs to other parts of the body. Red blood cells with normal hemoglobin (hemoglobin-A) are smooth and round and glide through blood vessels.

In people with sickle cell disease, abnormal hemoglobin molecules—hemoglobin S—stick to one another and form long, rod-like structures. These structures cause red blood cells to become stiff, assuming a sickle shape. Their shape causes these red blood cells to pile up, causing blockages and damaging vital organs and tissue.

Sickle cells are destroyed rapidly in the bodies of people with the disease, causing anemia. This anemia is what gives the disease its commonly known name—sickle cell anemia.

The sickle cells also block the flow of blood through vessels, resulting in lung tissue damage that causes acute chest syndrome, pain episodes, stroke, and priapism (painful, prolonged erection). It also causes damage to the spleen, kidneys, and liver. The damage to the spleen makes patients—especially young children—easily overwhelmed by bacterial infections.

A baby born with sickle cell disease inherits a gene for the disorder from both parents. When both parents have the genetic defect, there's a 25 percent chance that each child will be born with sickle cell disease.

If a child inherits only one copy of the defective gene (from either parent), there is a 50 percent chance that the child will carry the sickle cell trait. People who only carry the sickle cell trait typically don't get the disease, but can pass the defective gene on to their children.

New Treatments Prolong Life

Until recently, people with sickle cell disease were not expected to survive childhood. But today, due to preventive drug treatment, improved medical care, and aggressive research, half of sickle cell patients live beyond fifty years.

Treatments for sickle cell include antibiotics, pain management, and blood transfusions. A new drug treatment, hydroxyurea, which is an anti-tumor drug, appears to stimulate the production of fetal hemoglobin, a type of hemoglobin usually found only in newborns. Fetal hemoglobin helps prevent the "sickling" of red blood cells. Patients treated with hydroxyurea also have fewer attacks of acute chest syndrome and need fewer blood transfusions.

Bone Marrow Transplantation: The Only Cure

Currently the only cure for sickle cell disease is bone marrow transplantation. In this procedure a sick patient is transplanted with bone marrow from healthy, genetically compatible sibling donors. However only about 18 percent of children with sickle cell disease have a healthy, matched sibling donor. Bone marrow transplantation is a risky procedure with many complications.

Gene Therapy Offers Promise of a Cure

Researchers are experimenting with attempts to cure sickle cell disease by correcting the defective gene and inserting it into the bone marrow of those with sickle cell to stimulate production of normal hemoglobin. Recent experiments show promise. In December 2001, scientists at Harvard Medical School and Massachusetts Institute of Technology (MIT), supported by the National Institutes of Health (NIH), announced that they had corrected sickle cell disease in mice using gene therapy.

Researchers used bioengineering to create mice with a human gene that produces the defective hemoglobin causing sickle cell disease. Bone marrow containing the defective hemoglobin gene was removed from the mice and genetically "corrected" by the addition of the anti-sickling human beta-hemoglobin gene. The corrected marrow was then transplanted into other mice with sickle cell disease. The genetically corrected mice began producing high levels of normal red blood cells and showed a dramatic reduction in sickled cells. Scientists are hopeful that the techniques can be applied to human gene transplantation using autologous transplantation, in which some of the patient's own bone marrow cells would be removed and genetically corrected.

Is There a Test for Sickle Cell Disease?

Doctors diagnosis sickle cell through a blood test that checks for hemoglobin S—the defective form of hemoglobin. To confirm the diagnosis, a sample of blood is examined under a microscope to check for large numbers of sickled red blood cells—the hallmark trait of the disease.

In more than forty states, testing for the defective sickle cell gene is routinely performed on newborns.

Sickle cell disease can also be detected in an unborn baby. Amniocentesis, a procedure in which a needle is used to take fluid from around the baby for testing, can show whether the fetus has sickle cell disease or carries the sickle cell gene. If the test shows that the child will have sickle cell disease, some parents may choose not to continue the pregnancy. Genetic counselors can help parents make these difficult decisions.

A new technique used in conjunction with in vitro fertilization, called pre-implantation genetic diagnosis (PGD), enables parents who carry the sickle cell trait to test embryos for the defective gene before implantation, and to choose to implant only those embryos free of the sickle cell gene.

Section 9.4

Thalassemia

Thalassemias are genetic disorders that involve the decreased and defective production of hemoglobin, a molecule found inside all red blood cells (RBCs) that transports oxygen throughout the body.

As frightening as thalassemias can be, the outlook is encouraging. In the past twenty years, new therapies have greatly improved the quality of life and life expectancy in kids who have these diseases.

About Thalassemias

The two types of thalassemia are alpha-thalassemia and beta-thalassemia. Their names describe which part of the hemoglobin molecule that is affected, the alpha or the beta chain. Hemoglobin contains two different kinds of protein chains named alpha and beta chains. Any deficiency in these chains causes abnormalities in the formation, size, and shape of RBCs.

Thalassemia can cause ineffective production of RBCs and their destruction. As a result, people with thalassemia often have a reduced number of RBCs in the bloodstream (anemia), which can affect the transportation of oxygen to body tissues. In addition, thalassemia can cause RBCs to be smaller than normal or drop hemoglobin in the RBCs to below-normal levels.

Kids who have different forms of thalassemia have different kinds of health problems. Some only have mild anemia with little or no effects, while others require frequent serious medical treatment.

Causes

Thalassemia is always inherited, passed on from parents to children through their genes. A child cannot develop the disease unless both parents carry a thalassemia gene.

If only one parent passes a gene for thalassemia on to the child, then the child is said to have thalassemia trait. Thalassemia trait will not develop into the full-blown disease, and no medical treatment is necessary.

Many families have thalassemia carriers, but the trait often goes undiagnosed because it produces no or few symptoms. Frequently, thalassemia is not diagnosed in a family until a baby is born with it. So if someone in your family carries a thalassemia gene, it's wise to have genetic counseling if you're thinking of having children.

At one time it was believed that the disease affected only people of Italian or Greek descent, but it's now known that many people with thalassemia also come from or are descended from Africa, Malaysia, China, and many parts of Southeast Asia.

Because of a recent pattern of migration from Southeast Asia, there has been an increase in the past decade of thalassemia in North America. Testing for thalassemia is generally recommended for anyone from Southeast Asia with unexplained anemia.

If your doctor determines that your child is at risk for thalassemia, prenatal tests can find out if your unborn child is affected.

Alpha-Thalassemia

Children with alpha-thalassemia trait do not have thalassemia disease. People normally have four genes for alpha globin, two inherited from each parent. If one or two of these four genes are affected, the child is said to have alpha-thalassemia trait.

A specific blood test called a hemoglobin electrophoresis is used to screen for alpha-thalassemia trait and can be done in infancy. Sometimes, alpha-thalassemia trait can be detected through routine newborn blood screening, which is required in most states in the United States.

Often, results of the hemoglobin electrophoresis test are normal in people who have alpha-thalassemia trait and a diagnosis of alpha-thalassemia is done only after other conditions are ruled out and after the parents are screened. The disease can be harder to detect in older kids and adults.

Kids who have the alpha-thalassemia trait usually have no significant health problems except mild anemia, which can cause slight fatigue.

Alpha-thalassemia trait is often mistaken for an iron deficiency anemia because RBCs will appear small when viewed under a microscope.

Other cases can cause more severe anemia where three genes are affected. People with this form of alpha-thalassemia may require occasional blood transfusions during times of physical stress, like fevers or other illnesses, or when the anemia is severe enough to cause symptoms such as fatigue.

The most severe form of the disorder is called alpha-thalassemia major. This type is extremely rare, and women carrying fetuses with this form of thalassemia have a high incidence of miscarriage because the fetuses cannot survive.

Beta-Thalassemia

Beta-thalassemia, the most common form of the disorder seen in the United States, is grouped into three categories: beta-thalassemia minor (trait), intermedia, and major (Cooley anemia). A person who carries a beta-thalassemia gene has a 25 percent (1 in 4) chance of having a child with the disease if his or her partner also carries the trait.

Beta-thalassemia minor (trait): Beta-thalassemia minor often goes undiagnosed because kids with the condition have no real symptoms other than mild anemia and small red blood cells. It is often suspected based on routine blood tests such as a complete blood count (CBC) and can be confirmed with a hemoglobin electrophoresis. No treatment is usually needed.

As with alpha-thalassemia trait, the anemia associated with this condition may be misdiagnosed as an iron deficiency.

Beta-thalassemia intermedia: Children with beta-thalassemia intermedia have varying effects from the disease—mild anemia might be their only symptom or they might require regular blood transfusions.

The most common complaint is fatigue or shortness of breath. Some kids also experience heart palpitations, also due to the anemia, and mild jaundice, which is caused by the destruction of abnormal red blood cells that result from the disease. The liver and spleen may be enlarged, which can feel uncomfortable for a child. Severe anemia can also affect growth.

Another symptom of beta-thalassemia intermedia can be bone abnormalities. Because the bone marrow is working overtime to make more

RBCs to counteract the anemia, kids can experience enlargement of their cheekbones, foreheads, and other bones. Gallstones are a frequent complication because of abnormalities in bile production that involve the liver and the gallbladder.

Some kids with beta-thalassemia intermedia may require a blood transfusion only occasionally. They will always have anemia, but may not need transfusions except during illness, medical complications, or later on during pregnancy.

Other children with this form of the disease require regular blood transfusions. In these kids, low or falling hemoglobin levels greatly reduce the blood's ability to carry oxygen to the body, resulting in extreme fatigue, poor growth, and facial abnormalities. Regular transfusions can help alleviate these problems. Sometimes, kids who have this form of the disease have their spleens removed.

Beta-thalassemia intermedia is often diagnosed in the first year of life. Doctors may be prompted to test for it when a child has chronic anemia or a family history of the condition. As long as it is diagnosed while the child is still doing well and has not experienced any serious complications, it can be successfully treated and managed.

Beta-thalassemia major: Beta-thalassemia major, also called Cooley anemia, is a severe condition in which regular blood transfusions are necessary for the child to survive.

Although multiple lifelong transfusions save lives, they also cause a serious side effect: an overload of iron in the bodies of thalassemia patients. Over time, people with thalassemia accumulate deposits of iron, especially in the liver, heart, and endocrine (hormone-producing) glands. The deposits eventually can affect the normal functioning of the heart, and liver, in addition to delaying growth and sexual maturation.

To minimize iron deposits, kids must undergo chelation (iron-removing) therapy. This can be done by taking daily medication by mouth or by subcutaneous or intravenous administration.

Daily chelation therapy is given five to seven days a week and has been proven to prevent liver and heart damage from iron overload, allow for normal growth and sexual development, and increase life span. Iron concentrations are monitored every few months. Sometimes liver biopsies are needed to get a more accurate picture of the body's iron load.

Children on regular transfusions are monitored closely for iron levels and complications of iron overload on the chelation medications.

Other risks associated with chronic blood transfusions for thalassemia major include blood-borne diseases like hepatitis B and C. Blood banks screen for such infections, in addition to rarer infections such as human immunodeficiency virus (HIV). In addition, kids who have many transfusions can develop allergic reactions that can prevent further transfusions and cause serious illnesses.

For kids and teens with thalassemia, adolescence can be a difficult time, particularly because of the amount of time required for transfusions and chelation therapy.

Recently, some kids have successfully undergone bone marrow transplants to treat thalassemia major; however, this is considered only in cases of severely disabling thalassemia disease. There is considerable risk to bone marrow transplants: the procedure involves the destruction of all of the blood-forming cells in the bone marrow and repopulating the marrow space with donor cells that must match perfectly (the closest match is usually from a sibling).

The procedure is usually done in children younger than sixteen years of age who have no existing evidence of liver scarring or serious liver disease. Results have been encouraging so far, with disease-free survival in many patients.

Blood-forming stem cells taken from umbilical cord blood have also been successfully transplanted, and research using this technique is expected to increase. Currently bone marrow treatment is the only known cure for the disease.

Talking to the Doctor

If you know the thalassemia trait exists in your family, it's important to meet with your doctor, particularly if you notice any of the symptoms of thalassemia major—anemia, listlessness, or bone abnormalities—in your child.

If you're thinking of having children, speak with a genetic counselor to determine your risk of passing on the disease.

Chapter 10

CHARGE Syndrome

What is CHARGE syndrome?

CHARGE syndrome is a disorder that affects many areas of the body. CHARGE stands for coloboma, heart defect, atresia choanae (also known as choanal atresia), retarded growth and development, genital abnormality, and ear abnormality. The pattern of malformations varies among individuals with this disorder, and infants often have multiple life-threatening medical conditions. The diagnosis of CHARGE syndrome is based on a combination of major and minor characteristics.

The major characteristics of CHARGE syndrome are more specific to this disorder than are the minor characteristics. Many individuals with CHARGE syndrome have a hole in one of the structures of the eye (coloboma), which forms during early development. A coloboma may be present in one or both eyes and can affect a person's vision, depending on its size and location. Some people also have small eyes (microphthalmia). One or both nasal passages may be narrowed (choanal stenosis) or completely blocked (choanal atresia). Individuals with CHARGE syndrome frequently have cranial nerve abnormalities. The cranial nerves emerge directly from the brain and extend to various areas of the head and neck, controlling muscle movement and transmitting sensory information. Abnormal function of certain cranial nerves can cause swallowing problems, facial paralysis, a sense

Reprinted from "CHARGE Syndrome," *Genetics Home Reference*, a service of the U.S. National Library of Medicine, May 2008.

of smell that is diminished (hyposmia) or completely absent (anosmia), and mild to profound hearing loss. People with CHARGE syndrome also typically have middle and inner ear abnormalities and unusually shaped ears.

The minor characteristics of CHARGE syndrome are not specific to this disorder; they are frequently present in people without CHARGE syndrome. The minor characteristics include heart defects, slow growth starting in late infancy, developmental delay, and an opening in the lip (cleft lip) with or without an opening in the roof of the mouth (cleft palate). Individuals frequently have hypogonadotropic hypogonadism, which affects the production of hormones that direct sexual development. Males are often born with an unusually small penis (micropenis) and undescended testes (cryptorchidism). External genitalia abnormalities are seen less often in females with CHARGE syndrome. Puberty can be incomplete or delayed. Individuals may have a tracheoesophageal fistula, which is an abnormal connection (fistula) between the esophagus and the trachea. People with CHARGE syndrome also have distinctive facial features, including a square-shaped face and difference in the appearance between the right and left sides of the face (facial asymmetry). Individuals have a wide range of cognitive function, from normal intelligence to major learning disabilities with absent speech and poor communication.

How common is CHARGE syndrome?

CHARGE syndrome occurs in approximately 1 in 8,500 to 10,000 individuals.

What genes are related to CHARGE syndrome?

Mutations in the CHD7 gene cause more than half of all cases of CHARGE syndrome. The CHD7 gene provides instructions for making a protein that most likely regulates gene activity (expression) by a process known as chromatin remodeling. Chromatin is the complex of deoxyribonucleic acid (DNA) and protein that packages DNA into chromosomes. The structure of chromatin can be changed (remodeled) to alter how tightly DNA is packaged. Chromatin remodeling is one way gene expression is regulated during development. When DNA is tightly packed, gene expression is lower than when DNA is loosely packed.

Most mutations in the CHD7 gene lead to the production of an abnormally short, nonfunctional CHD7 protein, which presumably disrupts chromatin remodeling and the regulation of gene expression. Changes in gene expression during embryonic development likely cause the signs and symptoms of CHARGE syndrome.

About one-third of individuals with CHARGE syndrome do not have an identified mutation in the CHD7 gene. Researchers suspect that other genetic and environmental factors may be involved in these individuals.

How do people inherit CHARGE syndrome?

CHARGE syndrome is inherited in an autosomal dominant pattern, which means one copy of the altered gene in each cell is sufficient to cause the disorder. Most cases result from new mutations in the CHD7 gene and occur in people with no history of the disorder in their family. In rare cases, an affected person inherits the mutation from an affected parent.

Chapter 11

Connective Tissue Disorders

Chapter Contents

Section 11.1

What Are Heritable Disorders of Connective Tissue?

Reprinted from "What Are Heritable Disorders of Connective Tissue," National Institute of Arthritis and Musculoskeletal and Skin Diseases, National Institutes of Health, August 2007.

More than two hundred heritable disorders of connective tissue (HDCTs) affect the tissues between the cells of your body. The disorders are called "heritable," because they are passed on from parent to child. HDCTs come from changes to genes that build tissues.

Some HDCTs change the look and growth of skin, bones, joints, heart, blood vessels, lungs, eyes, and ears. Others change how these tissues work. Many, but not all, HDCTs are rare.

What are genes?

Genes carry our hereditary (family) information. We each have two copies of most genes: one set from each parent. Genes are what make you look like your biological family.

What is connective tissue?

Connective tissue supports many parts of the body (skin, eyes, heart, etc.). Think of it as "cellular glue" that does the following:

- Helps bring nutrients to the tissue

- Gives tissue form and strength

- Helps some of the tissues do their work

Connective tissue is made of many kinds of proteins. Sometimes genes that have changed make proteins that don't do their job right. This can change how the connective tissues work. Sometimes this leads to an HDCT.

What are some kinds of heritable disorders of connective tissue?

Common HDCTs include the following:

- **Ehlers-Danlos syndrome (EDS):** This group of HDCTs mostly affects the skin and joints. With EDS, connective tissue becomes weak. This can cause fragile, sagging skin, and loose joints.

- **Epidermolysis bullosa (EB):** With these disorders, the skin blisters when it is stressed. For example, a hug could cause a blister.

- **Marfan syndrome:** This disorder can affect the heart, blood vessels, lungs, eyes, bones, and ligaments. People with this syndrome may be unusually tall and thin, with long arms and legs.

- **Osteogenesis imperfecta (OI):** With this disorder, bones break easily. Sometimes they break for no obvious reason.

Who gets heritable disorders of connective tissue?

By one estimate, more than a half million people in the United States could have an HDCT. It can affect anyone. Some of these disorders are obvious at birth. Others don't become obvious until later in life.

Does anything increase the chances of having a genetic disease?

Several things make people more likely to get or pass on a genetic disease:

- Parents who have a genetic disease

- A family history of a genetic disease

- Parents who are closely related

- Parents who come from an ethnic group or region where the disease is common

- Parents who don't have disease symptoms but "carry" a certain gene (sometimes this gene is found through genetic testing)

What are the symptoms of heritable disorders of connective tissue?

Each HDCT has its own symptoms. Some examples are as follows:

- **Bone growth problems:** People with bone growth disorders can have brittle bones. They can also have bones that are too long or too short.

- **Joint issues:** Some HDCTs cause joints to be too loose or too tight.

- **Skin problems:** There are HDCTs that cause loose skin, skin that hangs in folds, or blistered skin.

- **Blood vessel damage:** Some HDCTs lead to weak blood vessels. Other HDCTs can close off or block blood vessels.

- **Height issues:** Some HDCTs cause people to be unusually tall or short.

- **Head and facial structural problems:** Certain HDCTs can make the head and face look different from others.

How do doctors diagnose heritable disorders of connective tissue?

To diagnose HCDTs, doctors look at the following things:

- Family history
- Medical history
- Results from a physical exam

Some people may also see a medical geneticist (someone who studies how genes affect people). Lab tests can confirm many HDCTs, but not all.

What treatments are available?

There are certain ways to manage and treat each disorder. But in general, people with HDCTs should do the following:

- Take care of their health
- Stay in touch with doctors who will know about new treatments
- Have regular checkups so doctors can check for changes or problems

What research is being done on heritable disorders of connective tissue?

Experts are trying to do the following:

- Figure out where changes (mutations) are in the connective tissue genes
- Find out which changes cause the HDCTs
- Try to find out how these changes cause the HDCT
- Use all the new knowledge to plan and test new kinds of therapy

Other research looks at the following things:

- Ways to use gene therapy
- Gene changes that cause bone disease
- Groups of proteins that cause tissue to be stiff
- Cells that form the body's tissues
- Aneurysms (weak spots in blood vessel walls that can burst)
- Drugs that can be used to treat brittle bones
- Mind-body therapy for chronic pain
- Bone growth that isn't normal
- Gene defects that cause elastin to not work right (elastin is what lets tissues stretch)

Section 11.2

Beals Syndrome
(Congenital Contractural Arachnodactyly)

"Beals Syndrome/CCA," © 2009 National Marfan Foundation
(www.marfan.org). Reprinted with permission.

What is Beals syndrome?

Beals syndrome, or congenital contractural arachnodactyly (CCA), is a genetic condition caused by an alteration (mutation) in a gene (FBN2) that is closely related to the gene (FBN1) that causes Marfan syndrome. It is similar but distinct from Marfan syndrome.

Beals syndrome can cause contractures of the joints (an inability to fully extend a joint) and abnormally shaped ears. People with Beals syndrome have many of the skeletal problems and aortic enlargement that affect people with Marfan syndrome, and the treatment of these problems is the same. The eyes are not affected.

What are the symptoms of Beals syndrome?

Following are features commonly associated with Beals syndrome:

- Inability to fully extend multiple joints such as fingers, elbows, knees, toes, and hips (contractures)

- Delay in motor development often occurs (due to congenital contractures)

- Crumpled appearance to the top of the ear

- Long, slender fingers and toes (arachnodactyly)

- Curvature of the spine (scoliosis)

- Backward and lateral curvature of the spine at birth or early childhood (kyphoscoliosis)

- Reduced bone mass (osteopenia)

- Long, narrow body type (dolichostenomelia)

112

- Chest abnormalities—concave chest (pectus excavatum) or pigeon chest (pectus carinatum)
- Underdevelopment of muscles—particularly calves (muscular hypoplasia)
- Facial abnormalities, such as unusually small jaws (micrognathia) and highly arched palate
- Occasionally aortic enlargement and/or mitral valve regurgitation

What is the treatment for Beals syndrome?

People with Beals syndrome benefit from physical therapy that can improve mobility of joints. Sometimes braces are used to provide stability.

People with Beals syndrome should have their heart monitored on a yearly basis to check for cardiovascular complications that may arise.

Section 11.3

Ehlers-Danlos Syndrome

"Ehlers-Danlos Syndrome,"
© 2009 A.D.A.M., Inc. Reprinted with permission.

Ehlers-Danlos syndrome is a group of inherited disorders marked by extremely loose joints, hyperelastic skin that bruises easily, and easily damaged blood vessels.

Causes

There are six major types and at least five minor types of Ehlers-Danlos syndrome (EDS).

A variety of gene mutations (changes) cause problems with collagen, the material that provides strength and structure to skin, bone, blood vessels, and internal organs.

The abnormal collagen leads to the symptoms associated with EDS. In some forms of the condition this can include rupture of internal organs or abnormal heart valves.

Family history is a risk factor in some cases.

Symptoms

Symptoms of EDS include:

- Double-jointedness;
- Easily damaged, bruised, and stretchy skin;
- Easy scarring and poor wound healing;
- Flat feet;
- Increased joint mobility, joints popping, early arthritis;
- Joint dislocation;
- Joint pain;
- Premature rupture of membranes during pregnancy;
- Very soft and velvety skin;
- Vision problems.

Exams and Tests

Examination by the health care provider may show:

- Deformed surface of the eye (cornea);
- Excess joint laxity and joint hypermobility;
- Mitral valve prolapse;
- Periodontitis;
- Rupture of intestines, uterus, or eyeball (seen only in vascular EDS, which is rare);
- Signs of platelet aggregation failure (platelets do not clump together properly);
- Soft, thin, or very stretchy (hyperextensible) skin.

Tests performed to diagnose EDS include:

- Collagen typing (performed on a skin biopsy sample);

- Collagen gene mutation testing;
- Echocardiogram (heart ultrasound);
- Lysyl hydroxylase or oxidase activity.

Treatment

There is no specific cure for Ehlers-Danlos syndrome. Individual problems and symptoms are evaluated and cared for appropriately. Frequently, physical therapy or evaluation by a doctor specializing in rehabilitation medicine is needed.

Outlook (Prognosis)

People with EDS generally have a normal life span. Intelligence is normal.

Those with the rare vascular type of EDS are at significantly increased risk for rupture of a major organ or blood vessel. These individuals, therefore, have a high risk of sudden death.

Possible Complications

Possible complications of Ehlers-Danlos syndrome include:

- Chronic joint pain;
- Early-onset arthritis;
- Failure of surgical wounds to close (or stitches tear out);
- Premature rupture of membranes during pregnancy;
- Rupture of major vessels, including a ruptured aortic aneurysm (only in vascular EDS);
- Rupture of a hollow organ such as the uterus or bowel (only in vascular EDS);
- Rupture of the eyeball.

When to Contact a Medical Professional

Call for an appointment with your health care provider if you have a family history of Ehlers-Danlos syndrome and you are concerned about your risk or are planning to start a family.

Call for an appointment with your health care provider if you or your child have symptoms of EDS.

Prevention

Genetic counseling is recommended for prospective parents with a family history of Ehlers-Danlos syndrome. Those planning to start a family should be aware of the type of EDS they have and its mode of inheritance (how it is passed down to children). This can be determined through testing and evaluation suggested by your health care provider or genetic counselor.

Identifying any significant health risks may help prevent severe complications by vigilant screening and lifestyle alterations.

References

Pyeritz RE. Inherited diseases of connective tissue. In: Goldman L, Ausiello D, eds. *Cecil Medicine.* 23rd ed. Philadelphia, Pa: Saunders Elsevier; 2007: chap 281.

Section 11.4

Marfan Syndrome

Reprinted from "Questions and Answers about Marfan Syndrome,"
National Institute of Arthritis and Musculoskeletal and Skin Diseases,
National Institutes of Health, NIH Publication No. 072-5000, August 2007.

What is Marfan syndrome?

Marfan syndrome is a heritable condition that affects the connective tissue. The primary purpose of connective tissue is to hold the body together and provide a framework for growth and development. In Marfan syndrome, the connective tissue is defective and does not act as it should. Because connective tissue is found throughout the body, Marfan syndrome can affect many body systems, including the skeleton, eyes, heart and blood vessels, nervous system, skin, and lungs.

Marfan syndrome affects men, women, and children, and has been found among people of all races and ethnic backgrounds. It is estimated that at least one in five thousand people in the United States have the disorder.

What are the symptoms of Marfan syndrome?

Marfan syndrome affects different people in different ways. Some people have only mild symptoms, while others are more severely affected. In most cases, the symptoms progress as the person ages. The body systems most often affected by Marfan syndrome are the skeleton, the eyes, the heart and blood vessels, the nervous system, the skin, and the lungs.

Skeleton: People with Marfan syndrome are typically very tall, slender, and loose-jointed. Because Marfan syndrome affects the long bones of the skeleton, a person's arms, legs, fingers, and toes may be disproportionately long in relation to the rest of the body. A person with Marfan syndrome often has a long, narrow face, and the roof of the mouth may be arched, causing the teeth to be crowded. Other skeletal problems include a sternum (breastbone) that is either protruding or indented, curvature of the spine (scoliosis), and flat feet.

Eyes: More than half of all people with Marfan syndrome experience dislocation of one or both lenses of the eye. The lens may be slightly higher or lower than normal, and may be shifted off to one side. The dislocation may be minimal, or it may be pronounced and obvious. One serious complication that may occur with this disorder is retinal detachment. Many people with Marfan syndrome are also nearsighted (myopic), and some can develop early glaucoma (high pressure within the eye) or cataracts (the eye's lens loses its clearness).

Heart and blood vessels (cardiovascular system): Most people with Marfan syndrome have problems associated with the heart and blood vessels. Because of faulty connective tissue, the wall of the aorta (the large artery that carries blood from the heart to the rest of the body) may be weakened and stretch, a process called aortic dilatation. Aortic dilatation increases the risk that the aorta will tear (aortic dissection) or rupture, causing serious heart problems or sometimes sudden death. Sometimes, defects in heart valves can also cause problems. In some cases, certain valves may leak, creating a "heart murmur," which a doctor can hear with a stethoscope. Small leaks may not result in any symptoms, but larger ones may cause shortness of breath, fatigue, and palpitations (a very fast or irregular heart rate).

Nervous system: The brain and spinal cord are surrounded by fluid contained by a membrane called the dura, which is composed of connective tissue. As someone with Marfan syndrome gets older, the dura often weakens and stretches, then begins to weigh on the vertebrae in the lower spine and wear away the bone surrounding the spinal cord. This is called dural ectasia. These changes may cause only mild discomfort; or they may lead to radiated pain in the abdomen; or to pain, numbness, or weakness in the legs.

Skin: Many people with Marfan syndrome develop stretch marks on their skin, even without any weight change. These stretch marks can occur at any age and pose no health risk. However, people with Mar-fan syndrome are also at increased risk for developing an abdominal or inguinal hernia, in which a bulge develops that contains part of the intestines.

Lungs: Although connective tissue problems make the tiny air sacs within the lungs less elastic, people with Marfan syndrome generally do not experience noticeable problems with their lungs. If, however, these tiny air sacs become stretched or swollen, the risk of lung collapse may increase. Rarely, people with Marfan syndrome may have sleep-related breathing disorders such as snoring, or sleep apnea (which is characterized by brief periods when breathing stops).

What causes Marfan syndrome?

Marfan syndrome is caused by a defect, or mutation, in the gene that determines the structure of fibrillin-1, a protein that is an important part of connective tissue. A person with Marfan syndrome is born with the disorder, even though it may not be diagnosed until later in life.

The defective gene that causes Marfan syndrome can be inherited: The child of a person who has Marfan syndrome has a 50 percent chance of inheriting the disease. Sometimes a new gene defect occurs during the formation of sperm or egg cells, making it possible for two parents without the disease to have a child with the disease. But this is rare. Two unaffected parents have only a one in ten thousand chance of having a child with Marfan syndrome. Possibly 25 percent of cases are due to a spontaneous mutation at the time of conception.

Although everyone with Marfan syndrome has a defect in the same gene, different mutations are found in different families, and not everyone experiences the same characteristics to the same degree. In

118

other words, the defective gene expresses itself in different ways in different people. This phenomena is known as variable expression. Scientists do not yet understand why variable expression occurs in people with Marfan syndrome.

How is Marfan syndrome diagnosed?

There is no specific laboratory test, such as a blood test or skin biopsy, to diagnose Marfan syndrome. The doctor and/or geneticist (a doctor with special knowledge about inherited diseases) relies on observation and a complete medical history, including the following:

- Information about any family members who may have the disorder or who had an early, unexplained, heart-related death

- A thorough physical examination, including an evaluation of the skeletal frame for the ratio of arm/leg size to trunk size

- An eye examination, including a "slit lamp" evaluation

- Heart tests such as an echocardiogram (a test that uses ultrasound waves to examine the heart and aorta)

The doctor may diagnose Marfan syndrome if the patient has a family history of the disease, and if there are specific problems in at least two of the body systems known to be affected. For a patient with no family history of the disease, at least three body systems must be affected before a diagnosis is made. Moreover, two of the systems must show clear signs that are relatively specific for Marfan syndrome.

In some cases, a genetic analysis may be useful in making a diagnosis of Marfan syndrome, but such analyses are often time consuming and may not provide any additional helpful information. Family members of a person diagnosed with Marfan syndrome should not assume they are not affected if there is no knowledge that the disorder existed in previous generations of the family. After a clinical diagnosis of a family member, a genetic study might identify the specific mutation for which a test can be performed to determine if other family members are affected.

Recently, doctors discovered a connective tissue disorder known as Loeys-Dietz syndrome, which has several characteristics that overlap with those of Marfan syndrome. When making a diagnosis, it is important to distinguish between the two disorders: Loeys-Dietz is more likely to cause fatal aortic aneurysms, and treatment for the two is different. A diagnostic test for Loeys-Dietz syndrome is available.

What types of doctors treat Marfan syndrome?

Because a number of body systems may be affected, a person with Marfan syndrome should be cared for by several different types of doctors. A general practitioner or pediatrician may oversee routine health care and refer the patient to specialists such as a cardiologist (a doctor who specializes in heart disorders), an orthopedist (a doctor who specializes in bones), or an ophthalmologist (a doctor who specializes in eye disorders), as needed. Some people with Marfan syndrome also go to a geneticist.

What treatment options are available?

There is no cure for Marfan syndrome. To develop one, scientists may have to identify and change the specific gene responsible for the disorder before birth. However, a range of treatment options can minimize and sometimes prevent complications. The appropriate specialists will develop an individualized treatment program; the approach the doctors use depends on which systems have been affected.

Skeletal: Annual evaluations are important to detect any changes in the spine or sternum. This is particularly important in times of rapid growth, such as adolescence. A serious malformation not only can be disfiguring, but also can prevent the heart and lungs from functioning properly. In some cases, an orthopedic brace or surgery may be recommended to limit damage and disfigurement.

Eyes: Early, regular eye examinations are essential for identifying and correcting any vision problems associated with Marfan syndrome. In most cases, eyeglasses or contact lenses can correct the problem, although surgery may be necessary in some cases.

Heart and blood vessels: Regular checkups and echocardiograms help the doctor evaluate the size of the aorta and the way the heart is working. The earlier a potential problem is identified and treated, the lower the risk of life-threatening complications. Those with heart problems are encouraged to wear a medical alert bracelet and to go to the emergency room if they experience chest, back, or abdominal pain. Some heart-valve problems can be managed with drugs such as beta-blockers, which may help decrease stress on the aorta. In other cases, surgery to replace a valve or repair the aorta may be necessary.

Surgery should be performed before the aorta reaches a size that puts it at high risk for tear or rupture. Because blood clots can form around artificial heart valves, people who have a valve replaced must take the blood-thinning drug warfarin (Coumadin®) for the rest of their lives. They must also take extreme care to prevent endocarditis (inflammation of the lining of the heart cavity and valves). Dentists should be alerted to this risk; they are likely to recommend that the patient be prescribed protective medicines before they perform dental work.

Because warfarin carries a risk of some serious side effects, including excessive bleeding, and because it is dangerous to unborn babies, doctors are increasingly opting for a newer aortic root replacement procedure that enables people to keep their own valves. The procedure involves removing and replacing the enlarged part of the aorta with a Dacron tube, and resuspending the natural valve into the tube so that the tube supports the valve. The procedure is often performed at an earlier stage than traditional valve replacement. It may also be offered to women with aortic enlargement who are considering becoming pregnant, because it can prevent the rapid aortic growth and possible tearing that sometimes occur during pregnancy.

Nervous system: If dural ectasia (swelling of the covering of the spinal cord) develops, medication may help minimize any associated pain.

Lungs: It is especially important that people with Marfan syndrome not smoke, as they are already at increased risk for lung damage. Any problems with breathing during sleep should be assessed by a doctor.

Pregnancy poses a particular concern due to the stress on the body, particularly the heart. A pregnancy should be undertaken only under conditions specified by obstetricians and other specialists familiar with Marfan syndrome. The pregnancy should be monitored as a high-risk condition. Women with an aortic measurement of four centimeters or greater may want to discuss the possibility of a valve-sparing aortic root replacement with their doctors before becoming pregnant. Women with Marfan syndrome may also seek genetic counseling concerning the likelihood that they will pass the disease on to their children.

While eating a balanced diet is important for maintaining a healthy lifestyle, no vitamin or dietary supplement has been shown to help slow, cure, or prevent Marfan syndrome.

For most people with Marfan syndrome, engaging in moderate aerobic exercise is important for promoting skeletal and cardiovascular health and a sense of well-being. However, because of the risk of aortic dissection, people with the syndrome should not engage in contact sports, competitive athletics, or isometric exercise.

What are some of the emotional and psychological effects of Marfan syndrome?

Being diagnosed and learning to live with a genetic disorder can cause social, emotional, and financial stress. It often requires a great deal of adjustment in outlook and lifestyle. A person who is an adult when Marfan syndrome is diagnosed may feel angry or afraid. There may also be concerns about passing the disorder to future generations or about its physical, emotional, and financial implications.

The parents and siblings of a child diagnosed with Marfan syndrome may feel sadness, anger, and guilt. It is important for parents to know that nothing that they did caused the fibrillin-1 gene to mutate. Parents may be concerned about the genetic implications for siblings or have questions about the risk to future children.

Some children with Marfan syndrome are advised to restrict their activities. This may require a lifestyle adjustment that is hard for a child to understand or accept.

For both children and adults, appropriate medical care, accurate information, and social support make it easier to live with the disease. Genetic counseling may also be helpful for understanding the disease and its potential impact on future generations.

While Marfan syndrome is a lifelong disorder, the outlook has improved in recent years. As recently as the 1970s, the life expectancy of a person with Marfan syndrome was two-thirds that of a person without the disease; however, with improvements in recognition and treatment, people with Marfan syndrome now have a life expectancy similar to that of the average person.

What research is being conducted to help people with Marfan syndrome?

Numerous studies are underway that should lead to a better understanding of Marfan syndrome and its treatment. They include a plan to identify the factors responsible for the cardiovascular manifestations of Marfan syndrome, a study to better understand the process that leads to skeletal manifestations, and studies to clarify the role of a chemical messenger called transforming growth factor-beta in the disorder.

Scientists are conducting research on Marfan syndrome from a variety of perspectives. One approach is to better understand what happens once the genetic defect or mutation occurs. How does it change the way connective tissue develops and functions in the body? Why are people with Marfan syndrome affected differently? Scientists are searching for the answers to these questions both by studying the genes themselves and by studying large family groups affected by the disease. Mouse models that carry mutations in the fibrillin-1 gene may help scientists better understand the disorder. Animal studies that can provide preliminary information for gene therapy are also underway.

Other scientists are focusing on ways to treat some of the complications that arise in people with Marfan syndrome. Clinical studies are being conducted to evaluate the usefulness of certain medications in preventing or reducing problems with the aorta.

For example, research has shown that the blood pressure medication losartan prevents aortic aneurysms in a mouse model of Marfan syndrome. New studies receiving funding from the National Heart, Lung and Blood Institute are now underway to determine whether the drug has the same beneficial effect in people.

Section 11.5

Osteogenesis Imperfecta

Reprinted from "Learning about Osteogenesis Imperfecta," National Human Genome Research Institute, National Institutes of Health, May 2, 2008.

What is osteogenesis imperfecta?

Osteogenesis imperfecta (OI) is a genetic disorder that causes a person's bones to break easily, often from little or no apparent trauma. OI is also called "brittle bone disease." OI varies in severity from person to person, ranging from a mild type to a severe type that causes death before or shortly after birth. In addition to having fractures, people with OI also have teeth problems (dentinogenesis imperfecta), and hearing loss when they are adults. People who have OI may also have muscle weakness, loose joints (joint laxity), and skeletal malformations.

OI occurs in approximately 1 in 20,000 individuals, including people diagnosed after birth. OI occurs with equal frequency among males and females and among racial and ethnic groups. Life expectancy varies depending on how severe the OI is, ranging from very brief (lethal form, OI type II) to average.

There are four well-known types of OI. These types are distinguished mostly by fracture frequency and severity and by characteristic features. Three additional types of OI (type V, VI, and VII) have also been identified.

The vast majority (90 percent) of OI is caused by a single dominant mutation in one of two type I collagen genes: COL1A1 or COL1A2. The COL1A1 and COL1A2 genes provide instructions for making proteins that are used to create a larger molecule called type I collagen. This type of collagen is the most common protein in bone, skin, and other tissues that provide structure and strength to the body (connective tissues). OI type VII is caused by recessive mutations in the CRTAP gene.

What are the symptoms of osteogenesis imperfecta?

Osteogenesis imperfecta (OI) causes bones to be fragile and easily broken and is also responsible for other health problems.

Type I OI is the mildest form of the condition. People who have type I OI have bone fractures during childhood and adolescence often due to minor trauma. When these individuals reach adulthood they have fewer fractures.

Type II OI is the most severe form of OI. Infants with type II have bones that appear bent or crumpled and fractured before birth. Their chest is narrow and they have fractured and misshapen ribs and underdeveloped lungs. These infants have short, bowed arms and legs; hips that turn outward; and unusually soft skull bones. Most infants with type II OI are stillborn or die shortly after birth, usually from breathing failure.

Type III OI also has relatively severe signs and symptoms. Infants with OI type III have very soft and fragile bones that may begin to fracture before birth or in early infancy. Some infants have rib fractures that can cause life-threatening problems with breathing. Bone abnormalities tend to get worse over time and often interfere with the ability to walk.

Type IV OI is the most variable form of OI. Symptoms of OI type IV can range from mild to severe. About 25 percent of infants with OI type IV are born with bone fractures. Others may not have broken bones until later in childhood or adulthood. Infants with OI type IV have leg bones that are bowed at birth, but bowing usually lessens as they get older.

Some types of OI are also associated with progressive hearing loss, a blue or grey tint to the part of the eye that is usually white (the sclera), teeth problems (dentinogenesis imperfecta), abnormal curvature of the spine (scoliosis), and loose joints. People with this condition may have other bone abnormalities and are often shorter in stature than average.

How is osteogenesis imperfecta diagnosed?

OI is often inherited from an affected parent. The diagnosis of OI is made on the basis of family history and/or clinical presentation. Frequent fractures, short stature, a blue hue to the white part of the eye (blue sclera), teeth problems (dentinogenesis imperfecta), and hearing loss that progresses after puberty may be present.

X-rays are also used to diagnose OI. X-ray findings include fractures that are at different stages of healing; an unexpected skull bone pattern called wormian bones; and bones in the spine called "codfish vertebrae."

Laboratory testing for OI may include either biochemical testing or deoxyribonucleic acid (DNA)–based sequencing of COL1A1 and

COL1A2. Biochemical testing involves studying collagens taken from a small skin biopsy. Changes in type I collagen are an indication of OI.

DNA sequencing of COL1A1 and COL1A2 is used to identify the type I collagen gene mutation responsible for the altered collagen protein. DNA testing requires a blood sample for DNA extraction. Both tests are relatively sensitive, detecting approximately 90 percent and 95 percent, respectively, of individuals with the clinical diagnosis of OI. Normal biochemical and molecular testing in a child with OI warrants additional testing of less common collagen genes (CRTAP and P3H [LEPRE1]) responsible for some of the rare recessive forms of OI.

What is the treatment for osteogenesis imperfecta?

There is currently no cure for OI. Treatment involves supportive therapy to decrease the number of fractures and disabilities, help with independent living, and maintain overall health. OI is best managed by a medical team including the child's own doctor and genetic, orthopedic, and rehabilitation medicine. Supportive therapy is unique to each individual depending on the severity of their condition and their age.

Physical and occupational therapies to help improve their ability to move, to prevent fractures, and to increase muscle strength are often useful.

Fractures are treated as they would be in children and adults who do not have OI. An orthopedic treatment called intramedullary rodding (placing rods in the bones) is used to help with positioning of legs that helps with more normal functioning when necessary.

A newer treatment with medication called bisphosphonates is being used to help with bone formation and to decrease the need for surgery.

Is osteogenesis imperfecta inherited?

Most types of OI are inherited in an autosomal dominant pattern. Almost all infants with the severe type II OI are born into families without a family history of the condition. Usually, the cause in these families is a new mutation in the egg or sperm or very early embryo in the COL1A1 or COL1A2 gene. In the milder forms of OI, 25 to 30 percent of cases occur as a result of new mutations. The other cases are inherited from a parent who has the condition. Whether a person has OI due to a new mutation or an inherited genetic change, an adult with the disorder can pass the condition down to future generations.

In autosomal dominant inherited OI, a parent who has OI has one copy of a gene mutation that causes OI. With each of his/her pregnancies, there is a 1 in 2 (50 percent) chance to pass on the OI gene mutation to a child who would have OI, and a 1 in 2 (50 percent) chance to pass on the normal version of the gene to a child who would not have OI.

Rarely, OI can be inherited in an autosomal recessive pattern. Most often, the parents of a child with an autosomal recessive disorder are not affected but are carriers of one copy of the altered gene. Autosomal recessive inheritance means two copies of the gene must be altered for a person to be affected by the disorder. The autosomal recessive form of type III OI usually results from mutations in genes other than COL1A1 and COL1A2.

Section 11.6

Stickler Syndrome

What is Stickler syndrome?

Stickler syndrome may be the most common tissue disorder in the United States, possibly affecting one in ten thousand persons.

People with Stickler syndrome have the following characteristics:

- Some degree of cleft palate
- Cataracts and/or retinal detachment at an early age
- A flat face
- A small jaw
- Skeletal abnormalities

Why did this happen?

Doctors believe it is the result of a mutation of the genes during fetal development. Three genes have been identified as causing Stickler syndrome: COL11A1, COL11A2, and COL2A1. Other genes may also cause Stickler syndrome that have not yet been identified.

Will this happen to children I have in the future?

Stickler syndrome tends to run in families. There is a 50 percent chance of passing it on to future children if you carry the trait.

What kinds of problems could my child have?

In addition to the physical characteristics common to Stickler syndrome, your child may have the following problems:

- Joint pain
- Scoliosis
- Hearing loss
- Mitral valve prolapse

Will my child need surgery?

Depending on the severity of the Stickler syndrome, your child may need some or all of the following surgeries:

- Repair to the cleft palate
- Surgery to correct retinal detachment and/or to remove cataracts
- Regular hearing and eye exams
- Corrective dentistry due to the small jaw

New advances in procedures to correct Stickler syndrome continue to be made. Be an advocate for your child!

Chapter 12

Cornelia de Lange Syndrome

What is Cornelia de Lange syndrome?

Cornelia de Lange syndrome is a developmental disorder that affects many parts of the body. The features of this disorder vary widely among affected individuals and range from relatively mild to severe.

Cornelia de Lange syndrome is characterized by slow growth before and after birth, mental retardation that is usually severe to profound, abnormalities involving the arms and hands, and distinctive facial features. The facial differences include thin, arched eyebrows; long eyelashes; low-set ears; small, widely spaced teeth; and a small, upturned nose. Many affected individuals also have behavior problems similar to autism, a developmental condition that affects communication and social interaction.

Additional signs and symptoms of Cornelia de Lange syndrome can include excessive body hair (hirsutism), an unusually small head (microcephaly), hearing loss, and problems with the digestive tract. Some people with this condition are born with an opening in the roof of the mouth called a cleft palate. Seizures, heart defects, eye problems, and skeletal abnormalities also have been reported in people with this condition.

Reprinted from "Cornelia de Lange Syndrome," *Genetics Home Reference*, a service of the U.S. National Library of Medicine, March 2007.

How common is Cornelia de Lange syndrome?

Although the exact incidence is unknown, Cornelia de Lange syndrome likely affects 1 in 10,000 to 30,000 newborns.

What genes are related to Cornelia de Lange syndrome?

Mutations in the NIPBL, SMC1A, and SMC3 genes cause Cornelia de Lange syndrome.

Mutations in the NIPBL gene have been identified in about half of all cases of Cornelia de Lange syndrome. This gene provides instructions for making a protein called delangin. Although the exact function of this protein is unknown, it appears to play an essential role in directing development before birth. Delangin regulates the activity of other genes in the developing limbs, face, and other parts of the body. NIPBL mutations lead to the production of an abnormal or nonfunctional version of this protein. These changes disrupt the regulation of genes involved in normal development, leading to the varied signs and symptoms of Cornelia de Lange syndrome.

Mutations in the SMC1A gene appear to be a less common cause of Cornelia de Lange syndrome. Although individuals with mutations in this gene have many of the major features of the condition, the signs and symptoms tend to be milder than those seen with NIPBL mutations. The SMC1A gene provides instructions for making a protein that helps regulate the structure and organization of chromosomes. Like delangin, this protein probably also controls the activity of certain genes that are important for normal development. Mutations in the SMC1A gene may cause features of Cornelia de Lange syndrome by disrupting the regulation of critical genes during early development.

Rare cases of Cornelia de Lange syndrome are caused by mutations in the SMC3 gene. Like mutations in the SMC1A gene, SMC3 mutations tend to cause a relatively mild form of the condition. This gene provides instructions for making a protein that interacts with the SMC1A protein to regulate chromosome structure. Scientists are working to determine how SMC3 mutations result in the developmental problems characteristic of Cornelia de Lange syndrome.

Researchers are looking for additional changes in the NIPBL, SMC1A, and SMC3 genes, as well as mutations in other genes, that may be responsible for this condition.

How do people inherit Cornelia de Lange syndrome?

When Cornelia de Lange syndrome is caused by mutations in the NIPBL or SMC3 gene, this condition is considered to have an autosomal dominant pattern of inheritance. Autosomal dominant inheritance means one copy of the altered gene in each cell is sufficient to cause the disorder. Almost all cases result from new mutations in the gene and occur in people with no history of the condition in their family.

Cases of Cornelia de Lange syndrome caused by SMC1A mutations have an X-linked pattern of inheritance. A condition is considered X-linked if the mutated gene that causes the disorder is located on the X chromosome, one of the two sex chromosomes. Studies of X-linked Cornelia de Lange syndrome indicate that one copy of the altered gene in each cell may be sufficient to cause the condition. Unlike most X-linked conditions, in which males are more frequently affected or experience more severe symptoms than females, X-linked Cornelia de Lange syndrome appears to affect males and females similarly. Most cases result from new mutations in the SMC1A gene and occur in people with no history of the condition in their family.

Chapter 13

Cystic Fibrosis

Cystic fibrosis (CF) is a genetic disorder that particularly affects the lungs and digestive system and makes kids who have it more vulnerable to repeated lung infections. Now, thanks to high-tech medical advances in drug therapy and genetics, children born with CF can look forward to longer and more comfortable lives. In the last ten years, research into all aspects of CF has helped doctors to understand the illness better and to develop new therapies. Ongoing research may someday lead to a cure.

What Is Cystic Fibrosis?

Currently affecting more than thirty thousand children and young adults in the United States, cystic fibrosis makes kids sick by disrupting the normal function of epithelial cells—cells that make up the sweat glands in the skin and that also line passageways inside the lungs, liver, pancreas, and digestive and reproductive systems.

The inherited CF gene directs the body's epithelial cells to produce a defective form of a protein called CFTR (or cystic fibrosis transmembrane conductance regulator) found in cells that line the lungs,

133

digestive tract, sweat glands, and genitourinary system. When the CFTR protein is defective, epithelial cells can't regulate the way chloride (part of the salt called sodium chloride) passes across cell membranes. This disrupts the essential balance of salt and water needed to maintain a normal thin coating of fluid and mucus inside the lungs, pancreas, and passageways in other organs. The mucus becomes thick, sticky, and hard to move.

Normally, mucus in the lungs traps germs, which are then cleared out of the lungs. But in CF, the thick, sticky mucus and the germs it has trapped remain in the lungs, which become infected.

In the pancreas, thick mucus blocks the channels that would normally carry important enzymes to the intestines to digest foods. When this happens, the body can't process or absorb nutrients properly, especially fats. Kids with CF have problems gaining weight, even with a normal diet and a good appetite.

A Family's Risk for CF

Humans have twenty-three pairs of chromosomes made of the inherited genetic chemical deoxyribonucleic acid (DNA). The CF gene is found on chromosome number 7. It takes two copies of a CF gene—one inherited from each parent—for a child to show symptoms of CF. People born with only one CF gene (inherited from only one parent) and one normal gene are CF carriers. CF carriers do not show CF symptoms themselves, but can pass the problem CF gene to their children. Scientists estimate that about twelve million Americans are currently CF carriers. If two CF carriers have a child, there is a one in four chance that the child will have CF.

Almost 1,400 different mutations of the CF gene can lead to cystic fibrosis (some mutations cause milder symptoms than others). About 70 percent of people with CF have the disease because they inherited the mutant gene Delta F508 from both of their parents. This can be detected by genetic testing, which can be done in kids both before and after birth and in adults thinking about starting or enlarging their families.

Of all ethnic groups, Caucasians have the highest inherited risk for CF, and Asian Americans have the lowest. In the United States today, about 1 of every 3,600 Caucasian children is born with CF. This compares with 1 of every 17,000 African Americans and only 1 of every 90,000 Asian Americans. Although the chances of inherited risk may vary, CF has been described in every geographic area of the world among every ethnic population.

Scientists don't know exactly why the CF gene evolved in humans, but they have some evidence to show that it helped to protect earlier generations from the bacteria that cause cholera, a severe intestinal infection.

How CF Affects Kids

The diagnosis of CF is being made earlier and earlier, usually in infancy. However, about 15 percent of those with CF are diagnosed later in life (even adulthood). Symptoms usually center around the lungs and digestive organs and can be more or less severe.

A few kids with CF begin having symptoms at birth. Some are born with a condition called meconium ileus. Although all newborns have meconium—the thick, dark, putty-like substance that usually passes from the rectum in the first few days of life—in CF, the meconium can be too thick and sticky to pass and can completely block the intestines.

More commonly, though, babies born with CF don't gain weight as expected. They fail to thrive in spite of a normal diet and a good appetite. In these children, mucus blocks the passageways of the pancreas and prevents pancreatic digestive juices from entering the intestines. Without these digestive juices, the intestines can't absorb fats and proteins completely, so nutrients pass out of the body unused rather than helping the body grow. Poor fat absorption makes the stools appear oily and bulky and increases the child's risk for deficiencies of the fat-soluble vitamins (vitamins A, D, E, and K). Unabsorbed fats may also cause excessive intestinal gas, an abnormally swollen belly, and abdominal pain or discomfort.

Because CF also affects epithelial cells in the skin's sweat glands, kids with CF may have a salty "frosting" on their skin or taste "salty" when their parents kiss them. They may also lose abnormally large amounts of body salt when they sweat on hot days.

Cystic fibrosis is the most common cause of pancreatic insufficiency in children, but a condition called Shwachman-Diamond syndrome (SDS) is the second most common cause. SDS is a genetic condition that causes a reduced ability to digest food because digestive enzymes don't work properly. Some of the symptoms of SDS are similar to those of CF, so it may be confused with cystic fibrosis. However, in children with SDS, the sweat test is normal.

Because CF produces thick mucus within the respiratory tract, a child with CF may suffer from nasal congestion, sinus problems, wheezing, and asthma-like symptoms. As CF symptoms progress, the child may develop a chronic cough that produces globs of thick, heavy, discolored mucus. They may also suffer from repeated lung infections.

As chronic infections reduce lung function, the ability to breathe often decreases. A person with CF may eventually begin to feel short of breath, even when resting. Despite aggressive medical therapy, lung disease develops in nearly all patients with CF and is a common cause of disability and shortened life span.

Identifying a Child with CF

By performing genetic tests during pregnancy, parents can now learn whether their unborn children may have CF. But even when genetic tests confirm CF, there's still no way to predict beforehand whether a specific child's CF symptoms will be severe or mild. Genetic testing can also be done on a child after birth, and can be performed on parents, siblings, and other relatives who are considering having a family.

After birth, the standard diagnostic test for CF is called the sweat test—an accurate, safe, and painless way to diagnose CF. In the sweat test, a small electric current is used to carry the chemical pilocarpine into the skin of the forearm. This stimulates sweat glands in the area to produce sweat. Over a period of thirty to sixty minutes, sweat is collected on filter paper or gauze and tested for chloride.

To diagnose CF, two sweat tests are generally performed in a lab accredited by the Cystic Fibrosis Foundation. A child must have a sweat chloride result of greater than 60 on two separate sweat tests to make the diagnosis of CF. Sweat test normal values for infants are lower.

Several other tests are standard parts of the routine care used to monitor a child's CF:

- Chest x-rays

- Blood tests to evaluate nutritional status

- Bacterial studies that confirm the growth of *Pseudomonas aeruginosa*, *Staphylococcus aureus*, or *Haemophilus influenzae* bacteria in the lungs (these bacteria are common in CF but may not affect healthy people exposed to CF)

- Pulmonary function tests (PFTs) to measure the effects of CF on breathing (PFTs are done as soon as the child is old enough to be able to cooperate in the testing procedure; infant PFTs are currently being studied)

Treating Kids with CF

When kids are first diagnosed with CF, they may or may not have to spend some time in the hospital, depending on their condition. If they do, they'll have diagnostic tests, especially baseline measurements of their breathing (lung function) and a nutritional assessment. Before they leave, their doctors will make sure that their lungs are clear and that they've started a diet with digestive enzymes and vitamins that will help them to gain weight normally. Afterward, they'll probably see their doctor for follow-up visits at least once every one to three months.

The basic daily care program varies from child to child, but usually includes pulmonary therapy (treatments to maintain lung function) and nutritional therapy (a high-calorie, high-fat diet with vitamin supplements). Kids with CF can also take oral doses of pancreatic enzymes to help them digest food better. They may also occasionally need oral or inhaled antibiotics to treat lung infections and mucolytic medication (a mucus-thinning drug) to keep mucus fluid and flowing.

A new treatment for CF, which is still being researched, is an inhaled spray containing normal copies of the CF gene. These normal genes deliver the correct copy of the CF gene into the lungs of CF patients. Since 1993, more than one hundred CF patients have been treated with CF gene therapy, and test trials are underway in at least nine different U.S. medical centers and other centers around the world. Another new therapy, called protein repair therapy, aims at repairing the defective CFTR protein. Numerous medications, including a spice called curcumin, are also being tested.

Caring for a child with CF can be tough at times, but parents need not feel alone. Doctors can usually refer them to a local support group linked to the Cystic Fibrosis Foundation.

Chapter 14

Endocrine Disorders

Chapter Contents

Section 14.1

Congenital Adrenal Hyperplasia (21-Hydroxylase Deficiency)

Reprinted from "Facts about CAH: Congenital Adrenal Hyperplasia," National Institutes of Health Clinical Center, 2006.

What are the adrenal glands?

The adrenal glands are a pair of walnut-sized organs above the kidneys. They make hormones, which act like chemical messengers to affect other organs in the body. An organ at the base of the brain, called the pituitary gland, helps regulate the adrenal glands. Each adrenal gland has two parts: the medulla (the inner part), and the cortex (the outer part).The medulla makes the hormone adrenaline. The cortex makes the hormones cortisol, aldosterone, and androgens.

Congenital adrenal hyperplasia (CAH) affects how the adrenal cortex works. In severe cases, the adrenal medulla may also not function normally.

What do adrenal hormones do?

Hormones made by the adrenal glands are important for the body's normal function. Cortisol affects energy levels, sugar levels, blood pressure, and the body's response to illness or injury. Aldosterone helps maintain the proper salt level. Androgens are male- like hormones needed for normal growth and development in both boys and girls. Adrenalin affects blood sugar levels, blood pressure, and the body's response to physical stress.

What is CAH?

The adrenal glands help keep the body in balance by making the right amounts of cortisol, aldosterone, and androgens. But in CAH, production of cortisol is blocked. Some children with CAH also lack aldosterone. These imbalances cause the adrenal gland to make too much androgen.

Symptoms: Too little cortisol may cause tiredness and nausea. During illness or injury, low cortisol levels can lead to low blood pressure and even death.

Lack of aldosterone, which occurs in three out of four patients with classic CAH, upsets salt levels. This imbalance may cause dehydration (too little fluid within the body), and possibly death. Chronic salt imbalance may also cause abnormal growth.

Too much androgen causes abnormal physical development in children. Boys and girls with CAH may grow too fast, develop early pubic hair and acne, and stop growing too soon, causing short stature. Girls exposed to high levels of androgens before birth may have abnormal external genitalia at birth. Although their internal female organs are normal, excess androgens may also affect puberty and cause irregular menstrual periods.

Too much cortisol replacement also causes abnormal development in children. Side effects include obesity and short stature. Also, too much hydrocortisone, the medicine given to replace cortisol in the body, can cause decreased bone density (osteoporosis) and high cholesterol levels.

Are there different types of CAH?

There are many types of CAH. The severe form is called classic CAH, while the mild form is called nonclassic CAH.

Classic CAH: The most common is 21-hydroxylase deficiency (95 percent of cases). A child with this type of CAH has adrenal glands that cannot make enough cortisol and may or may not make aldosterone. As a result, the glands overwork trying to make these hormones and end up making too much of what they can make: androgens.

The second most common form of CAH is 11-hydroxylase deficiency. A child with this type of CAH has adrenal glands that make too much androgen and not enough cortisol. Children with this type of CAH may also have high blood pressure. These patients do not have aldosterone deficiency.

Rare other types of CAH include 3-beta-hydroxy-steroid dehydrogenase deficiency, lipoid CAH, and 17-hydroxylase deficiency.

Nonclassic (late-onset) CAH: This type of CAH is a mild form of CAH and is almost always due to 21-hydroxylase deficiency. Only a handful of people have been described as having nonclassic (mild) CAH due to other causes. People with nonclassic 21-hydroxylase deficiency

141

make enough cortisol and aldosterone, but they make excess androgens. Symptoms come and go, beginning at any time but typically in late childhood or early adulthood. Boys often do not need treatment. Girls usually need treatment to suppress their excess androgens.

Nonclassic CAH is common. One in every one thousand people has nonclassic 21-hydroxylase deficiency. Incidence is higher in certain ethnic groups including Ashkenazi Jews, Hispanics, Yugoslavs, and Italians.

How is CAH inherited?

An inherited disorder is one that can be passed from the parents to their children. CAH is a type of inherited disorder called "autosomal recessive."

For a child to have CAH, each parent must either have CAH or carry a genetic mutation. This means that if two parents are CAH carriers (that is, they have the gene for CAH but not the disorder), their children have a 25 percent chance (1 in 4) of being born with CAH. Each sibling without CAH has two chances in three of being a carrier. Tests can be done to find out if someone is a carrier.

Classic CAH occurs in one in fifteen thousand births.

How is CAH treated?

The standard treatment for classic 21- hydroxylase deficiency is hydrocortisone which replaces cortisol, and fludrocortisone (Florinef®) which replaces aldosterone. For 11-hydroxylase deficiency, the treatment is only hydrocortisone. Patients can be started on longer-acting forms of hydrocortisone (i.e. prednisone or dexamethasone) when they are done growing.

Because replacement medications cannot mimic the body's exact needs, patients, on average, are about four inches shorter than their peers.

Patients with the nonclassic form of CAH need only hydrocortisone (or a longer acting form of hydrocortisone). Some patients with nonclassic CAH are able to come off medication as adults, but patients with classic CAH need lifelong treatment.

What if a child with CAH has an illness, surgery, or a major injury?

During these times, a child with CAH needs closer medical attention and should be under a doctor's care. More cortisol is needed to meet the body's increased needs for this hormone. Higher doses of hydrocortisone are given by mouth or sometimes by intramuscular injection. Intravenous medication is needed before surgery.

Medical alert identification: In an emergency, it is important to alert medical personnel about the diagnosis of adrenal insufficiency, so wearing a medical alert identification bracelet or necklace is recommended. The information on the medic alert should include, "adrenal insufficiency, requires Cortef." It is also important for the adult or parent to learn how to administer an intramuscular injection of Cortef® in case of emergency.

How long can people live with CAH?

People with CAH have a normal life expectancy.

Can a woman with CAH become pregnant and have a baby?

Increased androgens may cause irregular menstrual periods and make it harder for a woman with CAH to conceive a child. But if she takes her medications as directed, she can become pregnant and have a baby.

Do men with CAH have fertility problems?

Men who take medications as directed usually have normal fertility. Rarely, however, they may develop "adrenal rest tissue" in their testicles. This is when adrenal tissue grows in other parts of the body such as the testicles or scrotum. Having adrenal rest tissue may affect a man's ability to father a child. The tissue does not turn to cancer, but it can grow enough to cause discomfort or infertility. Large growths are rare, and surgery is usually not needed.

Do children with CAH outgrow it?

CAH cannot be outgrown. Classic CAH requires treatment for life. Some patients with nonclassic CAH may not require treatment as adults. Treatment is tailored for each patient and adjusted during childhood for growth.

Can CAH be diagnosed prenatally?

CAH can be diagnosed before birth. Amniocentesis or chorionic villus sampling during pregnancy can check for the disorder.

Neonatal screening: Testing for classic CAH is part of the routine newborn screen done in most states.

Can CAH be treated prenatally?

Experimental prenatal treatment is available for fetuses at risk for classic CAH. For this treatment, mothers take dexamethasone, a potent form of hydrocortisone. This drug suppresses androgens in the fetus and allows female genitalia to develop more normally. This treatment lessens or eliminates the need for surgery in girls. It does not, however, treat other aspects of the disorder. Children with CAH still need to take hydrocortisone and Florinef for life. (Florinef is a brand name for fludrocortisone. It is easier to say than fludrocortisone.)

What research is being done?

Researchers are working on many aspects of CAH including discovering new ways to diagnose and treat the disorder and finding the precise genetic defects that cause CAH. At the National Institutes of Health (NIH), scientists are learning more about CAH. They are also searching for better treatments for children and adults with CAH.

Section 14.2

Congenital Hypothyroidism

"Congenital Hypothyroidism," © 2008 MAGIC Foundation
(www.magicfoundation.org). Reprinted with permission.

You have just learned that your baby has congenital hypothyroidism. Suddenly, you have a lot of confusion and certainly may be frightened regarding the wellbeing of your new infant. As a concerned parent, you probably wish to learn as much as you can about the condition and what you and your health care professional can do to help your baby's condition as your child grows and develops.

Ask Questions

As you learn about congenital hypothyroidism, it is probable that you will have questions that may be specific to your child. Leave no questions unanswered, even if you think the questions are simple or silly. A greater understanding of this condition will allow you to provide optimal care for your child.

What Is Congenital Hypothyroidism?

This is a disorder that affects infants from birth (congenital), resulting from the loss of thyroid function (hypothyroidism), normally due to failure of the thyroid gland to develop correctly. Sometimes the thyroid gland is absent, or ectopic (in an abnormal location). As a result, the thyroid gland does not produce enough thyroxine/T4 after birth. This may result in abnormal growth and development, as well as slower mental function.

What Is the Thyroid Gland?

The thyroid is a bowtie-shaped gland located in the neck, below the Adam's apple. The thyroid gland is part of the endocrine system. This gland is responsible for secreting a hormone called thyroxine (T4) which plays a vital role in normal growth and development in children.

This gland, like other glands in the endocrine system is controlled by the pituitary gland. It works very much like a thermostat. The brain senses the amount of T4 and then signals the thyroid with another hormone, thyroid-stimulating hormone (TSH), to produce more or less T4. When the thyroid gland produces enough T4, no extra stimulation is needed and the TSH level remains at a normal level. When there is not enough T4, the TSH rises. These characteristics of the T4 and TSH hormones allow for screening of newborns to assess whether or not they have hypothyroidism (an underactive thyroid gland).

Why Did My Child Develop Congenital Hypothyroidism?

In most hypothyroid babies, there is no specific reason why the thyroid gland did not develop normally, although some of these children have an inherited form of this disorder. Congenital hypothyroidism is present in about one in four thousand infants in North America. There are a small proportion of children who have temporary (transient) congenital hypothyroidism for a period of time after birth. It is impossible to distinguish these transient hypothyroid babies from those with true congenital hypothyroidism and so these infants will be treated as well. Often, after the age of two or three, in children for whom transient or temporary hypothyroidism is suspected the medication can be gradually discontinued for a short amount of time on a trial basis. The child will be retested to see if they can remain off medicine. This is not the case for true congenital hypothyroidism, where L-thyroxine is necessary throughout your child's life.

Symptoms of Congenital Hypothyroidism

Often these babies appear perfectly normal at birth, which is why screening is so vital. However, some may have one or more of the following symptoms:

- Large, despite having poor feeding habits, increased birth weight
- Puffy face, swollen tongue
- Hoarse cry
- Low muscle tone
- Cold extremities
- Persistent constipation, bloated or full to the touch

- Lack of energy, sleeps most of the time, appears tired even when awake

- Little to no growth

Children born with symptoms have a greater risk of developmental delay than children born without symptoms.

What Tests Are Used to Find Congenital Hypothyroidism?

The usual way to discover congenital hypothyroidism is by a screening process done on all newborns between twenty-four and seventy-two hours old. The reason this is done so early is that infants with congenital hypothyroidism usually appear normal at birth and many do not show any of the signs or symptoms noted before. For the screening test, blood is obtained from your baby's heel and is placed on a filter paper. At a laboratory the T4 and/or TSH level is measured. If the T4 is low and/or the TSH is elevated, indicating hypothyroidism, your pediatrician is contacted immediately so treatment can begin without delay. It is likely that the blood test will be repeated to confirm the diagnosis. The physicians may also take an x-ray of the legs to look at the ends of the bones. In babies with hypothyroidism, the bones have an immature appearance which helps to confirm diagnosis of congenital hypothyroidism. A thyroid scan should be done to determine the location or absence of the thyroid gland. These tests, bone age and thyroid scan, can be done at the time of diagnosis.

How Does One Treat Congenital Hypothyroidism?

Treatment for congenital hypothyroidism is replacement of the missing thyroid hormone in pill form. It is extremely important that these pills be taken daily for life because thyroxine/T4 is essential for all the body's functions. In general, the average starting dose for L-thyroxine or Levothyroxine (synthetic T4) in a newborn is between 25 and 50 mcg per day or 10 mcg to 15 mcg/kg of body weight. This value increases dependent upon the individual needs of the child. The pill can be crushed, then administered in a small amount of water/ formula or breast milk while your child is still an infant. Please be aware that L-thyroxine should not be mixed with Soy formula as this product interferes with absorption. Blood tests will be done on a regular basis to ensure that the hormone levels are in a normal range.

Thyroid hormone is necessary for normal brain and intellectual development and such development can be delayed when there is a lack of L-thyroxine. With early replacement of adequate thyroid hormone and proper follow-up and care, the outlook for most children with congenital hypothyroidism is excellent.

What Type of Medical Attention Should My Child Receive?

Generally, children are seen every two to three months for the first three years, once normal levels have been established. The goal is to maintain the concentration of T4 in the mid to upper half of the normal range (10 mg/dL to 16 mg/dL) for the first years of life. The TSH level should be maintained within the normal reference range for infants. The treatment for hypothyroidism is safe, simple, and effective. Successful treatment, however, depends on lifelong daily medication with close follow-up of hormone levels. Making this procedure of taking medication on a routine basis needs to become a part of the lifestyle of you and your child in order to assure optimal growth and development.

Section 14.3

Kallmann Syndrome

Reprinted from "Kallmann Syndrome," *Genetics Home Reference*,
a service of the U.S. National Library of Medicine, August 2008.

What is Kallmann syndrome?

Kallmann syndrome is a condition characterized by delayed or absent puberty and an impaired sense of smell.

This disorder is a form of hypogonadotropic hypogonadism (HH), which is a condition affecting the production of hormones that direct sexual development. Males with hypogonadotropic hypogonadism are often born with an unusually small penis (micropenis) and undescended testes (cryptorchidism). At puberty, most affected individuals do not develop secondary sex characteristics, such as the growth of facial hair and deepening of the voice in males. Affected females usually do not begin menstruating at puberty and have little or no breast development. In some people, puberty is incomplete or delayed.

In Kallmann syndrome, the sense of smell is either diminished (hyposmia) or completely absent (anosmia). This feature distinguishes Kallmann syndrome from most other forms of hypogonadotropic hypogonadism, which do not affect the sense of smell. Many people with Kallmann syndrome are not aware that they are unable to detect odors until the impairment is discovered through testing.

The features of Kallmann syndrome vary, even among affected people in the same family. Additional signs and symptoms can include a failure of one kidney to develop (unilateral renal agenesis), a cleft lip with or without an opening in the roof of the mouth (a cleft palate), abnormal eye movements, hearing loss, and abnormalities of tooth development. Some affected individuals have a condition called bimanual synkinesis, in which the movements of one hand are mirrored by the other hand. Bimanual synkinesis can make it difficult to do tasks that require the hands to move separately, such as playing a musical instrument.

Researchers have identified four forms of Kallmann syndrome, designated types 1 through 4, which are distinguished by their genetic cause. The four types are each characterized by hypogonadotropic hypogonadism and an impaired sense of smell. Additional features, such as a cleft palate, seem to occur only in types 1 and 2.

How common is Kallmann syndrome?

Kallmann syndrome is estimated to affect 1 in 10,000 to 86,000 people and occurs more often in males than in females. Kallmann syndrome 1 is the most common form of the disorder.

What genes are related to Kallmann syndrome?

Mutations in the KAL1, FGFR1, PROKR2, and PROK2 genes cause Kallmann syndrome. KAL1 mutations are responsible for Kallmann syndrome 1. Kallmann syndrome 2 results from mutations in the FGFR1 gene. Mutations in the PROKR2 and PROK2 genes cause Kallmann syndrome types 3 and 4, respectively.

The genes associated with Kallmann syndrome play a role in the development of certain areas of the brain before birth. Although some of their specific functions are unclear, these genes appear to be involved in the formation and movement (migration) of a group of nerve cells that are specialized to process smells (olfactory neurons). These nerve cells come together into a bundle called the olfactory bulb, which is critical for the perception of odors. The KAL1, FGFR1, PROKR2, and PROK2 genes also play a role in the migration of neurons that produce a hormone called gonadotropin-releasing hormone (GnRH). GnRH controls the production of several other hormones that direct sexual development before birth and during puberty. These hormones are important for the normal function of the gonads (ovaries in women and testes in men).

Studies suggest that mutations in the KAL1, FGFR1, PROKR2, or PROK2 gene disrupt the migration of olfactory nerve cells and GnRH-producing nerve cells in the developing brain. If olfactory nerve cells do not extend to the olfactory bulb, a person's sense of smell will be impaired or absent. Misplacement of GnRH-producing neurons prevents the production of certain sex hormones, which interferes with normal sexual development and causes the characteristic features of hypogonadotropic hypogonadism. It is unclear how gene mutations lead to the other possible signs and symptoms of Kallmann syndrome. Because the features of this condition vary among individuals, researchers suspect that additional genetic and environmental factors may be involved.

Together, mutations in the KAL1, FGFR1, PROKR2, and PROK2 genes account for 25 to 30 percent of all cases of Kallmann syndrome. In cases without an identified mutation in one of these genes, the cause of the condition is unknown. Researchers are looking for other genes that can cause this disorder.

How do people inherit Kallmann syndrome?

Kallmann syndrome 1 (caused by KAL1 mutations) has an X-linked recessive pattern of inheritance. The KAL1 gene is located on the X chromosome, which is one of the two sex chromosomes. In males (who have only one X chromosome), one altered copy of the gene in each cell is sufficient to cause the condition. In females (who have two X chromosomes), a mutation must be present in both copies of the gene to cause the disorder. Males are affected by X-linked recessive disorders much more frequently than females. A striking characteristic of X-linked inheritance is that fathers cannot pass X-linked traits to their sons.

Most cases of Kallmann syndrome 1 are described as simplex, which means only one person in a family is affected. Some affected people inherit a KAL1 mutation from their mothers, who carry a single mutated copy of the gene in each cell. Other people have the condition as a result of a new mutation in the KAL1 gene.

Other forms of Kallmann syndrome can be inherited in an autosomal dominant pattern, which means one copy of the altered gene in each cell is sufficient to cause the disorder. In some cases, an affected person inherits the mutation from one affected parent. Other cases result from new mutations in the gene and occur in people with no history of the disorder in their family.

In several families, Kallmann syndrome has shown an autosomal recessive pattern of inheritance. Autosomal recessive inheritance means both copies of the gene in each cell have mutations. The parents of an individual with an autosomal recessive condition each carry one copy of the mutated gene, but they typically do not show signs and symptoms of the condition.

Chapter 15

Familial Hypercholesterolemia

What is familial hypercholesterolemia?

Familial hypercholesterolemia is an inherited condition that causes high levels of LDL (low density lipoprotein) cholesterol levels beginning at birth, and heart attacks at an early age. Cholesterol is a fatlike substance that is found in the cells of the body. Cholesterol is also found in some foods. The body needs some cholesterol to work properly and uses cholesterol to make hormones, vitamin D, and substances that help with food digestion. However, if too much cholesterol is present in the bloodstream, it builds up in the wall of the arteries and increases the risk of heart disease.

Cholesterol is carried in the bloodstream in small packages called lipoproteins. These small packages are made up of fat (lipid) on the inside and proteins on the outside. There are two main kinds of lipoprotein that carry cholesterol throughout the body. These are: low-density lipoprotein (LDL) and high-density lipoprotein (HDL).

The cholesterol carried by LDL is some times called the "bad cholesterol." People who have familial hypercholesterolemia have high levels of LDL cholesterol because they cannot remove the LDL from the bloodstream properly. The organ responsible for the removal of the LDL is the liver. High levels of LDL cholesterol in the blood increase the risk for heart attacks and heart disease.

Reprinted from "Learning about Familial Hypercholesterolemia," National Human Genome Research Institute, National Institutes of Health, November 7, 2008.

The cholesterol carried by HDL is sometimes called the "good cholesterol." HDL carries cholesterol from other parts of the body to the liver. The liver removes cholesterol from the body. Higher levels of HDL cholesterol lower a person's chance for getting heart disease.

Men who have familial hypercholesterolemia have heart attacks in their forties to fifties, and 85 percent of men with the disorder have a heart attack by age sixty. Women who have familial hypercholesterolemia also have an increased risk for heart attack, but it happens ten years later than in men (so in their fifties and sixties).

Familial hypercholesterolemia is inherited in families in an autosomal dominant manner. In autosomal dominant inherited conditions, a parent who carries an altered gene that causes the condition has a one in two (50 percent) chance to pass on that altered gene to each of his or her children.

The altered gene (gene mutation) that causes familial hypercholesterolemia is located on chromosome number 19. It contains the information for a protein called LDL receptor that is responsible to clear up LDL from the blood stream. One in five hundred individuals carries one altered gene causing familial hypercholesterolemia. These individuals are called heterozygotes. More rarely, a person inherits the gene mutation from both parents, making them genetically homozygous. Individuals who are homozygous have a much more severe form of hypercholesterolemia, with heart attack and death often occurring before age thirty.

What are the symptoms of familial hypercholesterolemia?

The major symptoms and signs of familial hypercholesterolemia are as follows:

- High levels of total cholesterol and LDL cholesterol
- A strong family history of high levels of total and LDL cholesterol and/or early heart attack
- Elevated and therapy-resistant levels of LDL in either or both parents
- Xanthomas (waxy deposits of cholesterol in the skin or tendons)
- Xanthelasmas (cholesterol deposits in the eyelids)
- Corneal arcus (cholesterol deposit around the cornea of the eye)

If angina (chest pain) is present may be sign that heart disease is present.

Individuals who have homozygous familial hypercholesterolemia develop xanthomas beneath the skin over their elbows, knees, and buttocks as well as in the tendons at a very early age, sometime in infancy. Heart attacks and death may occur before thirty.

How is familial hypercholesterolemia diagnosed?

Diagnosis of familial hypercholesterolemia is based on physical examination and laboratory testing. Physical examination may find xanthomas and xanthelasmas (skin lesions caused by cholesterol-rich lipoprotein deposits), and cholesterol deposits in the eye called corneal arcus.

Laboratory testing includes blood testing of cholesterol levels, studies of heart function, and genetic testing. Blood testing of cholesterol levels may show: increased total cholesterol usually above 300 mg/dl (total cholesterol of more than 250 mg/dl in children) and LDL levels usually above 200 mg/dl. Studies of heart function, such as a stress test, may be abnormal. Genetic testing may show an alteration (mutation) in the LDL receptor gene.

What is the treatment for familial hypercholesterolemia?

The overall goal of treatment is to lower the risk for atherosclerotic heart disease by lowering the LDL cholesterol levels in the blood stream. Atherosclerosis is a condition in which fatty material collects along the walls of arteries. This fatty material thickens, hardens, and may eventually block the arteries. Atherosclerosis happens when fat and cholesterol and other substances build up in the arteries and form a hardened material called plaque. The plaque deposits make the arteries less flexible and make it more difficult for blood to flow, leading to heart attack and stroke.

The first step in treatment for an individual who has heterozygous familial hypercholesterolemia is changing the diet to reduce the total amount of fat eaten to 30 percent of the total daily calories. This can be done by limiting the amount of beef, pork, and lamb in the diet; cutting out butter, whole milk, and fatty cheeses as well as some oils like coconut and palm oils; and eliminating egg yolks, organ meats, and other sources of saturated fat from animals. Dietary counseling is often recommended to help people to make these changes in their eating habits.

Exercise, especially to lose weight, may also help in lowering cholesterol levels.

Drug therapy is usually necessary in combination with diet, weight loss, and exercise, as these interventions may not be able to lower cholesterol levels alone. There are a number of cholesterol-lowering medications that are currently used. The first and more effective choice are drugs called "statins." Other drugs that may be used in combination with or instead of the statins are: bile acid sequestrant resins (for example, cholestyramine), ezetimibe, nicotinic acid (niacin), gemfibrozil, and fenofibrate.

Individuals who have homozygous familial hypercholesterolemia need more aggressive therapies to treat their significantly elevated levels of cholesterol. Often drug therapies are not sufficient to lower LDL cholesterol levels at the desired goal and these individuals may require periodical LDL apheresis, a procedure to "clean up" LDL from the bloodstream, or highly invasive surgery such as a liver transplant.

Is familial hypercholesterolemia inherited?

Familial hypercholesterolemia is inherited in an autosomal dominant manner. This means that to have this condition it is sufficient that the altered (mutated) gene is present on only one of the person's two number 19 chromosomes. A person who inherits one copy of the gene mutation causing familial hypercholesterolemia from one of his or her parents is said to have heterozygous familial hypercholesterolemia. This person has a one in two (50 percent) chance to pass on the mutated gene to each of his or her children.

A person who inherits a mutated copy of the gene causing familial hypercholesterolemia from both parents is said to have homozygous familial hypercholesterolemia. This is a much more severe form of familial hypercholesterolemia than heterozygous familial hypercholesterolemia. Each of this person's children will inherit one copy of the mutated gene and will have heterozygous familial hypercholesterolemia.

Chapter 16

Growth Disorders

Chapter Contents

Section 16.1

Achondroplasia

Reprinted from "Learning about Achondroplasia," National Human
Genome Research Institute, National Institutes of Health, August 12, 2008.

What is achondroplasia?

Achondroplasia is a disorder of bone growth. It is the most common form of disproportionate short stature. It occurs in one in every fifteen thousand to one in forty thousand live births. Achondroplasia is caused by a gene alteration (mutation) in the FGFR3 gene. The FGFR3 gene makes a protein called fibroblast growth factor receptor 3 that is involved in converting cartilage to bone. FGFR3 is the only gene known to be associated with achondroplasia. All people who have only a single copy of the normal FGFR3 gene and a single copy of the FGFR3 gene mutation have achondroplasia.

Most people who have achondroplasia have average-size parents. In this situation, the FGFR3 gene mutation occurs in one parent's egg or sperm cell before conception. Other people with achondroplasia inherit the condition from a parent who has achondroplasia.

What are the symptoms of achondroplasia?

People who have achondroplasia have abnormal bone growth that causes the following clinical symptoms: short stature with disproportionately short arms and legs, short fingers, a large head (macrocephaly), and specific facial features with a prominent forehead (frontal bossing) and mid-face hypoplasia.

The intelligence and life span in individuals with achondroplasia is usually normal.

Infants born with achondroplasia typically have weak muscle tone (hypotonia). Because of the hypotonia, there may be delays in walking and other motor skills. Compression of the spinal cord and/or upper airway obstruction increases the risk of death in infancy.

People with achondroplasia commonly have breathing problems in which breathing stops or slows down for short periods (apnea). Other health issues include obesity and recurrent ear infections. Adults with achondroplasia may develop a pronounced and permanent sway of the lower back (lordosis) and bowed legs. The problems with the lower back can cause back pain leading to difficulty with walking.

How is achondroplasia diagnosed?

Achondroplasia is diagnosed by characteristic clinical and x-ray findings in most affected individuals. In individuals who may be too young to make a diagnosis with certainty or in individuals who do not have the typical symptoms, genetic testing can be used to identify a mutation in the FGFR3 gene.

Genetic testing can identify mutations in 99 percent of individuals who have achondroplasia. Testing for the FGFR3 gene mutation is available in clinical laboratories.

What is the treatment for achondroplasia?

No specific treatment is available for achondroplasia. Children born with achondroplasia need to have their height, weight, and head circumference monitored using special growth curves standardized for achondroplasia. Measures to avoid obesity at an early age are recommended.

A magnetic resonance imaging (MRI) or computed tomography (CT) scan may be needed for further evaluation of severe muscle weakness (hypotonia) or signs of spinal cord compression. To help with breathing, surgical removal of the adenoids and tonsils, continuous positive airway pressure (CPAP) by nasal mask, or a surgical opening in the airway (tracheostomy) may be needed to correct obstructive sleep apnea.

When there are problems with the lower limbs, such as hyperreflexia, clonus, or central hypopnea, then surgery called suboccipital decompression is performed to decrease pressure on the brain.

Children who have achondroplasia need careful monitoring and support for social adjustment.

Is achondroplasia inherited?

Most cases of achondroplasia are not inherited. When achondroplasia is inherited, it is inherited in an autosomal dominant manner.

Over 80 percent of individuals who have achondroplasia have parents with normal stature and are born with achondroplasia as a result of a new (de novo) gene alteration (mutation). These parents have a small chance of having another child with achondroplasia.

A person who has achondroplasia who is planning to have children with a partner who does not have achondroplasia has a 50 percent chance, with each pregnancy, of having a child with achondroplasia. When both parents have achondroplasia, the chance for them, together, to have a child with normal stature is 25 percent. Their chance of having a child with achondroplasia is 50 percent. Their chance for having a child who inherits the gene mutation from both parents (called homozygous achondroplasia—a condition that leads to death) is 25 percent.

Section 16.2

Dwarfism

There's been a lot of discussion over the years about the proper way to refer to a child with dwarfism. Many people who have the condition prefer the term "little person" or "person of short stature." For some, "dwarf" is acceptable. For most, "midget" definitely is not. But here's an idea everyone can agree on: Why not simply call a person with dwarfism by his or her name?

Being of short stature is only one of the characteristics that make a little person who he or she is. If you're the parent or loved one of a little person, you know this to be true. But here are some facts that other people may not realize about dwarfism and those who have it.

Dwarfism:

- is a condition characterized by short stature. Technically, that means an adult height of 4 feet 10 inches or under, according to the advocacy group Little People of America (LPA).

- can be caused by any one of more than two hundred conditions, most of which are genetic. The most common type, accounting for 70 percent of all cases of short stature, is called achondroplasia.

- can and most often does occur in families where both parents are of average height. In fact, 85 percent of children with achondroplasia are born to average-size parents.

Dwarfism isn't:

- an intellectual disability. A person who has dwarfism is typically of normal intelligence.

- a disease that requires a "cure." Most people with the condition can live long, fulfilling lives.

- a reason to assume someone is incapable. Little people go to school, go to work, marry, and raise children, just like their average-size peers.

What Causes Short Stature?

More than two hundred conditions are known to cause short stature in a child. Most are caused by a spontaneous genetic mutation in the egg or sperm cells prior to conception. Other conditions are caused by genes inherited from one or both parents. In either of these cases, two average-size parents can have a child with short stature (though this is far more likely to occur with a spontaneous mutation). Similarly, depending on the type of condition causing the short stature, it is possible for little people to have an average-size child.

What prompts a gene to mutate is not yet clearly understood. The change is seemingly random and unpreventable, and can occur in any pregnancy. Generally, when average-size parents have a child with short stature due to a spontaneous mutation, it is rare to have a second child who is also of short stature. However, if parents have some form of dwarfism themselves, the odds are much greater that their children will have it as well. A genetic counselor can help determine the likelihood of passing on the condition in these cases.

Dwarfism has other causes, including metabolic or hormonal disorders in infancy or childhood. Chromosomal abnormalities, pituitary gland disorders (which influence growth and metabolism), absorptive problems (when the body can't absorb nutrients adequately), and kidney disease can all lead to short stature if a child fails to grow at a normal rate.

Types of Short Stature

Most types of dwarfism are known as skeletal dysplasias, which are conditions of abnormal bone growth. They're divided into two types: short-trunk and short-limb dysplasias. People with short-trunk dysplasia have a shortened trunk with longer limbs, whereas those with short-limb dysplasia have an average-sized trunk but small arms and legs.

By far, the most common skeletal dysplasia is achondroplasia, a short-limb dysplasia that occurs in about 1 of every 26,000 to 40,000 babies of all races and ethnicities. It can be caused by a spontaneous mutation in one gene or a child can inherit the gene from a parent who has achondroplasia. People with achondroplasia have a relatively long trunk and shortened upper parts of their arms and legs. They may share other features as well, such as a large head with a prominent forehead, a flattened bridge of the nose, shortened hands and fingers, and reduced muscle tone. The average adult height for someone with achondroplasia is about four feet.

Diastrophic dysplasia is another, less common form of short-limb dwarfism. It occurs in about 1 in 100,000 births, and is also sometimes characterized by cleft palate, clubfeet, and ears with a cauliflower appearance. People who have it tend to have shortened forearms and calves (this is known as mesomelic shortening).

Spondyloepiphyseal dysplasias (SED) refers to a group of short-trunk skeletal conditions that affect about 1 in 95,000 babies. Along with achondroplasia and diastrophic dysplasia, it is one of the most common forms of dwarfism. In some forms, a lack of growth in the trunk area may not become apparent until the child is between five and ten years old; other forms are apparent at birth. Often, kids with this disorder also have clubfeet, cleft palate, and a barrel-chested appearance.

In general, dwarfism caused by skeletal dysplasias results in what is known as disproportionate short stature—meaning the limbs are short in comparison with the rest of the body. Metabolic or hormonal disorders typically cause proportionate dwarfism, meaning a person's arms, legs, and trunk are all shortened but remain in proportion to overall body size.

Diagnosis

Some types of dwarfism can be identified through prenatal testing if a doctor suspects a particular condition and tests for it. But most cases are not identified until after the child is born. In those instances, the doctor makes a diagnosis based on the child's appearance, failure to grow, and x-rays of the bones. Depending on the type of dwarfism the child has, diagnosis often can be made almost immediately after birth.

Once a diagnosis is made, there is no "treatment" for most of the conditions that lead to short stature. Hormonal or metabolic problems may be treated with hormone injections or special diets to spark a child's growth, but skeletal dysplasias cannot be "cured." People with these types of dwarfism can, however, get medical care for some of the health complications that are associated with short stature. Problems associated with the different forms of dwarfism involve other body systems—such as vision or hearing—and require careful monitoring.

Possible Complications and Treatments

Short stature is the one quality all people with dwarfism have in common. After that, each of the many conditions that cause dwarfism has its own set of characteristics and possible complications. Fortunately, many of these complications are treatable, so that people of short stature can lead healthy, active lives.

For example, some babies with achondroplasia may experience hydrocephalus (excess fluid around the brain). They may also have a greater risk of developing apnea—a temporary stop in breathing during sleep—because of abnormally small or misshapen airways or, more likely, because of airway obstruction by the adenoids or the tonsils. Occasionally, a part of the brain or spinal cord is compressed. With close monitoring by doctors, however, these potentially serious problems can be detected early and surgically corrected.

As a child with dwarfism grows, other issues may also become apparent, including:

- delayed development of some motor skills, such as sitting up and walking;

- a greater susceptibility to ear infections and hearing loss;

- breathing problems caused by small chests;

- weight problems;

- curvature of the spine (scoliosis);

- bowed legs;

- trouble with joint flexibility and early arthritis;

- lower back pain or leg numbness;

- crowding of teeth in the jaw.

Proper medical care can alleviate many of these problems. For example, surgery can often bring relief from the pain of joints that wear out under the stress of bearing weight differently with limited flexibility. Surgery also can be used to improve some of the leg, hip, and spine problems people with short stature sometimes face.

Nonsurgical options may help, too—for instance, excessive weight can worsen many orthopedic problems, so a nutritionist might help develop a healthy plan for shedding extra pounds. And doctors or physical therapists can recommend ways to increase physical activity without putting extra stress on the bones and joints.

Helping Your Child

Although types of dwarfism, and their severity and complications, vary from person to person, in general a child's life span is not affected by the dwarfism. Though the Americans with Disabilities Act protects the rights of people with dwarfism, many members of the short-statured community don't feel that they have a disability.

You can help your child with dwarfism lead the best life possible by building his or her sense of independence and self-esteem right from the start. Here are some tips to keep in mind:

- Treat your child according to his or her age, not size. If you expect a six-year-old to clean up his or her room, don't make an exception simply because your child is small.

- Adapt to your child's limitations. Something as simple as a light switch extender can give a short-statured child a sense of independence around the house.

- Present your child's condition—both to your child and to others—as a difference rather than a hindrance. Your attitude and expectations can have a significant influence on your child's self-esteem.

- Learn to deal with people's reactions, whether it's simple curiosity or outright ignorance, without anger. Address questions or comments as directly as possible, then take a moment to point out something special about your child. If your child is with you, this approach shows that you notice all the other qualities that make him or her unique. It will also help prepare your child for dealing with these situations when you're not there.

- If your child is teased at school, don't overlook it. Talk to teachers and administrators to make sure your child is getting the support he or she needs.

- Encourage your child to find a hobby or activity to enjoy. If sports aren't going to be your child's forte, then maybe music, art, computers, writing, or photography will be.

- Finally, get involved with support associations like the Little People of America. Getting to know other people with dwarfism— both as peers and mentors—can show your child just how much he or she can achieve.

Section 16.3

Multiple Epiphyseal Dysplasia

Reprinted from "Multiple Epiphyseal Dysplasia," *Genetics Home Reference*, a service of the U.S. National Library of Medicine, February 2008.

What is multiple epiphyseal dysplasia?

Multiple epiphyseal dysplasia is a disorder of cartilage and bone development primarily affecting the ends of the long bones in the arms and legs (epiphyses). There are two types of multiple epiphyseal dysplasia, which can be distinguished by their pattern of inheritance. Both the dominant and recessive types have relatively mild signs and symptoms, including joint pain that most commonly affects the hips and knees, early-onset arthritis, and a waddling walk. Although some people with multiple epiphyseal dysplasia have mild short stature as adults, most are of normal height. The majority of individuals are diagnosed during childhood; however, some mild cases may not be diagnosed until adulthood.

Recessive multiple epiphyseal dysplasia is distinguished from the dominant type by malformations of the hands, feet, and knees and abnormal curvature of the spine (scoliosis). About 50 percent of individuals with recessive multiple epiphyseal dysplasia are born with at least one abnormal feature, including an inward- and downward-turning foot (clubfoot), an opening in the roof of the mouth (cleft palate), an unusual curving of the fingers or toes (clinodactyly), or ear swelling. An abnormality of the kneecap called a double-layered patella is also relatively common.

How common is multiple epiphyseal dysplasia?

The incidence of dominant multiple epiphyseal dysplasia is estimated to be at least one in ten thousand newborns. The incidence of recessive multiple epiphyseal dysplasia is unknown. Both forms of this disorder may actually be more common because some people with mild symptoms are never diagnosed.

What genes are related to multiple epiphyseal dysplasia?

Mutations in the COMP, COL9A1, COL9A2, COL9A3, or MATN3 gene can cause dominant multiple epiphyseal dysplasia. These genes provide instructions for making proteins that are found in the spaces between cartilage-forming cells (chondrocytes). These proteins interact with each other and play an important role in cartilage and bone formation. Cartilage is a tough, flexible tissue that makes up much of the skeleton during early development. Most cartilage is later converted to bone, except for the cartilage that continues to cover and protect the ends of bones and is present in the nose and external ears.

The majority of individuals with dominant multiple epiphyseal dysplasia have mutations in the COMP gene. About 10 percent of affected individuals have mutations in the MATN3 gene. Mutations in the COMP or MATN3 gene prevent the release of the proteins produced from these genes into the spaces between the chondrocytes. The absence of these proteins leads to the formation of abnormal cartilage, which can cause the skeletal problems characteristic of dominant multiple epiphyseal dysplasia.

The COL9A1, COL9A2, and COL9A3 genes provide instructions for making a protein called type IX collagen. Collagens are a family of proteins that strengthen and support connective tissues, such as skin, bone, cartilage, tendons, and ligaments. Mutations in the COL9A1, COL9A2, or COL9A3 gene are found in less than 5 percent of individuals with dominant multiple epiphyseal dysplasia. It is not known how mutations in these genes cause the signs and symptoms of this disorder. Research suggests that mutations in these genes may cause type IX collagen to accumulate inside the cell or interact abnormally with other cartilage components.

Some people with dominant multiple epiphyseal dysplasia do not have a mutation in the COMP, COL9A1, COL9A2, COL9A3, or MATN3 gene. In these cases, the cause of the condition is unknown.

Mutations in the SLC26A2 gene cause recessive multiple epiphyseal dysplasia. This gene provides instructions for making a protein that is essential for the normal development of cartilage and for its conversion to bone. Mutations in the SLC26A2 gene alter the structure of developing cartilage, preventing bones from forming properly and resulting in the skeletal problems characteristic of recessive multiple epiphyseal dysplasia.

How do people inherit multiple epiphyseal dysplasia?

Multiple epiphyseal dysplasia can have different inheritance patterns.

This condition can be inherited in an autosomal dominant pattern, which means one copy of the altered gene in each cell is sufficient to cause the disorder. In some cases, an affected person inherits the mutation from one affected parent. Other cases may result from new mutations in the gene. These cases occur in people with no history of the disorder in their family.

Multiple epiphyseal dysplasia can also be inherited in an autosomal recessive pattern, which means both copies of the gene in each cell have mutations. Most often, the parents of an individual with an autosomal recessive condition each carry one copy of the mutated gene, but do not show signs and symptoms of the condition.

Section 16.4

Russell-Silver Syndrome

In 1953 and 1954, Dr. Silver and Dr. Russell independently described groups of small-for-gestational-age (SGA) children whose pregnancies had been complicated by intrauterine growth restriction (IUGR). Their common findings were short stature without catch-up growth, normal head size for age, a distinctive triangular face, low-set ears, and incurving fifth fingers. These two groups of patients are now considered to have had variations of the same disorder that we now call Russell-Silver syndrome (RSS) in the United States and Silver-Russell syndrome (SRS) in Europe.

One interesting and important aspect of the Russell-Silver syndrome is its variation in phenotype. In this context, a phenotype is all the physical characteristics and abnormalities found in an individual patient that are attributed specifically to Russell-Silver syndrome. Some individuals with Russell-Silver syndrome have many traits, thus a severe phenotype, while others have very few traits, thus a mild phenotype.

When first described, Russell-Silver syndrome was *not* thought to be a genetic disorder because it recurred within families rarely, and when it did recur, its pattern of transmission failed to follow a consistent genetic mode of inheritance. More recent understandings of genetic mechanisms have led scientists to conclude that Russell-Silver syndrome is genetic, but its genetics are not simple. Scientists now believe that the RSS phenotype is associated with more than one genotype.

A genotype is the status of a specific gene at a specific location on a specific chromosome. Therefore, an abnormal genotype means there has been a specific alteration, such as a deletion, duplication, insertion, substitution, or imprinting error within the code of a specific gene located at a specific site in an individual's genetic code.

Since our genotype is responsible for our phenotype, abnormal genotypes result in abnormal phenotypes. If we assume several genotypes for Russell-Silver syndrome, then we should not be surprised at a variety of phenotypes. We view this as one reason for the marked variability within the group of patients considered to have Russell-Silver syndrome (RSS). But deciding which child should be considered to have Russell-Silver syndrome is not always easy. When more is known about the genetics of Russell-Silver syndrome, we will find that some patients were incorrectly included while others were incorrectly excluded.

How is Russell-Silver syndrome diagnosed?

The diagnosis of Russell-Silver syndrome is still a judgment call on a physician's part because there is no definitive laboratory test that can answer yes or no in a specific case. Doctors generally base their diagnosis on characteristic, clinical findings that make up the RSS phenotype. It is easy to diagnose the "textbook" RSS phenotype. A small-for-gestational-age child, however, who lacks catch-up growth, has low weight for height, normal head size for age, and few, if any, features that make him look different, is much more difficult to classify.

What is the typical Russell-Silver syndrome (RSS) phenotype?

The RSS phenotype includes a number of physical and developmental characteristics. One of these, asymmetry, is unique to Russell-Silver syndrome, while others, like low birth weight and length, are shared by RSS and SGA children in general.

Characteristics considered to distinguish Russell-Silver syndrome children from other small-for-gestational-age children are as follows:

- Body asymmetry (large side is "normal" side)
- Inadequate catch-up growth in first two years
- Persistently low weight for height
- Lack of interest in eating
- Lack of muscle mass and/or poor muscle tone
- Broad forehead
- Large head size for body size
- Hypoplastic (underdeveloped) chin and mid-face
- Downturned corners of mouth and thin upper lip
- High-arched palate
- Small, crowded teeth

- Low-set, posteriorly rotated and/or prominent ears
- Unusually high-pitched voice in early years
- Clinodactyly (inward curving) of the fifth finger
- Syndactyly (webbing) of the second and third toes
- Hypospadias (abnormal opening of the penis)
- Cryptorchidism (undescended testicles)
- Café-au-lait (coffee-with-milk) birthmarks
- Dimples in the posterior shoulders and hips
- Narrow, flat feet
- Scoliosis (curved spine, associated with spinal asymmetry and accentuated by a short leg)

Characteristics of small-for-gestational-age patients in general that are seen more often in Russell-Silver syndrome patients are as follows:

- Fasting hypoglycemia and mild metabolic acidosis
- Generalized intestinal movement abnormalities:
  - Esophageal reflux resulting in movement of food up from stomach into food tube
  - Delayed stomach emptying resulting in vomiting or frequent spitting up
  - Slow movement of the small intestine and/or large intestine (constipation)
- Blue sclera (bluish tinge in white of eye)
- Late closure of the anterior fontanel (soft spot)
- Frequent ear infections or chronic fluid in ears
- Congenital absence of the second premolars
- Delay of gross and fine motor development
- Delay of speech and oral motor development
- Kidney abnormalities
- Delayed bone age early, later fast advancement
- Early pubic hair and underarm odor (adrenarche)

- Early puberty or rarely true precocious puberty

- Classical or neurosecretory growth hormone deficiency

- Attention deficit disorder (ADD) and specific learning disabilities

What should I do if I think my small-for-gestational-age child has Russell-Silver syndrome?

- Have your child's diagnosis confirmed by a doctor who is familiar with RSS-SGA patients.

- Make sure your child is measured carefully and frequently. Keep your own records.

- Find an endocrinologist who knows how to treat SGA children's growth failure and discuss the options.

- Find a pediatrician who is willing to learn from experts about RSS-SGA children, and will coordinate care and opinions with consulting specialists.

- Get adequate calories into your child. Insufficient nutrition and low blood sugar damage the developing brain and compound the growth failure.

- Take necessary measures to prevent hypoglycemia in young RSS children. Pay special attention to the night when everyone is asleep, anytime your child is ill or not eating normally, and when your child is unusually active or stressed.

Know clues that hypoglycemia is occurring:

- Waking to feed at night past early infancy

- Excessive sweating

- Extreme crankiness improved by feeding

- Difficulty waking up in the morning

- Ketones in the urine

Prevent hypoglycemia by doing the following:

- Feeding frequently during the day and night

- Keeping snacks with you at all times

- Feeding through a gastrostomy tube

- Adding glucose polymer in infant's, and cornstarch in child's, bed- and nighttime feeding

- Keeping glucose gel with you at all times

- Making prior arrangements with your doctor and local emergency room to start intravenous (IV) glucose if feeding is impossible

- Having urine ketone sticks at home

Treat your child his age, not his size. Arrange safe, age-appropriate activities; buy age-appropriate clothes; and expect age-appropriate behavior and responsibility.

Watch your child's psychosocial and motor development. All states have developmental evaluation and intervention services for children less than three. These programs are based on the child's needs, not parental income. For children over three years, the school district becomes responsible for providing these services. Take advantage of this; intervention can make a world of difference for your child!

Seek appropriate consultation for recurrent ear infections, hypospadias, undescended testicles, leg length discrepancies, etc. But remember the following:

- Only emergency surgery should be done until the child is gaining weight well.

- A young SGA child should *never* be fasted or kept NPO (having nothing by mouth) for more than four hours for *any* reason without glucose-running IV.

- For surgery, IV glucose should be given during the procedure and continued in the recovery room.

Why does my child have Russell-Silver syndrome?

It is not your fault! You could have done nothing to prevent it! Russell-Silver syndrome occurs through complicated genetic mechanisms and could never be caused by what you as parents did or did not do.

What can I expect regarding my child's cognitive abilities?

An infant with Russell-Silver syndrome is generally born with normal intelligence. Learning disabilities and attention deficit disorder (ADD) appear to be increased in incidence in RSS. Autism and similar disorders like pervasive developmental disorder (PDD) may also be increased. It is unclear whether these problems just appear to be increased in RSS, are innate to RSS, or are acquired through early malnutrition and hypoglycemia, both of which are preventable.

What treatments are available for Russell-Silver syndrome?

For RSS and non-RSS/SGA patients, the prospect for a normal life with a normal adult height is closer than ever before. By understanding the importance of aggressively feeding these children, no matter what it takes, we are able to avoid the malnutrition and low blood sugar that in the past has so negatively affected their growth and development. With the recent U.S. Food and Drug Administration's approval of growth hormone for the treatment of the growth failure associated with being born small for gestational age, these young children can start the first grade with a normal height if treated early. By taking medications to postpone puberty, called LHRH analogues (LHRHa), the older children can recover growth potential lost in utero, in infancy, and in early childhood. By continuing growth hormone until growth is finished, the teenagers have a better growth spurt during puberty.

Section 16.5

Thanatophoric Dysplasia

Reprinted from "Thanatophoric Dysplasia," *Genetics Home Reference*, a service of the U.S. National Library of Medicine, June 2006.

What is thanatophoric dysplasia?

Thanatophoric dysplasia is a severe skeletal disorder characterized by extremely short limbs and folds of extra (redundant) skin on the arms and legs. Other features of this condition include a narrow chest, short ribs, underdeveloped lungs, and an enlarged head with a large forehead and prominent, wide-spaced eyes.

Researchers have described two major forms of thanatophoric dysplasia, type I and type II. Type I thanatophoric dysplasia is distinguished by the presence of curved thigh bones and flattened bones of the spine (platyspondyly). Type II thanatophoric dysplasia is characterized by straight thigh bones and a moderate to severe skull abnormality called a cloverleaf skull.

The term "thanatophoric" is Greek for "death bearing." Infants with thanatophoric dysplasia are usually stillborn or die shortly after birth from respiratory failure; however, a few affected individuals have survived into childhood with extensive medical help.

How common is thanatophoric dysplasia?

This condition occurs in one in twenty thousand to fifty thousand newborns. Type I thanatophoric dysplasia is more common than type II.

What genes are related to thanatophoric dysplasia?

Mutations in the FGFR3 gene cause thanatophoric dysplasia.

Both types of thanatophoric dysplasia result from mutations in the FGFR3 gene. This gene provides instructions for making a protein that is involved in the development and maintenance of bone and brain tissue. Mutations in this gene cause the FGFR3 protein to be overly active, which leads to the severe disturbances in bone growth that are characteristic of thanatophoric dysplasia. It is not known how FGFR3 mutations cause the brain and skin abnormalities associated with this disorder.

How do people inherit thanatophoric dysplasia?

Thanatophoric dysplasia is considered an autosomal dominant disorder because one mutated copy of the FGFR3 gene in each cell is sufficient to cause the condition. Virtually all cases of thanatophoric dysplasia are caused by new mutations in the FGFR3 gene and occur in people with no history of the disorder in their family. No affected individuals are known to have had children; therefore, the disorder has not been passed to the next generation.

Chapter 17

Heart Rhythm Disorders

Chapter Contents

Section 17.1

Brugada Syndrome

Excerpted from "The Brugada Syndrome," © Masonic Medical Research Laboratory (www.mmrl.edu). Reprinted with permission. The full text of this document may be accessed online at http://www.mmrl.edu/Pubs/ TheBrugadaSyndrome.pdf; accessed January 9, 2009.

What is the Brugada syndrome?

The clinical entity now known as Brugada syndrome was first described by Drs. Pedro and Josep Brugada in 1992 and named "Brugada syndrome" by scientists at the Masonic Medical Research Laboratory (MMRL) in 1996 in honor of the Brugada brothers. The cellular basis for the life-threatening abnormal heart rhythms associated with this syndrome was discovered by Dr. Antzelevitch and co-workers at the MMRL in the early 1990s. Brugada syndrome is a form of sudden cardiac death that tragically takes the lives of young adults. It is an inherited syndrome that can lead to life-threatening ventricular tachycardia and fibrillation. Ventricular fibrillation occurs when the electrical activity in the main pumping chambers of the heart (ventricles) goes into disarray, causing the muscle of the heart to beat in an uncoordinated fashion, thus preventing the normal flow of blood to the rest of the body. If not corrected by the administration of an electrical shock to the victim's heart within several minutes, the patient could sustain brain damage (due to lack of oxygen) or death can result.

How common is the Brugada syndrome?

Because of its recent identification, the true incidence of the syndrome is not well established. We do know that in Southeast Asia and Japan it occurs in five out of ten thousand individuals. Available data indicates that there are numerous cases in the United States and Europe as well.

Can I inherit the syndrome from my parents?

Yes. Several arrhythmia diseases may be inherited, including the Brugada syndrome, long QT syndrome, short QT syndrome, and atrial fibrillation. A parent with the Brugada syndrome usually has a 50 percent chance of transmitting the disease to his son or daughter.

How do I know if I have the disease?

An electrocardiogram (ECG) can often provide a definitive diagnosis. If the diagnosis is not clear, additional tests can be performed using sodium channel blockers to unmask the typical ECG features of the disease. Genetic testing is useful in confirming the diagnosis and in identifying family members with the disease.

Is there any treatment or cure for the Brugada syndrome?

There is no cure. The only proven effective treatment at present is the implantation of an implantable cardioverter defibrillator (ICD). This device automatically senses when the heart experiences a dangerous arrhythmia and automatically provides an electrical shock to restore normal sinus rhythm.

However, research is ongoing and the future is promising. Investigations conducted at the MMRL have delineated the ionic and cellular mechanism responsible for the arrhythmias that cause sudden death in patients with the Brugada syndrome. This work has identified a class of drugs known as transient outward current blockers (e.g., quinidine) that are useful as adjuncts to ICDs or as alternatives in those cases in which an ICD is not an option or in regions of the world where an ICD is not affordable. Clinical studies have shown quinidine to be effective in preventing arrhythmias in a small cohorts of patients with Brugada syndrome. Placebo-controlled blinded studies to evaluate the effectiveness of quinidine have not been performed as yet. Studies at the MMRL also identified other agents such as isoproterenol that have proven useful in quieting "electrical storms" sometimes encountered in patients with this disease. MMRL investigators are working with pharmaceutical companies to develop more cardioselective and specific transient outward current blockers to treat the Brugada syndrome.

What is an arrhythmia?

In very simple terms, an arrhythmia is an abnormal heart rhythm resulting from the electrical instability within the heart. Some arrhythmias, such as extra beats, are commonly benign, whereas others, like atrial fibrillation, if left untreated can result in stroke, and still others, like ventricular tachycardia and fibrillation, are still more ominous. Ventricular fibrillation is the arrhythmia usually responsible for sudden death.

Should certain drugs or conditions be avoided in patients with the Brugada syndrome?

Drugs that are known to block the sodium channels in the heart, including some antidepressant drugs, should be avoided because they can aggravate the syndrome and precipitate life-threatening arrhythmias. Work at the MMRL conducted in 1998 identified fever as another important risk factor that should be avoided and closely monitored, particularly in children with the syndrome.

What is molecular genetics research?

Genetics is a science that plays a role in all fields of medicine, from cancer to cardiology. We have approximately thirty to thirty-five thousand genes in our bodies that encode for all of the proteins responsible for the functions of our organs. These include proteins such as insulin, which controls our blood sugar, to angiotensin II, which controls our blood pressure. These genes can malfunction and cause diseases such as diabetes and hypertension. The branch of genetics in which we have interest is directed towards the identification of defective genes, with the aim of understanding the specific cause of disease, which provides us the capability to design specific treatments and cures. Genetics holds the key to better diagnosis, prevention, and treatment of disease and hopefully a longer, healthier and more fruitful life.

In 1998, working together with colleagues worldwide, our scientists showed for the first time that a faulty gene that encodes the sodium channel (SCN5A) in the heart contributes to the development of this syndrome. Defects in six different genes have been associated with the Brugada syndrome. Four of the six were discovered by MMRL scientists.

What happens once a defective gene has been identified as causing a life-threatening arrhythmia?

The first step is the identification of a defective gene. Once this has been detected, the mutated gene is isolated and studied in special cell types that allow us to assess how the function of the cell is affected. This provides us an understanding of how the defective gene causes the disease. The next step is to try to correct this malfunction by designing specific drugs or other treatments.

Section 17.2

Familial Atrial Fibrillation

Excerpted from "Familial Atrial Fibrillation," *Genetics Home Reference*, a service of the U.S. National Library of Medicine, January 2007.

What is familial atrial fibrillation?

Familial atrial fibrillation is an inherited condition that disrupts the heart's normal rhythm. This condition is characterized by uncoordinated electrical activity in the heart's upper chambers (the atria), which causes the heartbeat to become fast and irregular. If untreated, this abnormal heart rhythm can lead to dizziness, chest pain, a sensation of fluttering or pounding in the chest (palpitations), shortness of breath, or fainting (syncope). Atrial fibrillation also increases the risk of stroke and sudden death. Complications of familial atrial fibrillation can occur at any age, although some people with this heart condition never experience any health problems associated with the disorder.

How common is familial atrial fibrillation?

Atrial fibrillation is the most common type of sustained abnormal heart rhythm (arrhythmia), affecting more than three million people in the United States. The risk of developing this irregular heart rhythm increases with age. The incidence of the familial form of atrial fibrillation is unknown; however, recent studies suggest that up to 30 percent of all people with atrial fibrillation may have a history of the condition in their family.

What genes are related to familial atrial fibrillation?

Mutations in the KCNQ1 gene cause familial atrial fibrillation.

The KCNE2 and KCNJ2 genes are associated with familial atrial fibrillation.

A small percentage of all cases of familial atrial fibrillation are associated with changes in the KCNE2, KCNJ2, and KCNQ1 genes. These genes provide instructions for making proteins that act as channels across the cell membrane. These channels transport positively charged atoms (ions) of potassium into and out of cells. In heart (cardiac) muscle, the ion channels produced from the KCNE2, KCNJ2, and KCNQ1 genes play critical roles in maintaining the heart's normal rhythm. Mutations in these genes have been identified in only a few families worldwide. These mutations increase the activity of the channels, which changes the flow of potassium ions between cells. This disruption in ion transport alters the way the heart beats, increasing the risk of syncope, stroke, and sudden death.

Most cases of atrial fibrillation are not caused by mutations in a single gene. This condition is often related to structural abnormalities of the heart or underlying heart disease. Additional risk factors for atrial fibrillation include high blood pressure (hypertension), diabetes mellitus, a previous stroke, or an accumulation of fatty deposits and scar-like tissue in the lining of the arteries (atherosclerosis). Although most cases of atrial fibrillation are not known to run in families, studies suggest that they may arise partly from genetic risk factors. Researchers are working to determine which genetic changes may influence the risk of atrial fibrillation.

How do people inherit familial atrial fibrillation?

Familial atrial fibrillation appears to be inherited in an autosomal dominant pattern, which means one copy of the altered gene in each cell is sufficient to cause the disorder.

Section 17.3

Long QT Syndrome

What Is the Long QT Syndrome?

The long QT syndrome is a rare disorder of the heart's electrical system that can affect otherwise healthy people. Although the heart's mechanical function is normal, there are defects in ion channels, which are cell structures in the heart muscle. These electrical defects can cause a very fast heart rhythm (arrhythmia) called torsade de pointes. This abnormal rhythm (a form of ventricular tachycardia) is too fast for the heart to beat effectively, and so the blood flow to the brain falls dramatically, causing sudden loss of consciousness, or syncope (fainting).

Why Is It Called Long QT Syndrome?

The name long QT syndrome comes from the measurement of the heart's contractions by electrocardiogram (EKG or ECG). When the heart contracts, it emits an electrical signal that can be recorded on the ECG. This signal produces a waveform, and different parts of this waveform are designated by letters P, Q, R, S, and T. The Q–T interval marks the time for electrical activation and inactivation of the ventricles, which are the lower chambers of the heart. In people with the long QT syndrome, the Q–T interval takes longer than normal to occur. It should be noted, however, that tests do not always reveal long QT syndrome. People with the disorder do not necessarily have a prolonged Q–T interval all the time, and at the time they have an ECG, the Q–T interval may be normal.

Symptoms of the Long QT Syndrome

People with the long QT syndrome may have no symptoms at all. Among those who do, fainting (syncope) and an abnormal heartbeat (arrhythmia) are common. Symptoms occur especially during physical exercise, intense emotion (such as fright, anger, or pain), or when awakened or startled by a noise such as an alarm clock, telephone, or thunder. Syncope is commonly misdiagnosed as a common faint, but it can be fatal. Usually, there is no warning before syncope.

What Causes the Long QT Syndrome?

The long QT syndrome is commonly inherited. There are at least two inherited variants, and in one type, individuals with long QT syndrome are deaf. The majority of people with long QT syndrome have family members with the disorder and have had at least one episode of fainting by age ten. Even if the disorder has not been diagnosed in the family (as relatives may have died of sudden unknown causes), any history of fainting or sudden loss of consciousness during exercise or strong emotion necessitates medical tests.

The long QT syndrome can also be acquired, most often through the administration of medications that are contraindicated in patients with long QT syndrome.

How is the Long QT Syndrome Treated?

Beta-blocker medications are effective for about 90 percent of patients. A small group of patients may also benefit from other drugs, either instead of or in addition to the beta-blockers. In patients who do not respond to medication, the insertion of a pacemaker or defibrillator may be effective. Surgical cutting of certain nerves in the neck, called cervicothoracic sympathectomy, can be effective as well. All patients with the long QT syndrome should be treated, including asymptomatic patients and especially children, because sudden death often occurs with the first episode of syncope and it is not possible to predict which patients are vulnerable.

Drugs to Avoid with the Long QT Syndrome

Many drugs can prolong the Q–T interval and cause heart rhythm abnormalities. It is very important to inquire about the risk of any medication, whether it is a prescription or over-the-counter drug, that is recommended to a long QT patient. Some common medications that should be avoided include anesthetics and asthma medications (adrenaline), antihistamines, certain antibiotics, numerous heart medications, the gastrointestinal drug Propulsid®, some antifungal drugs, psychotropic medications, the diuretic Lozol®, and others. It should also be noted that many diuretics cause potassium loss (as does extensive vomiting and diarrhea), and low potassium levels can worsen long QT syndrome.

Editor's Note:

Since the original publication of this article, Propulsid has been withdrawn from the market due to concerns about causing long QT syndrome even in previously healthy people. Additionally, newer-generation antipsychotic drugs have been increasingly recognized as impacting on QT intervals. A comprehensive and regularly updated list of medications that affect the QT interval is available on the web at www.azcert.org.

Chapter 18

Hereditary Deafness

Chapter Contents

Section 18.1

Usher Syndrome

Reprinted from "Usher Syndrome," National Institute on
Deafness and Other Communication Disorders, National Institutes
of Health, NIH Publication No. 98-4291, February 2008.

What is Usher syndrome?

Usher syndrome is the most common condition that affects both
hearing and vision. A syndrome is a disease or disorder that has more
than one feature or symptom. The major symptoms of Usher syndrome
are hearing loss and an eye disorder called retinitis pigmentosa, or
RP. RP causes night-blindness and a loss of peripheral vision (side
vision) through the progressive degeneration of the retina. The retina
is a light-sensitive tissue at the back of the eye and is crucial for vision. As RP progresses, the field of vision narrows—a condition known
as "tunnel vision"—until only central vision (the ability to see straight
ahead) remains. Many people with Usher syndrome also have severe
balance problems.

There are three clinical types of Usher syndrome: type 1, type 2,
and type 3. In the United States, types 1 and 2 are the most common
types. Together, they account for approximately 90 to 95 percent of
all cases of children who have Usher syndrome.

Who is affected by Usher syndrome?

Approximately 3 to 6 percent of all children who are deaf and another 3 to 6 percent of children who are hard of hearing have Usher
syndrome. In developed countries such as the United States, about
four babies in every one hundred thousand births have Usher syndrome.

What causes Usher syndrome?

Usher syndrome is inherited, which means that it is passed from
parents to their children through genes. Genes are located in almost

every cell of the body. Genes contain instructions that tell cells what to do. Every person inherits two copies of each gene, one from each parent. Sometimes genes are altered, or mutated. Mutated genes may cause cells to act differently than expected.

Usher syndrome is inherited as an autosomal recessive trait. The term *autosomal* means that the mutated gene is not located on either of the chromosomes that determine a person's sex; in other words, both males and females can have the disorder and can pass it along to a child. The word recessive means that, to have Usher syndrome, a person must receive a mutated form of the Usher syndrome gene from each parent. If a child has a mutation in one Usher syndrome gene but the other gene is normal, he or she is predicted to have normal vision and hearing. People with a mutation in a gene that can cause an autosomal recessive disorder are called carriers, because they "carry" the gene with a mutation, but show no symptoms of the disorder. If both parents are carriers of a mutated gene for Usher syndrome, they will have a one-in-four chance of having a child with Usher syndrome with each birth.

Usually, parents who have normal hearing and vision do not know if they are carriers of an Usher syndrome gene mutation. Currently, it is not possible to determine whether a person who does not have a family history of Usher syndrome is a carrier. Scientists at the National Institute on Deafness and Other Communication Disorders are hoping to change this, however, as they learn more about the genes responsible for Usher syndrome.

What are the characteristics of the three types of Usher syndrome?

Type 1: Children with type 1 Usher syndrome are profoundly deaf at birth and have severe balance problems. Many of these children obtain little or no benefit from hearing aids. Parents should consult their doctor and other hearing health professionals as early as possible to determine the best communication method for their child. Intervention should be introduced early, during the first few years of life, so that the child can take advantage of the unique window of time during which the brain is most receptive to learning language, whether spoken or signed. If a child is diagnosed with type 1 Usher syndrome early on, before he or she loses the ability to see, that child is more likely to benefit from the full spectrum of intervention strategies that can help him or her participate more fully in life's activities.

Because of the balance problems associated with type 1 Usher syndrome, children with this disorder are slow to sit without support and typically don't walk independently before they are eighteen months old. These children usually begin to develop vision problems in early childhood, almost always by the time they reach age ten. Vision problems most often begin with difficulty seeing at night, but tend to progress rapidly until the person is completely blind.

Type 2: Children with type 2 Usher syndrome are born with moderate to severe hearing loss and normal balance. Although the severity of hearing loss varies, most of these children can benefit from hearing aids and can communicate orally. The vision problems in type 2 Usher syndrome tend to progress more slowly than those in type 1, with the onset of RP often not apparent until the teens.

Type 3: Children with type 3 Usher syndrome have normal hearing at birth. Although most children with the disorder have normal to near-normal balance, some may develop balance problems later on. Hearing and sight worsen over time, but the rate at which they decline can vary from person to person, even within the same family. A person with type 3 Usher syndrome may develop hearing loss by the teens, and he or she will usually require hearing aids by mid- to late adulthood. Night blindness usually begins sometime during puberty. Blind spots appear by the late teens to early adulthood, and by mid-adulthood the person is usually legally blind.

How is Usher syndrome diagnosed?

Because Usher syndrome affects hearing, balance, and vision, diagnosis of the disorder usually includes the evaluation of all three senses. Evaluation of the eyes may include a visual field test to measure a person's peripheral vision, an electroretinogram (ERG) to measure the electrical response of the eye's light-sensitive cells, and a retinal examination to observe the retina and other structures in the back of the eye. A hearing (audiologic) evaluation measures how loud sounds at a range of frequencies need to be before a person can hear them. An electronystagmogram (ENG) measures involuntary eye movements that could signify a balance problem.

Early diagnosis of Usher syndrome is very important. The earlier that parents know if their child has Usher syndrome, the sooner that child can begin special educational training programs to manage the loss of hearing and vision.

Table 18.1. Characteristics of Usher Syndrome

	Type 1	**Type 2**	**Type 3**
Hearing	Profound deafness in both ears from birth	Moderate to severe hearing loss from birth	Normal at birth; progressive loss in childhood or early teens
Vision	Decreased night vision before age ten	Decreased night vision begins in late childhood or teens	Varies in severity; night vision problems often begin in teens
Vestibular function (balance)	Balance problems from birth	Normal	Normal to near-normal, chance of later problems

Is genetic testing for Usher syndrome available?

So far, eleven genetic loci (a segment of chromosome on which a certain gene is located) have been found to cause Usher syndrome, and nine genes have been pinpointed that cause the disorder. They are as follows:

- **Type 1 Usher syndrome:** MY07A, USH1C, CDH23, PCDH15, SANS

- **Type 2 Usher syndrome:** USH2A, VLGR1, WHRN

- **Type 3 Usher syndrome:** USH3A

With so many possible genes involved in Usher syndrome, genetic tests for the disorder are not conducted on a widespread basis. Diagnosis of Usher syndrome is usually performed through hearing, balance, and vision tests. Genetic testing for a few of the identified genes is clinically available. Genetic testing for additional Usher syndrome genes may be available through clinical research studies.

How is Usher syndrome treated?

Currently, there is no cure for Usher syndrome. The best treatment involves early identification so that educational programs can begin as soon as possible. The exact nature of these programs will depend on the severity of the hearing and vision loss as well as the age and abilities of the person. Typically, treatment will include hearing aids, assistive listening devices, cochlear implants, or other communication methods such as American Sign Language; orientation and mobility training; and communication services and independent-living training that may include Braille instruction, low-vision services, or auditory training.

Some ophthalmologists believe that a high dose of vitamin A palmitate may slow, but not halt, the progression of retinitis pigmentosa. This belief stems from the results of a long-term clinical trial supported by the National Eye Institute and the Foundation for Fighting Blindness. Based on these findings, the researchers recommend that most adult patients with the common forms of RP take a daily supplement of 15,000 IU (international units) of vitamin A in the palmitate form under the supervision of their eye care professional. (Because people with type 1 Usher syndrome did not take part in the study, high-dose vitamin A is not recommended for these patients.) People who are considering taking vitamin A should discuss this treatment option with their health care provider before proceeding. Other guidelines regarding this treatment option include the following:

- Do not substitute vitamin A palmitate with a beta-carotene supplement.

- Do not take vitamin A supplements greater than the recommended dose of 15,000 IU or modify your diet to select foods with high levels of vitamin A.

- Women who are considering pregnancy should stop taking the high-dose supplement of vitamin A three months before trying to conceive due to the increased risk of birth defects.

- Women who are pregnant should stop taking the high-dose supplement of vitamin A due to the increased risk of birth defects.

In addition, according to the same study, people with RP should avoid using supplements of more than 400 IU of vitamin E per day.

What research is being conducted on Usher syndrome?

Researchers are currently trying to identify all of the genes that cause Usher syndrome and determine the function of those genes. This research will lead to improved genetic counseling and early diagnosis, and may eventually expand treatment options.

Scientists also are developing mouse models that have the same characteristics as the human types of Usher syndrome. Mouse models will make it easier to determine the function of the genes involved in Usher syndrome. Other areas of study include the early identification of children with Usher syndrome, treatment strategies such as the use of cochlear implants for hearing loss, and intervention strategies to help slow or stop the progression of RP.

What are some of the latest research findings?

Researchers from the National Institute on Deafness and Communication Disorders (NIDCD), along with collaborators from universities in New York and Israel, pinpointed a mutation, named R245X, of the PCDH15 gene that accounts for a large percentage of type 1 Usher syndrome in today's Ashkenazi Jewish population. (The term "Ashkenazi" describes Jewish people who originate from Eastern Europe.) Based on this finding, the researchers conclude that Ashkenazi Jewish infants with bilateral, profound hearing loss who lack another known mutation that causes hearing loss should be screened for the R245X mutation.

Section 18.2

Waardenburg Syndrome

Excerpted from "Waardenburg Syndrome," *Genetics Home Reference*, a service of the U.S. National Library of Medicine, April 2006.

What is Waardenburg syndrome?

Waardenburg syndrome is a group of genetic conditions that can cause hearing loss and changes in coloring (pigmentation) of the hair, skin, and eyes. Although most people with Waardenburg syndrome have normal hearing, moderate to profound hearing loss can occur in one or both ears. People with this condition often have very pale blue eyes or different colored eyes, such as one blue eye and one brown eye. Sometimes one eye has segments of two different colors. Distinctive hair coloring (such as a patch of white hair or hair that prematurely turns gray) is another common sign of the condition. The features of

Waardenburg syndrome vary among affected individuals, even among people in the same family.

The four known types of Waardenburg syndrome are distinguished by their physical characteristics and sometimes by their genetic cause. Types I and II have very similar features, although people with type I almost always have eyes that appear widely spaced and people with type II do not. In addition, hearing loss occurs more often in people with type II than in those with type I. Type III (sometimes called Klein-Waardenburg syndrome) includes abnormalities of the upper limbs in addition to hearing loss and changes in pigmentation. Type IV (also known as Waardenburg-Shah syndrome) has signs and symptoms of both Waardenburg syndrome and Hirschsprung disease, an intestinal disorder that causes severe constipation or blockage of the intestine.

How common is Waardenburg syndrome?

Waardenburg syndrome affects an estimated one in ten thousand to twenty thousand people. In schools for the deaf, 2 to 3 percent of students have this condition. Types I and II are the most common forms of Waardenburg syndrome, while types III and IV are rare.

What genes are related to Waardenburg syndrome?

Mutations in the EDN3, EDNRB, MITF, PAX3, SNAI2, and SOX10 genes cause Waardenburg syndrome.

The genes that cause Waardenburg syndrome are involved in the formation and development of several types of cells, including pigment-producing cells called melanocytes. Melanocytes make a pigment called melanin, which contributes to skin, hair, and eye color and plays an essential role in the normal function of the inner ear. Mutations in any of these genes disrupt the normal development of melanocytes, leading to abnormal pigmentation of the skin, hair, and eyes and problems with hearing.

Types I and III Waardenburg syndrome are caused by mutations in the PAX3 gene. Mutations in the MITF and SNAI2 genes are responsible for type II Waardenburg syndrome.

Mutations in the SOX10, EDN3, or EDNRB genes cause type IV Waardenburg syndrome. In addition to melanocyte development, these genes are important for the development of nerve cells in the large intestine. Mutations in any of these genes result in hearing loss, changes in pigmentation, and intestinal problems related to Hirschsprung disease.

How do people inherit Waardenburg syndrome?

Waardenburg syndrome is usually inherited in an autosomal dominant pattern, which means one copy of the altered gene in each cell is sufficient to cause the disorder. In most cases, an affected person has one parent with the condition. A small percentage of cases result from new mutations in the gene; these cases occur in people with no history of the disorder in their family.

Some cases of type II and type IV Waardenburg syndrome appear to have an autosomal recessive pattern of inheritance, which means both copies of the gene in each cell have mutations. Most often, the parents of an individual with an autosomal recessive condition each carry one copy of the mutated gene, but do not show signs and symptoms of the condition.

Chapter 19

Huntington Disease

Alternative Names

Huntington chorea

Definition

Huntington disease is a disorder passed down through families in which nerve cells in the brain waste away, or degenerate.

Causes

American doctor George Huntington first described the disorder in 1872.

Huntington disease is caused by a genetic defect on chromosome number 4. The defect causes a part of deoxyribonucleic acid (DNA), called a CAG repeat, to occur many more times than it is supposed to. Normally, this section of DNA is repeated 10 to 35 times. But in persons with Huntington disease, it is repeated 36 to 120 times.

As the gene is passed on from one generation to the next, the number of repeats—called a CAG repeat expansion—tend to get larger. The larger the number of repeats, the greater your chance of developing symptoms at an earlier age.

There are two forms of Huntington disease. The most common is adult-onset Huntington disease. Persons with this form usually develop symptoms in their mid thirties and forties.

Early-onset form of Huntington disease is less common and begins in childhood or adolescence. Symptoms may resemble those of Parkinson disease with rigidity, slow movements, and tremor.

If one of your parents has Huntington disease, you have a 50 percent chance of getting the gene for the disease. If you get the gene from your parents, you will develop the disease at some point in your life, and can pass it onto your children. If you do not get the gene from your parents, you cannot pass the gene onto your children.

Symptoms

- Abnormal and unusual movements:
  - Head turning to shift eye position
  - Facial movements, including grimaces
  - Slow, uncontrolled movements
  - Quick, sudden, jerking movements of arms, legs, face, and other body parts
  - Unsteady gait
- Behavior changes:
  - Antisocial behaviors
  - Hallucinations
  - Irritability
  - Moodiness
  - Restlessness or fidgeting
  - Paranoia
  - Psychosis
- Dementia that slowly gets worse, including:
  - Loss of memory
  - Loss of judgment
  - Speech changes
  - Personality changes
  - Disorientation or confusion

Additional symptoms that may be associated with this disease:

- anxiety, stress, and tension;
- difficulty swallowing;
- speech impairment.

In children:

- rigidity;
- slow movements;
- tremor.

Exams and Tests

The doctor will perform a physical exam. The doctor may see signs of dementia and abnormal movements. Reflexes may be abnormal. The gait is often "prancing" and wide. Speech may be hesitant or enunciation poor.

A head computed tomography (CT) scan may show loss of brain tissue, especially deep in the brain.

Other tests that may show signs of Huntington disease include:

- head magnetic resonance imaging (MRI) scan;
- positron emission tomography (PET) or isotope scan of the brain.

DNA marker studies may be available to determine if you carry the gene for Huntington disease.

Treatment

There is no cure for Huntington disease, and there is no known way to stop the disease from getting worse. The goal of treatment is to slow down the course of the disease and help the person function for as long and as comfortably as possible.

Medications vary depending on the symptoms. Dopamine blockers may help reduce abnormal behaviors and movements. Drugs like tetrabenazine and amantadine are used to try to control extra movements. There has been some evidence to suggest that co-enzyme Q10 may also help slow down the course of the disease.

Depression and suicide are common among persons with Huntington disease. It is important for all those who care for a person with Huntington disease to monitor for symptoms and treat accordingly.

There is a progressive need for assistance and supervision, and twenty-four-hour care may eventually be needed.

Outlook (Prognosis)

Huntington disease causes progressive disability. Persons with this disease usually die within fifteen to twenty years. The cause of death is often infection, although suicide is also common.

It is important to realize that the disease affects everyone differently. The number of CAG repeats may determine the severity of symptoms. Persons with few repeats may have mild abnormal movements later in life and slow disease progression, while those with large repeats may be severely affected at a young age.

Possible Complications

- Loss of ability to care for self
- Loss of ability to interact
- Injury to self or others
- Increased risk of infection
- Depression
- Death

When to Contact a Medical Professional

Call your health care provider if symptoms of this disorder develop.

Prevention

Genetic counseling is advised if there is a family history of Huntington disease. Experts also recommend genetic counseling for couples with a family history of this disease who are considering having children.

Chapter 20

Hypohidrotic Ectodermal Dysplasia

What

Hypohidrotic ectodermal dysplasia (HED) is an inherited condition characterized by a reduced ability to sweat (hypohidrosis), missing teeth, and sparse hair.

Who

HED is estimated to occur in one out of twenty thousand children. The majority of affected children are boys but girls can also be affected, although somewhat less severely. All races and ethnicities are affected equally.

Signs and Symptoms

At birth, babies with HED may have excessively peeling skin. As they grow, they are noted to sweat less than other children. This is due to a reduced number of sweat glands. Sweating is important to help the body keep cool in hot environments. Decreased sweating puts children with HED at risk for hyperthermia (elevated body temperature). Signs of overheating include headache, irritability, lethargy, fainting, and muscle cramps. Teething is often delayed by six to twelve months and can be abnormally shaped (small cone-shaped teeth). Missing teeth and cavities are also common. Children with HED also have light-colored skin and reduced oil production by the skin. As a result, affected children have dry skin and even chronic eczema. The skin around the mouth and eyes may appear darkened and wrinkled. Children with HED have a dry mouth and a raspy voice because they don't make enough saliva and mucus. The interior lining of the nose can become dry, cracked and scabbed. Children with HED have flat, depressed noses, or "saddle" shaped noses. The child may also experience a decreased sense of smell and taste. A prominent forehead, large chin, and thick lips are also characteristic of people with HED. Scalp and body hair are sparse, light-colored, and slow growing. Hair tends to be brittle and breaks easily. Dandruff is common. Some children may develop no hair at all on their heads. The arms and legs may also be without hair, but facial hair is normally present. Nails are thin and brittle. The nipples are often underdeveloped and females may experience poor milk production later in life. The immune system is affected as well. Children with HED may have asthma and recurrent respiratory infections. Constipation may also occur. Children with HED have normal intelligence.

Possible Causes

HED is not contagious or preventable. It is an inherited genetic disorder. Ninety five percent of children with HED have the X-linked form, while the remaining 5 percent have either the autosomal recessive or autosomal dominant form. X-linked HED is caused by genetic changes (mutations) on the X chromosome. The autosomal recessive and dominant forms are caused by mutations on chromosomes 1 and 2, respectively. These genes are important for the proper development of skin tissues. X-linked HED largely affects boys, as girls carry two X chromosomes. Boys usually inherit the genetic mutation from their mothers, who typically have mild symptoms or none at all. When women are carriers of the mutated gene, 50 percent of their sons will have HED. All of the daughters of an affected male will be carriers, but none of the sons will be affected. In some cases, spontaneous mutations may be responsible for HED. Autosomally inherited HED affects boys and girls equally.

Diagnosis

An iodine sweat test may be used to diagnosis HED. In this test, iodine is applied to the skin and the temperature of the room is increased to induce sweating. The iodine solution changes color when exposed to sweat and can be used to determine the amount of sweating at its location. A skin biopsy is the best method to confirm the diagnosis of HED. Genetic testing and prenatal diagnosis are also available.

Treatment

There is no cure for HED. Treatment aims to preventing hyperthermia. Hot climates and exposure to heat must be minimized. Fevers must be treated promptly. Access to drinking water is essential in warm weather. An air conditioner and a humidifier are recommended to have in the home. The child may prefer to sleep naked. It is important to keep the skin well moisturized. Skin moisturizers are essential for the management of eczema and dry skin. Mild, nondrying soaps should be used. Artificial teardrops are important to use to keep the eyes from drying out. Rinsing the nose with salt water can prevent scabbing. Dental treatment must begin early. Dental implants, orthodontic therapy, and dentures may be necessary.

Prognosis

HED generally has a very good prognosis. Skin problems can vary in severity but they do not affect lifespan, which is normal in individuals with HED. Cosmetic complications can be reduced by aggressive daily skin care. Hyperthermia is the most feared complication because it can lead to heatstroke, which can be fatal. Participation in sports must often be reduced.

Chapter 21

Inborn Errors of Metabolism

Chapter Contents

Section 21.1

Biotinidase Deficiency

Excerpted from "Biotinidase Deficiency," *Genetics Home Reference*,
a service of the U.S. National Library of Medicine, January 2008.

What is biotinidase deficiency?

Biotinidase deficiency is an inherited disorder in which the body is unable to reuse and recycle the vitamin biotin. This disorder is classified as a multiple carboxylase deficiency, a group of disorders characterized by impaired activity of certain enzymes that depend on biotin.

The signs and symptoms of biotinidase deficiency typically appear within the first few months of life, but the age of onset varies. Children with profound biotinidase deficiency, the more severe form of the condition, often have seizures, weak muscle tone (hypotonia), breathing problems, and delayed development. If left untreated, the disorder can lead to hearing loss, eye abnormalities and loss of vision, problems with movement and balance (ataxia), skin rashes, hair loss (alopecia), and a fungal infection called candidiasis. Immediate treatment and lifelong management with biotin supplements can prevent many of these complications.

Partial biotinidase deficiency is a milder form of this condition. Affected children experience hypotonia, skin rashes, and hair loss, but these problems may appear only during illness, infection, or other times of stress.

How common is biotinidase deficiency?

Profound or partial biotinidase deficiency occurs in approximately one in sixty thousand newborns.

What genes are related to biotinidase deficiency?

Mutations in the BTD gene cause biotinidase deficiency.

The BTD gene provides instructions for making an enzyme called biotinidase. This enzyme helps the body reuse biotin, a B vitamin found in foods such as liver, egg yolks, and milk. Biotinidase removes biotin that is bound to proteins in food, leaving the vitamin in its free (unbound) state. The body needs free biotin to break down fats, proteins, and carbohydrates effectively. Biotinidase also recycles biotin within the body.

Mutations in the BTD gene reduce or eliminate the activity of biotinidase. Profound biotinidase deficiency results when the activity of biotinidase is reduced to less than 10 percent of normal. Partial biotinidase deficiency occurs when biotinidase activity is reduced to between 10 percent and 30 percent of normal. Without enough of this enzyme, biotin cannot be separated from proteins or recycled normally. As a result, the body is less able to process important nutrients. These defects underlie the potentially serious medical problems associated with biotinidase deficiency.

How do people inherit biotinidase deficiency?

This condition is inherited in an autosomal recessive pattern, which means both copies of the gene in each cell have mutations. The parents of an individual with an autosomal recessive condition each carry one copy of the mutated gene, but they typically do not show signs and symptoms of the condition.

Section 21.2

Fructose Intolerance

From "Hereditary Fructose Intolerance," © 2009 A.D.A.M., Inc.
Reprinted with permission.

Alternative Names

Fructosemia; fructose intolerance; fructose aldolase B-deficiency; fructose 1, 6 bisphosphate aldolase deficiency

Definition

Hereditary fructose intolerance is a disorder of metabolism in which a person lacks the protein needed to break down fructose. Fructose is a fruit sugar that naturally occurs in the body. Man-made fructose is used as a sweetener in many foods, including baby food and drinks.

Causes

This condition occurs when the body is missing a substance called aldolase B. This substance is needed to break down fructose.

If a person without this substance eats fructose and sucrose (cane or beet sugar, table sugar), complicated chemical changes occur in the body. The body cannot change its energy storage material, glycogen, into glucose. As a result, the blood sugar falls and dangerous substances build up in the liver.

Hereditary fructose intolerance is inherited, which means it is passed down through families. It may be as common as one in twenty thousand in some European countries.

Symptoms

Symptoms can be seen after a baby starts eating food or formula.

The early symptoms of fructose intolerance are similar to those of galactosemia. Later symptoms relate more to liver disease.

Symptoms may include:

- convulsions;
- excessive sleepiness;
- irritability;
- jaundice;
- poor feeding as a baby;
- problems after eating fruits and fructose/sucrose-containing foods;
- vomiting.

Exams and Tests

Physical examination may show:

- yellow skin or eyes;
- hepatosplenomegaly (enlarged liver and spleen).

Tests that confirm the diagnosis include:

- blood clotting tests;
- blood sugar test;
- enzyme studies;
- genetic testing;
- kidney function tests;
- liver function tests;
- liver biopsy;
- uric acid blood test;
- urinalysis.

Blood sugar will be low, especially after receiving fructose or sucrose. Uric acid levels will be high.

Treatment

Complete elimination of fructose and sucrose from the diet is an effective treatment for most patients. Individual complications are treated as appropriate. For example, some patients can take medication to lower the level of uric acid in their blood and thereby decrease their risk for gout.

Outlook (Prognosis)

Hereditary fructose intolerance may be relatively mild or a very severe disease.

Complete avoidance of fructose and sucrose produces good results in most children with this condition. A few children will go on to develop severe liver disease.

In the severe form, even eliminating fructose and sucrose from the diet may not prevent severe liver disease.

How well a person does depends on how soon the diagnosis is made and how soon fructose and sucrose can be eliminated from the diet.

Possible Complications

- Hypoglycemia
- Illness due to eating fructose- or sucrose-containing foods
- Strong avoidance of fructose-containing foods due to noxious effects
- Seizures
- Bleeding
- Gout
- Liver failure
- Death

When to Contact a Medical Professional

Call your health care provider if your child develops symptoms of this condition after feeding starts. If your child has this condition, experts recommend seeing a doctor who specializes in biochemical genetics or metabolism.

Prevention

Couples with a family history of fructose intolerance who wish to have a baby may consider genetic counseling.

Most of the damaging effects of the disease can be prevented by strict adherence to a fructose-free diet.

Section 21.3

Galactosemia

What is galactosemia?

Galactosemia is an inherited disorder that prevents a person from processing the sugar galactose, which is found in many foods. Galactose also exists as part of another sugar, lactose, found in all dairy products.

Normally when a person consumes a product that contains lactose, the body breaks the lactose down into galactose and glucose. Galactosemia means too much galactose builds up in the blood. This accumulation of galactose can cause serious complications such as an enlarged liver, kidney failure, cataracts in the eyes, or brain damage. If untreated, as many as 75 percent of infants with galactosemia will die.

Duarte galactosemia is a variant of classic galactosemia. Fortunately, the complications associated with classic galactosemia have not been associated with Duarte galactosemia.

There is some disagreement over the need for dietary restriction in the treatment of children with Duarte galactosemia. Consult your healthcare professional for his or her advice on this topic.

What are the symptoms of galactosemia?

Galactosemia usually causes no symptoms at birth, but jaundice, diarrhea, and vomiting soon develop and the baby fails to gain weight. Although galactosemic children are started on dietary restrictions at birth, there continues to be a high incidence of long-term complications involving speech and language, fine and gross motor skill delays, and specific learning disabilities. Ovarian failure may occur in girls.

What causes galactosemia?

Classic galactosemia is a rare genetic metabolic disorder. A child born with classic galactosemia inherits a gene for galactosemia from both parents, who are carriers. A child with Duarte galactosemia inherits a gene for classic galactosemia from one parent and a Duarte variant gene from the other parent.

How is galactosemia diagnosed?

Diagnosis for both classic and Duarte galactosemia is made usually within the first week of life by blood test from a heel prick as part of a standard newborn screening.

How is galactosemia treated?

Treatment requires the strict exclusion of lactose/galactose from the diet. A person with galactosemia will never be able to properly digest foods containing galactose. There is no chemical or drug substitute for the missing enzyme at this time. An infant diagnosed with galactosemia will simply be changed to a formula that does not contain galactose. With care and continuing medical advances, most children with galactosemia can now live normal lives.

If my child has been diagnosed with galactosemia, what should I ask our doctor?

Speak to your doctor about your child's dietary restrictions.

Who is at risk for galactosemia?

The gene defect for galactosemia is a recessive genetic trait. This faulty gene only emerges when two carriers have children together and pass it to their offspring. For each pregnancy of two such carriers, there is a 25 percent chance that the child will be born with the disease and a 50 percent chance that the child will be a carrier for the gene defect.

Section 21.4

Homocystinuria

"Homocystinuria: General Overview," © 2004 Washington State Department of Health Newborn Screening Program. Reprinted with permission. Editor's Note added July 2009 by David A. Cooke, MD, FACP.

What is homocystinuria?

Homocystinuria is a treatable disorder that affects the way the body processes protein. Children with homocystinuria cannot use a part of the protein called methionine. If left untreated, methionine and related molecules build up in the bloodstream and lead to brain damage and other disabilities.

Is there only one form of homocystinuria?

No, there are several forms of homocystinuria. Some people with homocystinuria are treated slightly differently than others because they respond to treatment with a specific vitamin.

How does the body normally process methionine?

The body normally converts methionine into a different form called cysteine, which is then used by the body in other metabolic functions.

What happens to methionine in a child with homocystinuria?

In a child with homocystinuria, methionine cannot be converted to cysteine because one of the needed enzymes does not work properly. This results in large amounts of methionine and related molecules, which are toxic to the brain and nervous system.

What are the effects of having homocystinuria if it is not treated?

Without treatment, about half of people with homocystinuria die, usually from blood clots that block normal blood flow. Untreated homocystinuria can result in mental retardation and other problems of the nervous system. It can also result in eye problems and skeletal abnormalities.

What is the treatment for homocystinuria?

Some people with homocystinuria respond to vitamin B_6 (pyridoxine). Those who do not respond to this treatment are placed on a special diet that is low in methionine. To prevent mental retardation and developmental disability, treatment must begin shortly after birth. People with homocystinuria require specialized treatment through a clinic with experience in treating this disorder.

Why would a child have homocystinuria?

Homocystinuria is an inherited disorder. It results when a baby receives a double dose of a specific nonworking gene involved in methionine conversion (one from each parent). For more information about this, contact your health care provider or a genetic counselor.

How common is homocystinuria?

About one in every two hundred thousand babies in the United States is born with homocystinuria.

Editor's note: A drug called trimethylglycine (also known as betaine or Cystadane®) is FDA-approved for reducing homocysteine levels in people with homocystinuria. However, this medication does not eliminate the need for dietary restriction of homocysteine.

Section 21.5

Maple Syrup Urine Disease

What Is Maple Syrup Urine Disease (MSUD)?

MSUD is a potentially deadly disorder that affects the way the body breaks down three amino acids, leucine, isoleucine, and valine. When they're not being used to build a protein, these three amino acids can either be recycled or broken down and used for energy. They are normally broken down by six proteins that act as a team and form a complex called BCKD (branched-chain alpha-ketoacid dehydrogenase).

People with MSUD have a mutation that results in a deficiency for one of the six proteins that make up this complex. Therefore, they can't break down leucine, isoleucine, and valine. They end up with dangerously high levels of these amino acids in their blood, causing the rapid degeneration of brain cells and death if left untreated.

Defects in any of the six subunits that make up the BCKD protein complex can cause the development of MSUD. The most common defect is caused by a mutation in a gene on chromosome 19 that encodes the alpha subunit of the BCKD complex (BCKDHA).

How Do People Get MSUD?

MSUD is inherited in an autosomal recessive pattern. For a child to get the disease, he or she must inherit a defective copy of the gene from each parent. If both parents carry the MSUD gene, each of their children has a 25 percent chance of getting the disorder, and a 50 percent chance of being a carrier.

What Are the Symptoms of MSUD?

There is a classic form of MSUD and several less common forms. Each form varies in its severity and characteristic features. However, all subtypes of the disorder can be caused by mutations in any of the six genes used to build the BCKD protein complex.

A baby who has the disorder may appear normal at birth. But within three to four days, the symptoms appear. These may include: loss of appetite, fussiness, and sweet-smelling urine. The elevated levels of amino acids in the urine generate the smell, which is reminiscent of maple syrup. This is how MSUD got its name. If left untreated, the condition usually worsens. The baby will have seizures, go into a coma, and die within the first few months of life.

How Do Doctors Diagnose MSUD?

In some states, all babies are screened for MSUD within twenty-four hours after birth. A blood sample taken from the baby's heel is analyzed for high leucine levels.

How Is MSUD Treated?

Treatment involves dietary restriction of the amino acids leucine, isoleucine, and valine. This treatment must begin very early to prevent brain damage. Babies with the disease must eat a special formula that does not contain the amino acids leucine, isoleucine, and valine. As the person grows to adulthood, he or she must always watch his or her diet, avoiding high-protein foods such as meat, eggs, and nuts.

If levels of the three amino acids still get too high, patients can be treated with an intravenous (given through a vein) solution that helps the body use up excess leucine, isoleucine, and valine for protein synthesis.

Gene therapy is also a potential future treatment for patients with MSUD. This would involve replacing the mutated gene with a good copy, allowing the patient's cells to generate a functional BCKD protein complex and break down the excess amino acids.

Interesting Facts about MSUD

MSUD is an extremely rare disorder; only 1 in 180,000 babies is born with MSUD. But in certain populations, the disease is much more common. Among the Mennonites in Pennsylvania, as many as 1 out of every 176 babies is born with the disorder.

Section 21.6

Medium Chain Acyl-Coenzyme A Dehydrogenase Deficiency

"Medium Chain Acyl-CoA Dehydrogenase (MCAD) Deficiency:
General Overview," © 2008 Washington State Department of Health
Newborn Screening Program. Reprinted with permission.

What is medium chain acyl-CoA dehydrogenase deficiency (MCADD)?

MCAD deficiency is a treatable disorder that affects the way the body breaks down fats. If left untreated, MCAD deficiency can cause life-threatening illness.

How does the body normally process fats?

The body normally uses carbohydrates and sugars from our diet for energy and uses fats as an energy reserve. When all of the carbohydrates and sugars in our bodies have been used, we break down fats for energy. One of the enzymes that helps break down fats is called MCAD.

What happens to fats in a child with MCAD deficiency?

In a child with MCAD deficiency, fats cannot be broken down normally because the MCAD enzyme does not work properly. This can result in high levels of partially broken down fats, which are toxic to the brain and nervous system.

What are the effects of having MCAD deficiency if it is not treated?

Untreated MCAD deficiency can result in mental retardation, other problems of the nervous system, and sometimes death.

What is the treatment for MCAD deficiency?

Treatment for MCAD deficiency is usually straightforward. Treatment involves avoiding long periods of time without eating and having meals that are high in carbohydrates and low in fats (breast milk and commercial formula are fine). Infants should have at least one night-time feeding, or a late night snack, to reduce the time they go without eating. Special care must be taken if a person with MCAD deficiency becomes ill and has trouble keeping food down. This is usually treated in the hospital with an intravenous feeding. It is important that children with MCAD deficiency receive specialized management through a clinic with experience in treating this disorder.

Why would a child have MCAD deficiency?

MCAD deficiency is an inherited disorder. It results when a baby receives a double-dose of a nonworking MCAD gene (one from each parent). For more information about this, contact your health care provider or a genetic counselor.

What are the chances that a child will be born with MCAD deficiency?

About one in every twenty thousand babies in the United States is born with MCAD deficiency.

Section 21.7

Methylmalonic Acidemia

"Methylmalonic Acidemias," reprinted with permission from the Missouri Department of Health and Senior Services (www.dhss.mo.gov). This information is not intended to replace the advice of a genetic metabolic medical professional. The full text of this document may be accessed online at www.dhss.mo.gov/NewbornScreening/MMA.pdf; accessed January 8, 2009.

What Is It?

Methylmalonic acidemias (also known as MUT, Cbl A,B) is an inherited organic acid disorder. People with organic acid disorders, like MUT, Cbl A,B, cannot properly break down certain components of protein and fats. This is because the body is lacking a specific chemical called an enzyme. Since the body cannot properly break down the proteins and fats, certain organic acids build up in the blood and urine and cause problems when a person eats normal amounts of protein, or becomes sick.

What Are the Symptoms?

A person with MUT, Cbl A,B can appear normal at birth. The symptoms of MUT, Cbl A,B can be very variable between people. Some people with MUT, Cbl A,B will have the following symptoms after a few days of life: poor feeding, lack of energy, vomiting, low muscle tone, seizures, and trouble breathing. Kidney failure may develop. People with MUT, Cbl A,B may also present with the following symptoms later in infancy: failure to thrive, developmental delay, and seizures. People with MUT, Cbl A,B may have no symptoms at all. Many symptoms of MUT, Cbl A,B can be prevented by immediate treatment and lifelong management. People with MUT, Cbl A,B typically receive follow-up care by a team of professionals that is experienced in treating people with metabolic disorders.

Inheritance and Frequency

MUT, Cbl A,B is inherited in an autosomal recessive manner. This means that for a person to be affected with MUT, Cbl A,B, he or she

217

must have inherited two nonworking copies of the gene responsible for causing MUT, Cbl A,B. Usually, both parents of a person affected with an autosomal recessive disorder are unaffected because they are carriers. This means that they have one working copy of the gene, and one nonworking copy of the gene. When both parents are carriers, there is a one in four (or 25 percent) chance that both parents will pass on the nonworking copies of their gene, causing the baby to have MUT, Cbl A,B. Typically, there is no family history of MUT, Cbl A,B in an affected person. About one in fifty thousand babies born have MUT, Cbl A,B.

How Is It Detected?

MUT, Cbl A,B may be detected through newborn screening. A recognizable pattern of elevated chemicals alerts the laboratory that a baby may be affected. Confirmation of newborn screening results is required to make a firm diagnosis. This is usually done by a physician that specializes in metabolic conditions, or a primary care physician.

How Is It Treated?

MUT, Cbl A,B is treated by eating a diet low in protein and drinking a special formula, and sometimes medication, as recommended by a genetic metabolic medical professional.

Section 21.8

Phenylketonuria (PKU)

Reprinted from "Learning about Phenylketonuria (PKU),"
National Human Genome Research Institute, National Institutes
of Health, May 28, 2008.

What is phenylketonuria (PKU)?

Phenylketonuria (PKU) is an inherited disorder of metabolism that causes an increase in the blood of a chemical known as phenylalanine. Phenylalanine comes from a person's diet and is used by the body to make proteins. Phenylalanine is found in all food proteins and in some artificial sweeteners. Without dietary treatment, phenylalanine can build up to harmful levels in the body, causing mental retardation and other serious problems.

Women who have high levels of phenylalanine during pregnancy are at high risk for having babies born with mental retardation, heart problems, small head size (microcephaly), and developmental delay. This is because the babies are exposed to their mother's very high levels of phenylalanine before they are born.

In the United States, PKU occurs in 1 in 10,000 to 1 in 15,000 newborn babies. Newborn screening has been used to detect PKU since the 1960s. As a result, the severe signs and symptoms of PKU are rarely seen.

What are the symptoms of PKU?

Symptoms of PKU range from mild to severe. Severe PKU is called classic PKU. Infants born with classic PKU appear normal for the first few months after birth. However, without treatment with a low-phenylalanine diet, these infants will develop mental retardation and behavioral problems. Other common symptoms of untreated classic PKU include seizures, developmental delay, and autism. Boys and girls who have classic PKU may also have eczema of the skin and lighter skin and hair than their family members who do not have PKU.

Babies born with less severe forms of PKU (moderate or mild PKU) may have a milder degree of mental retardation unless treated with

219

the special diet. If the baby has only a very slight degree of PKU, often called mild hyperphenylalaninemia, there may be no problems and the special dietary treatment may not be needed.

How is PKU diagnosed?

PKU is usually diagnosed through newborn screening testing that is done shortly after birth on a blood sample (heel stick). However, PKU should be considered at any age in a person who has developmental delays or mental retardation. This is because, rarely, infants are missed by newborn screening programs.

What is the treatment for PKU?

PKU is treated by limiting the amount of protein (that contains phenylalanine) in the diet. Treatment also includes using special medical foods as well as special low-protein foods and taking vitamins and minerals. People who have PKU need to follow this diet for their lifetime. It is especially important for women who have PKU to follow the diet throughout their childbearing years.

Is PKU inherited?

PKU is inherited in families in an autosomal recessive pattern. Autosomal recessive inheritance means that a person has two copies of the gene that is altered. Usually, each parent of an individual who has PKU carries one copy of the altered gene. Since each parent also has a normal gene, they do not show signs or symptoms of PKU.

Gene alterations (mutations) in the PAH gene cause PKU. Mutations in the PAH gene cause low levels of an enzyme called phenylalanine hydroxylase. These low levels mean that phenylalanine from a person's diet cannot be metabolized (changed), so it builds up to toxic levels in the bloodstream and body. Having too much phenylalanine can cause brain damage unless diet treatment is started.

Section 21.9

Tyrosinemia

Excerpted from "Tyrosinemia," *Genetics Home Reference*,
a service of the U.S. National Library of Medicine, January 2008.

What is tyrosinemia?

Tyrosinemia is a genetic disorder characterized by elevated blood
levels of the amino acid tyrosine, a building block of most proteins.
Tyrosinemia is caused by the shortage (deficiency) of one of the enzymes required for the multistep process that breaks down tyrosine.
If untreated, tyrosine and its byproducts build up in tissues and organs, which leads to serious medical problems.

There are three types of tyrosinemia. Each has distinctive symptoms and is caused by the deficiency of a different enzyme. Type I
tyrosinemia, the most severe form of this disorder, is caused by a shortage of the enzyme fumarylacetoacetate hydrolase. Symptoms usually
appear in the first few months of life and include failure to gain weight
and grow at the expected rate (failure to thrive), diarrhea, vomiting,
yellowing of the skin and whites of the eyes (jaundice), cabbage-like
odor, and increased tendency to bleed (particularly nosebleeds). Type
I tyrosinemia can lead to liver and kidney failure, problems affecting
the nervous system, and an increased risk of liver cancer.

Type II tyrosinemia is caused by a deficiency of the enzyme tyrosine
aminotransferase. This form of the disorder can affect the eyes, skin,
and mental development. Symptoms often begin in early childhood
and include excessive tearing, abnormal sensitivity to light (photophobia), eye pain and redness, and painful skin lesions on the palms
and soles. About 50 percent of individuals with type II tyrosinemia
have some degree of mental retardation.

Type III tyrosinemia is a rare disorder caused by a deficiency of
the enzyme 4-hydroxyphenylpyruvate dioxygenase. Characteristic
features include mild mental retardation, seizures, and periodic loss
of balance and coordination (intermittent ataxia).

About 10 percent of newborns have temporarily elevated levels of
tyrosine. In these cases, the cause is not genetic. The most likely causes

are vitamin C deficiency or immature liver enzymes due to premature birth.

How common is tyrosinemia?

Worldwide, type I tyrosinemia affects about 1 person in 100,000. This type of tyrosinemia is much more common in Quebec, Canada. The overall incidence in Quebec is about 1 in 16,000 individuals. In the Saguenay-Lac St. Jean region of Quebec, type I tyrosinemia affects 1 person in 1,846.

Type II tyrosinemia occurs in fewer than 1 in 250,000 individuals. Type III tyrosinemia is very rare; only a few cases have been reported.

What genes are related to tyrosinemia?

Mutations in the FAH, HPD, and TAT genes cause tyrosinemia.

In the liver, enzymes break down tyrosine in a five-step process into harmless molecules that are either excreted by the kidneys or used in reactions that produce energy. Mutations in the FAH, HPD, or TAT gene cause a shortage of one of the enzymes in this multistep process. The resulting enzyme deficiency leads to a toxic accumulation of tyrosine and its byproducts, which can damage the liver, kidneys, nervous system, and other organs and tissues.

How do people inherit tyrosinemia?

This condition is inherited in an autosomal recessive pattern, which means both copies of the gene in each cell have mutations. The parents of an individual with an autosomal recessive condition each carry one copy of the mutated gene, but they typically do not show signs and symptoms of the condition.

Section 21.10

Urea Cycle Defects

What is a urea cycle disorder?

A urea cycle disorder is a genetic disorder caused by a deficiency of one of the enzymes in the urea cycle which is responsible for removing ammonia from the bloodstream. The urea cycle involves a series of biochemical steps in which nitrogen, a waste product of protein metabolism, is removed from the blood and converted to urea. Normally, the urea is transferred into the urine and removed from the body. In urea cycle disorders, the nitrogen accumulates in the form of ammonia, a highly toxic substance, and is not removed from the body, resulting in hyperammonemia. Ammonia then reaches the brain through the blood, where it causes irreversible brain damage, coma, and/or death.

Urea cycle disorders are included in the category of inborn errors of metabolism. There is no cure. Inborn errors of metabolism represent a substantial cause of brain damage and death among newborns and infants. Because many cases of urea cycle disorders remain undiagnosed and/or infants born with the disorders die without a definitive diagnosis, the exact incidence of these cases is unknown and underestimated. It is believed that up to 20 percent of sudden infant death syndrome cases may be attributed to an undiagnosed inborn error of metabolism such a urea cycle disorder. In April 2000, research experts at the Urea Cycle Consensus Conference estimated the incidence of the disorders at one in ten thousand births. This represents a significant increase in case diagnosis in the last few years. Research studies have now been initiated to more accurately determine the incidence and prevalence of UCDs.

What are the symptoms?

The neonatal period: Children with severe urea cycle disorders typically show symptoms after the first twenty-four hours of life. The baby may be irritable at first, or refuse feedings, followed by vomiting and increasing lethargy. Soon after, seizures, hypotonia (poor muscle tone, floppiness), respiratory distress (respiratory alkalosis), and coma may occur. These symptoms are caused by rising ammonia levels in the blood. Sepsis and Reye syndrome are common misdiagnoses. If untreated, these severely affected infants will die. Severe neonatal symptoms are more commonly seen in both boys and girls with ornithine transcarbamylase (OTC) and carbamyl phosphate synthetase (CPS) deficiency, but can also occur with citrullinemia or argininosuccinate lyase deficiency (ASA).

Childhood: Children with mild or moderate urea cycle enzyme deficiencies may not show recognizable symptoms until early childhood. Earliest symptoms may include failure to thrive, inconsolable crying, agitation or hyperactive behavior, sometimes accompanied by screaming, self-injurious behavior, and refusal to eat meat or other high-protein foods. Later symptoms may include frequent episodes of vomiting, especially following high-protein meals, lethargy and delirium, and finally, if the condition is undiagnosed and untreated, hyperammonemic coma or death may occur. Undiagnosed children may be referred to child psychologists because of their behavior and eating problems. Childhood episodes of hyperammonemia (high ammonia levels in the blood) may be brought on by viral illnesses including chicken pox, colds or flu, teething, growth spurts, high-protein meals, or even exhaustion. Common misdiagnoses include Reye syndrome. Childhood onset can be seen in both boys and girls affected by any of the urea cycle disorders.

Early clinical manifestations of arginase deficiency (similar to those of the other disorders) may be seen as early as one year of age, but some children with AG remain asymptomatic at four years of age. AG symptoms are usually progressive and include growth failure, spastic tetraplegia (lower limbs more severely affected than upper limbs), seizures, psychomotor retardation, and hyperactivity.

Major characteristics of N-acetylglutamate synthetase (NAGS) deficiency, considered the rarest urea cycle disorder, include severe hyperammonemia, deep encephalopathy despite only mild hyperammonemia, recurrent diarrhea and acidosis, movement disorder, hypoglycemia, and hyperornithinemia.[1]

Adulthood: Recently, the number of adults being diagnosed with urea cycle disorders has increased at an alarming rate. These individuals have survived undiagnosed to adulthood, probably due to less severe enzyme deficiencies. These individuals exhibit stroke-like symptoms, episodes of lethargy, and delirium. These adults are likely to be referred to neurologists or psychiatrists because of their psychiatric symptoms. However, without proper diagnosis and treatment, these individuals are at risk for permanent brain damage, coma, and death. Adult-onset symptoms have been observed following viral illnesses, childbirth, dieting, use of valproic acid (an anti-epileptic drug which causes excess ammonia), and chemotherapy.

OTC carriers: Approximately 85 percent of adult female carriers (heterozygotes) for OTC deficiency are asymptomatic (exhibit no symptoms). The remainder show symptoms including protein intolerance, headache, episodes of confusion or inability to concentrate, behavioral or neurological abnormalities, cyclical vomiting, and episodes of hyperammonemia. Studies have shown carriers to be of normal to above-normal intelligence, but some have been shown to demonstrate subtle deficits in fine motor, visual-spatial, and nonverbal functions.[2] Concerns are beginning to emerge with carriers with regard to common health issues (diabetes, hypercholesterolemia, cancer) and effects that treatments or drugs used to treat these common conditions may have on urea cycle function.

What kinds of disorders are there?

There are six enzyme disorders of the urea cycle, collectively known as inborn errors of urea synthesis, or urea cycle enzyme defects. Each is referred to by the initials of the missing enzyme:

- **CPS:** Carbamyl phosphate synthetase
- **NAGS:** N-acetylglutamate synthetase
- **OTC:** Ornithine transcarbamylase
- **AS:** Argininosuccinic acid synthetase (citrullinemia)
- **AL/ASA:** Argininosuccinate lyase (argininosuccinic aciduria)
- **AG:** Arginase

Additionally, there are three transporter defects:

- Mitochondrial ornithine carrier (hyperornithinemia-hyperammonemia-homocitrullinuria or HHH syndrome)

- Mitochondrial aspartate/glutamate carrier (citrullinemia type II)

- Dibasic amino acid carrier (hyperdibasic amino aciduria or lysinuric protein intolerance)

Neonatal onset disorders represent severe enzyme deficiencies or complete absence of enzyme function. Individuals with childhood or adult onset disease have partial enzyme deficiency. The percentage, or amount of enzyme function, varies widely between individuals with partial enzyme deficiencies. All of these disorders are transmitted genetically as autosomal recessive genes—each parent contributes a defective gene to the child—except for ornithine transcarbamylase deficiency. OTC deficiency is acquired in one of three ways: as an X-linked trait from the mother, who may be an undiagnosed carrier; in some cases of female children, the disorder can also be inherited from the defect on the father's X-chromosome; and finally, OTC deficiency may be acquired as a "new" spontaneous mutation occurring in the fetus. Recent research has shown that some female carriers of the disease may become symptomatic with the disorder later in life, suffering high ammonia levels and experiencing classic symptoms. Several undiagnosed women have died during childbirth as a result of high ammonia levels and on autopsy were determined to have been unknown symptomatic carriers of the disorder.

What are the treatment options?

The treatment of urea cycle disorders consists of dietary management to limit ammonia production in conjunction with medications and/or supplements which provide alternative pathways for the removal of ammonia from the bloodstream. A careful balance of dietary protein, carbohydrates, and fats is necessary to insure that the body receives adequate calories for energy needs, as well as adequate essential amino acids (for cell growth and development). Dietary protein must be carefully monitored and some restriction is necessary; too much dietary protein causes excessive ammonia production. However, if protein intake is too restrictive or insufficient calories are provided, the body will break down lean muscle mass (called catabolism) to obtain the amino acids or energy it requires; this catabolism creates excessive ammonia. Therefore, the correct nutritional balance for each individual in each stage of growth is critical in avoiding hyperammonemic crises. Frequent blood tests (serum ammonia, plasma quantitative amino acids) are required to monitor the disorders and are an important tool for optimizing treatment.

Treatment may include supplementation with special amino acid formulas (Cyclinex®, UCD I&II), developed specifically for urea cycle disorders, which can be prescribed to provide approximately 50 percent of the daily dietary protein allowance. Some patients may require individual branched chain amino acid supplementation. Metabolic nutritionists routinely prescribe calorie modules such as Pro-Phree®, Polycose®, and Moducal® to be used in combination with the amino acid formulas. Pharmaceutical grade (not over-the-counter) L-citrulline (for OTC and CPS deficiency) or L-arginine free base (ASA and citrullinemia) is also required. These are not to be used in arginase deficiency. Multiple vitamins and calcium supplements are also recommended.

Sodium phenylbutyrate (trade name Buphenyl®) is the primary medication being used to treat urea cycle disorders. The National Urea Cycle Disorders Foundation played a key role in initiating and supporting the research at Johns Hopkins University to develop the medication. Sodium benzoate is also used in some patients, solely or in conjunction with Buphenyl; both are "ammonia scavengers"—providing alternative pathways for removal of ammonia from the bloodstream and helping to prevent hyperammonemia. One or both of these medications is administered three to four times per day in order to insure continual removal of toxic ammonia from the bloodstream.

Children with urea cycle disorders often lack appetite (due to excess serotonin in the brain suppressing appetite) and some may benefit from receiving medications and some feedings either via gastrostomy tube (G-tube, a tube surgically implanted in the stomach) or nasogastric tube (NG-tube, manually inserted through the nose into the stomach). The access these tubes provide often makes a critical difference in metabolic stability and in averting hyperammonemic crises; medications and formulas can still be administered when children have flu or colds, etc. Some centers have reported as much as 70 percent reduction in hospital admissions after placement of G-tubes or parents were trained to use NG-tubes.

Optimal treatment of urea cycle disorders requires a medical team consisting minimally of a geneticist/metabolic specialist and nutritionist specifically experienced in successful management of the disorders. These teams are usually found at university hospitals. Specialty consultation and second opinions from experts in the field of UCDs can be obtained by families who live in areas where optimal medical care is not available.

When optimal treatment fails, or for neonatal onset CPS and OTC deficiency, liver transplant becomes an option. Liver transplants have been done successfully as a cure for the disorder (although L-arginine supplementation is still necessary in argininosuccinate lyase deficiency posttransplant). The transplant alternative must be carefully considered and evaluated with medical professionals to determine the potential of success compared to the serious risks and potential for new medical concerns, including the possibility of fatal viruses (Epstein-Barr, cytomegalovirus [CMV]), risk of developmental delay, or lymphoproliferative disease as a side effect of immunosuppression/immunosuppressants.

References

1. S. Brusilow, A. Horwich, "Urea Cycle Enzymes," *The Metabolic and Molecular Bases of Inherited Disease*, Vol 2 p.1810–1962: McGraw Hill.

2. A. Gropman, M. Batshaw: Cognitive outcome in urea cycle disorders. *Molecular Genetics and Metabolism* Vol 81, Sup 1, Apr 2004, p. 58–62.

Chapter 22

Kidney and Urinary System Disorders

Chapter Contents

Section 22.1

Cystinuria

Alternative Names

Stones—cystine; cystine stones

Definition

Cystinuria is a condition passed down through families in which stones form in the kidney, ureter, and bladder. It is an autosomal recessive disorder.

Causes

Cystinuria is caused by excessive levels of an amino acid called cystine in the urine. After entering the kidneys, most cystine normally dissolves and goes back into the bloodstream. But persons with cystinuria have a genetic defect that interferes with this process. As a result, cystine builds up in the urine and forms crystals or stones, which may get stuck in the kidneys, ureters, or bladder.

Cystinuria affects approximately one out of ten thousand people. Cystine stones are most common in young adults under age forty. Less than 3 percent of known urinary tract stones are cystine stones.

Symptoms

- Blood in the urine
- Flank pain or pain in the side or back:
  - Usually on one side; rarely felt on both sides
  - Often severe
  - May get increasingly worse over days
  - Pain may also be felt in the pelvis, groin, genitals, or between the upper abdomen and the back

Exams and Tests

The disorder is usually diagnosed after an episode of stones. Analysis of the stones shows they are made of cystine.

Tests that may be done to detect stones and diagnose this condition include:

- abdominal computed tomography (CT) scan, magnetic resonance imaging (MRI), or ultrasound;
- intravenous pyelogram (IVP);
- twenty-four-hour urine collection (shows high levels of cystine);
- urinalysis (may show cystine crystals).

Treatment

The goal of treatment is to relieve symptoms and prevent the development of more stones. A person with severe symptoms may need to be admitted to a hospital.

Treatment involves drinking plenty of fluids, particularly water, so that large amounts of urine are produced. The patient should drink at least six to eight glasses per day.

In some cases, fluids may need to be given through a vein.

Medications may be prescribed to help dissolve the cystine crystals. Eating less salt can also decrease cystine excretion and stone formation.

Pain relievers may be needed to control pain in the kidney or bladder area associated with the passage of stones. The stones usually pass through the urine on their own. If they do not, surgery may be needed.

Lithotripsy may be an alternative to surgery. However, this procedure is not as successful for removal of cystine stones as it is for other types of stones.

Outlook (Prognosis)

Cystinuria is a chronic, lifelong condition. Stones commonly return. However, the condition rarely results in kidney failure, and it does not affect other organs.

Possible Complications

- Bladder injury from stone
- Ureteral obstruction

- Kidney injury from stone
- Kidney infection
- Urinary tract infection

When to Contact a Medical Professional

Call your health care provider if you have symptoms of urinary tract stones.

Prevention

There is no known prevention for cystinuria. Any person with a known history of stones in the urinary tract should drink plenty of fluids to regularly produce a high amount of urine. This allows stones and crystals to leave the body before they become large enough to cause symptoms.

Section 22.2

Polycystic Kidney Disease

Excerpted from "Polycystic Kidney Disease," National Institute of Diabetes and Digestive and Kidney Diseases, National Institutes of Health, NIH Publication No. 08-4008, November 2007.

Polycystic kidney disease (PKD) is a genetic disorder characterized by the growth of numerous cysts in the kidneys. The kidneys are two organs, each about the size of a fist, located in the upper part of a person's abdomen, toward the back. The kidneys filter wastes and extra fluid from the blood to form urine. They also regulate amounts of certain vital substances in the body. When cysts form in the kidneys, they are filled with fluid. PKD cysts can profoundly enlarge the kidneys while replacing much of the normal structure, resulting in reduced kidney function and leading to kidney failure.

When PKD causes kidneys to fail—which usually happens after many years—the patient requires dialysis or kidney transplantation.

About one-half of people with the most common type of PKD progress to kidney failure, also called end-stage renal disease (ESRD).

PKD can also cause cysts in the liver and problems in other organs, such as blood vessels in the brain and heart. The number of cysts as well as the complications they cause help doctors distinguish PKD from the usually harmless "simple" cysts that often form in the kidneys in later years of life.

In the United States, about six hundred thousand[1] people have PKD, and cystic disease is the fourth leading cause of kidney failure. Two major inherited forms of PKD exist:

- Autosomal dominant PKD is the most common inherited form. Symptoms usually develop between the ages of thirty and forty, but they can begin earlier, even in childhood. About 90 percent of all PKD cases are autosomal dominant PKD.

- Autosomal recessive PKD is a rare inherited form. Symptoms of autosomal recessive PKD begin in the earliest months of life, even in the womb.

Autosomal Dominant PKD

What is autosomal dominant PKD?

Autosomal dominant PKD is the most common inherited disorder of the kidneys. The phrase "autosomal dominant" means that if one parent has the disease, there is a 50 percent chance that the disease gene will pass to a child. In some cases—perhaps 10 percent—autosomal dominant PKD occurs spontaneously in patients. In these cases, neither of the parents carries a copy of the disease gene.

Many people with autosomal dominant PKD live for several decades without developing symptoms. For this reason, autosomal dominant PKD is often called "adult polycystic kidney disease." Yet, in some cases, cysts may form earlier in life and grow quickly, causing symptoms in childhood.

The cysts grow out of nephrons, the tiny filtering units inside the kidneys. The cysts eventually separate from the nephrons and continue to enlarge. The kidneys enlarge along with the cysts—which can number in the thousands—while roughly retaining their kidney shape. In fully developed autosomal dominant PKD, a cyst-filled kidney can weigh as much as twenty to thirty pounds. High blood pressure is common and develops in most patients by age twenty or thirty.

What are the symptoms of autosomal dominant PKD?

The most common symptoms are pain in the back and the sides—between the ribs and hips—and headaches. The pain can be temporary or persistent, mild or severe.

People with autosomal dominant PKD also can experience the following complications:

- Urinary tract infections—specifically, in the kidney cysts

- Hematuria—blood in the urine

- Liver and pancreatic cysts

- Abnormal heart valves

- High blood pressure

- Kidney stones

- Aneurysms—bulges in the walls of blood vessels—in the brain

- Diverticulosis—small pouches bulge outward through the colon

How is autosomal dominant PKD diagnosed?

Autosomal dominant PKD is usually diagnosed by kidney imaging studies. The most common form of diagnostic kidney imaging is ultrasound, but more precise studies, such as computerized tomography (CT) scans or magnetic resonance imaging (MRI) are also widely used. In autosomal dominant PKD, the onset of kidney damage and how quickly the disease progresses can vary. Kidney imaging findings can also vary considerably, depending on a patient's age. Younger patients usually have both fewer and smaller cysts. Doctors have therefore developed specific criteria for diagnosing the disease with kidney imaging findings, depending on patient age. For example, the presence of at least two cysts in each kidney by age thirty in a patient with a family history of the disease can confirm the diagnosis of autosomal dominant PKD. If there is any question about the diagnosis, a family history of autosomal dominant PKD and cysts found in other organs make the diagnosis more likely.

In most cases of autosomal dominant PKD, patients have no symptoms and their physical condition appears normal for many years, so the disease can go unnoticed. Physical checkups and blood and urine tests may not lead to early diagnosis. Because of the slow, undetected progression of cyst growth, some people live for many years without knowing they have autosomal dominant PKD.

Once cysts have grown to about one-half inch, however, diagnosis is possible with imaging technology. Ultrasound, which passes sound waves through the body to create a picture of the kidneys, is used most often. Ultrasound imaging does not use any injected dyes or radiation and is safe for all patients, including pregnant women. It can also detect cysts in the kidneys of a fetus, but large cyst growth this early in life is uncommon in autosomal dominant PKD.

More powerful and expensive imaging procedures such as CT scans and MRI also can detect cysts. Recently, MRI has been used to measure kidney and cyst volume and monitor kidney and cyst growth, which may serve as a way to track progression of the disease.

Diagnosis can also be made with a genetic test that detects mutations in the autosomal dominant PKD genes, called PKD1 and PKD2. Although this test can detect the presence of the autosomal dominant PKD mutations before large cysts develop, its usefulness is limited by two factors: detection of a disease gene cannot predict the onset of symptoms or ultimate severity of the disease, and if a disease gene is detected, no specific prevention or cure for the disease exists. However, a young person who knows of a PKD gene mutation may be able to forestall the loss of kidney function through diet and blood pressure control. The genetic test may also be used to determine whether a young member of a PKD family can safely donate a kidney to a family member with the disease. Individuals with a family history of PKD who are of childbearing age might also want to know whether they have the potential of passing a PKD gene to a child. Anyone considering genetic testing should receive counseling to understand all the implications of the test.

How is autosomal dominant PKD treated?

Although a cure for autosomal dominant PKD is not available, treatment can ease symptoms and prolong life.

Pain: Pain in the area of the kidneys can be caused by cyst infection, bleeding into cysts, kidney stones, or stretching of the fibrous tissue around the kidney with cyst growth. A doctor will first evaluate which of these causes are contributing to the pain to guide treatment. If it is determined to be chronic pain due to cyst expansion, the doctor may initially suggest over-the-counter pain medications, such as aspirin or acetaminophen (Tylenol). Consult your doctor before taking any over-the-counter medication because some may be harmful to the kidneys. For most but not all cases of severe pain due to cyst expansion, surgery to shrink cysts can relieve pain in the back and sides. However, surgery provides only temporary relief and does not slow the disease's progression toward kidney failure.

Headaches that are severe or that seem to feel different from other headaches might be caused by aneurysms—blood vessels that balloon out in spots—in the brain. These aneurysms could rupture, which can have severe consequences. Headaches also can be caused by high blood pressure. People with autosomal dominant PKD should see a doctor if they have severe or recurring headaches—even before considering over-the-counter pain medications.

Urinary tract infections: People with autosomal dominant PKD tend to have frequent urinary tract infections, which can be treated with antibiotics. People with the disease should seek treatment for urinary tract infections immediately because infection can spread from the urinary tract to the cysts in the kidneys. Cyst infections are difficult to treat because many antibiotics do not penetrate the cysts.

High blood pressure: Keeping blood pressure under control can slow the effects of autosomal dominant PKD. Lifestyle changes and various medications can lower high blood pressure. Patients should ask their doctors about such treatments. Sometimes proper diet and exercise are enough to keep blood pressure controlled.

End-stage renal disease: After many years, PKD can cause the kidneys to fail. Because kidneys are essential for life, people with ESRD must seek one of two options for replacing kidney functions: dialysis or transplantation. In hemodialysis, blood is circulated into an external filter, where it is cleaned before re-entering the body; in peritoneal dialysis, a fluid is introduced into the abdomen, where it absorbs wastes and is then removed. Transplantation of healthy kidneys into ESRD patients has become a common and successful procedure. Healthy—non-PKD—kidneys transplanted into PKD patients do not develop cysts.

Autosomal Recessive PKD

What is autosomal recessive PKD?

Autosomal recessive PKD is caused by a mutation in the autosomal recessive PKD gene, called PKHD1. Other genes for the disease might exist but have not yet been discovered by scientists. We all carry two copies of every gene. Parents who do not have PKD can have a child with the disease if both parents carry one copy of the abnormal gene and both pass that gene copy to their baby. The chance of the child having autosomal recessive PKD when both parents carry the abnormal gene is 25 percent. If only one parent carries the abnormal gene, the baby cannot get autosomal recessive PKD but could ultimately pass the abnormal gene to his or her children.

The signs of autosomal recessive PKD frequently begin before birth, so it is often called "infantile PKD." Children born with autosomal recessive PKD often, but not always, develop kidney failure before reaching adulthood. Severity of the disease varies. Babies with the worst cases die hours or days after birth due to respiratory difficulties or respiratory failure.

Some people with autosomal recessive PKD do not develop symptoms until later in childhood or even adulthood. Liver scarring occurs in all patients with autosomal recessive PKD and tends to become more of a medical concern with increasing age.

What are the symptoms of autosomal recessive PKD?

Children with autosomal recessive PKD experience high blood pressure, urinary tract infections, and frequent urination. The disease usually affects the liver and spleen, resulting in low blood cell counts, varicose veins, and hemorrhoids. Because kidney function is crucial for early physical development, children with autosomal recessive PKD and decreased kidney function are usually smaller than average size. Recent studies suggest that growth problems may be a primary feature of autosomal recessive PKD.

How is autosomal recessive PKD diagnosed?

Ultrasound imaging of the fetus or newborn reveals enlarged kidneys with an abnormal appearance, but large cysts such as those in autosomal dominant PKD are rarely seen. Because autosomal recessive PKD tends to scar the liver, ultrasound imaging of the liver also aids in diagnosis.

How is autosomal recessive PKD treated?

Medicines can control high blood pressure in autosomal recessive PKD, and antibiotics can control urinary tract infections. Eating increased amounts of nutritious food improves growth in children with autosomal recessive PKD. In some cases, growth hormones are used.

In response to kidney failure, autosomal recessive PKD patients must receive dialysis or transplantation. If serious liver disease develops, some people can undergo combined liver and kidney transplantation.

Genetic Diseases

Genes are segments of deoxyribonucleic acid (DNA), the long molecules that reside in each of a person's cells. The genes, through complex processes, build proteins for growth and maintenance of the body. At conception, DNA—or genes—from both parents are passed to the child.

A genetic disease occurs when one or both parents pass abnormal genes to a child at conception. If receiving an abnormal gene from just one parent is enough to produce a disease in the child, the disease is said to have dominant inheritance. If receiving abnormal genes from both parents is needed to produce disease in the child, the disease is said to be recessive. A genetic disease can also occur through a spontaneous mutation.

The chance of acquiring a dominant disease is higher than the chance of acquiring a recessive disease. A child who receives only one gene copy for a recessive disease at conception will not develop the genetic disease—such as autosomal recessive PKD—but could pass the gene to the following generation.

Hope through Research

Scientists have begun to identify the processes that trigger formation of PKD cysts. Advances in the field of genetics have increased our understanding of the abnormal genes responsible for autosomal dominant and autosomal recessive PKD. Scientists have located two genes associated with autosomal dominant PKD. The first was located in 1985 on chromosome 16 and labeled PKD1. PKD2 was localized to chromosome 4 in 1993. Within three years, scientists had isolated the proteins these two genes produce—polycystin-1 and polycystin-2.

When both the PKD1 and PKD2 genes are normal, the proteins they produce work together to foster normal kidney development and inhibit cyst formation. A mutation in either of the genes can lead to cyst formation, but evidence suggests that disease development also requires other factors, in addition to the mutation in one of the PKD genes.

Genetic analyses of most families with PKD confirm mutations in either the PKD1 or PKD2 gene. In about 10 to 15 percent of cases, however, families with autosomal dominant PKD do not show obvious abnormalities or mutations in the PKD1 and PKD2 genes, using current testing methods.

Researchers have also recently identified the autosomal recessive PKD gene, called PKHD1, on chromosome 6. Genetic testing for autosomal recessive PKD to detect mutations in PKHD1 is now offered by a limited number of molecular genetic diagnostics laboratories in the United States.

Researchers have bred rodents with a genetic disease that parallels both inherited forms of human PKD. Studying these mice will lead to greater understanding of the genetic and nongenetic mechanisms involved in cyst formation. In recent years, researchers have discovered several compounds that appear to inhibit cyst formation in mice with the PKD gene. Some of these compounds are in clinical testing in humans. Scientists hope further testing will lead to safe and effective treatments for humans with the disease.

Recent clinical studies of autosomal dominant PKD are exploring new imaging methods for tracking progression of cystic kidney disease. These methods, using MRI, are helping scientists design better clinical trials for new treatments of autosomal dominant PKD.

References

1. Grantham JJ, Nair V, Winklhoffer F. Cystic diseases of the kidney. In: Brenner BM, ed. *Brenner & Rector's The Kidney.* Vol. 2. 6th ed. Philadelphia: WB Saunders Company; 2000: 1699–1730.

Chapter 23

Leukodystrophies

Introduction

What is leukodystrophy?

Leukodystrophy refers to progressive degeneration of the white matter of the brain due to imperfect growth or development of the myelin sheath, the fatty covering that acts as an insulator around nerve fiber. Myelin, which lends its color to the white matter of the brain, is a complex substance made up of at least ten different chemicals. The leukodystrophies are a group of disorders that are caused by genetic defects in how myelin produces or metabolizes these chemicals. Each of the leukodystrophies is the result of a defect in the gene that controls one (and only one) of the chemicals. Specific leukodystrophies include metachromatic leukodystrophy, Krabbe disease, adrenoleukodystrophy, Pelizaeus-Merzbacher disease, Canavan disease,

This chapter includes excerpts from the following fact sheets produced by the National Institute of Neurological Disorders and Stroke (NINDS): "NINDS Leukodystrophy Information Page," reviewed July 18, 2008; "NINDS Adrenoleukodystrophy Information Page," reviewed October 2, 2007; "NINDS Alexander Disease Information Page," reviewed November 20, 2007; "NINDS Canavan Disease Information Page," reviewed July 2, 2008; "NINDS Infantile Refsum Disease Information Page," reviewed February 14, 2007; "NINDS Krabbe Disease Information Page," reviewed July 1, 2008; "NINDS Metachromatic Leukodystrophy Information Page," reviewed February 13, 2007; "NINDS Pelizaeus-Merzbacher Disease Information Page," reviewed September 16, 2008; and "NINDS Zellweger Syndrome Information Page," reviewed December 11, 2007.

241

childhood ataxia with central nervous system hypomyelination or CACH (also known as vanishing white matter disease), Alexander disease, Refsum disease, and cerebrotendinous xanthomatosis. The most common symptom of a leukodystrophy disease is a gradual decline in an infant or child who previously appeared well. Progressive loss may appear in body tone, movements, gait, speech, ability to eat, vision, hearing, and behavior. There is often a slowdown in mental and physical development. Symptoms vary according to the specific type of leukodystrophy, and may be difficult to recognize in the early stages of the disease.

Is there any treatment?

Treatment for most of the leukodystrophies is symptomatic and supportive, and may include medications; physical, occupational, and speech therapies; and nutritional, educational, and recreational programs. Bone marrow transplantation is showing promise for a few of the leukodystrophies.

What is the prognosis?

The prognosis for the leukodystrophies varies according to the specific type of leukodystrophy.

What research is being done?

The National Institute of Neurological Disorders and Stroke (NINDS) supports research on genetic disorders, including the leukodystrophies. The goals of this research are to increase scientific understanding of these disorders, and to find ways to prevent, treat, and, ultimately, cure them.

Adrenoleukodystrophy

What is adrenoleukodystrophy?

Adrenoleukodystrophy (ALD) is one of a group of genetic disorders called the leukodystrophies that cause damage to the myelin sheath, an insulating membrane that surrounds nerve cells in the brain. People with ALD accumulate high levels of saturated, very long chain fatty acids (VLCFA) in the brain and adrenal cortex because they do not produce the enzyme that breaks down these fatty acids in the normal manner. The loss of myelin and the progressive dysfunction of the adrenal gland are the primary characteristics of ALD. ALD has two subtypes. The most common is the X-linked form (X-ALD), which involves an abnormal gene located on the X chromosome. Women have two X chromosomes and are the carriers of the disease, but since men only have one X chromosome and lack the protective effect of the extra X chromosome, they are more severely affected. Onset of X-ALD can occur in childhood or in adulthood. The childhood form is the most severe, with onset between ages four and ten. The most common symptoms are usually behavioral changes such as abnormal withdrawal or aggression, poor memory, and poor school performance. Other symptoms include visual loss, learning disabilities, seizures, poorly articulated speech, difficulty swallowing, deafness, disturbances of gait and coordination, fatigue, intermittent vomiting, increased skin pigmentation, and progressive dementia. In the milder adult-onset form, which typically begins between ages twenty-one and thirty-five, symptoms may include progressive stiffness, weakness or paralysis of the lower limbs, and ataxia. Although adult-onset ALD progresses more slowly than the classic childhood form, it can also result in deterioration of brain function. A mild form of ALD is occasionally seen in women who are carriers of the disorder. Symptoms include progressive stiffness, weakness or paralysis of the lower limbs, ataxia, excessive muscle tone, mild peripheral neuropathy, and urinary problems.

Is there any treatment?

Adrenal function must be tested periodically in all patients with ALD. Treatment with adrenal hormones can be lifesaving. Symptomatic and supportive treatments for ALD include physical therapy, psychological support, and special education. Recent evidence suggests that a mixture of oleic acid and erucic acid, known as "Lorenzo's Oil," administered to boys with X-ALD can reduce or delay the appearance of symptoms. Bone marrow transplants can provide long-term benefit to boys who have early evidence of X-ALD, but the procedure carries risk of mortality and morbidity and is not recommended for those whose symptoms are already severe or who have the adult-onset or neonatal forms. Oral administration of docosahexaenoic acid (DHA) may help infants and children with neonatal ALD.

What is the prognosis?

Prognosis for patients with ALD is generally poor due to progressive neurological deterioration. Death usually occurs within one to ten years after the onset of symptoms.

What research is being done?

The NINDS supports research on genetic disorders such as ALD. The aim of this research is to find ways to prevent, treat, and cure these disorders. Intensive basic research has proposed two new approaches, 4-phenylbutyrate and lovastatin, which could potentially lower levels of VLCFA in the brain. Therapeutic trials for both agents are planned.

Alexander Disease

What is Alexander disease?

Alexander disease is one of a group of neurological conditions known as the leukodystrophies, disorders that are the result of abnormalities in myelin, the "white matter" that protects nerve fibers in the brain. Alexander disease is a progressive and usually fatal disease. The destruction of white matter is accompanied by the formation of Rosenthal fibers, which are abnormal clumps of protein that accumulate in non-neuronal cells of the brain called astrocytes. Rosenthal fibers are sometimes found in other disorders, but not in the same amount or area of the brain that are featured in Alexander disease. The infantile form is the most common type of Alexander disease. It has an onset during the first two years of life. Usually there are both mental and physical developmental delays, followed by the loss of developmental milestones, an abnormal increase in head size, and seizures. The juvenile form of Alexander disease is less common and has an onset between the ages of two and thirteen. These children may have excessive vomiting, difficulty swallowing and speaking, poor coordination, and loss of motor control. Adult-onset forms of Alexander disease are rare, but have been reported. The symptoms sometimes mimic those of Parkinson disease or multiple sclerosis. The disease occurs in both males and females, and there are no ethnic, racial, geographic, or cultural/economic differences in its distribution.

Is there any treatment?

There is no cure for Alexander disease, nor is there a standard course of treatment. Treatment of Alexander disease is symptomatic and supportive.

What is the prognosis?

The prognosis for individuals with Alexander disease is generally poor. Most children with the infantile form do not survive past the age of six. Juvenile and adult-onset forms of the disorder have a slower, more lengthy course.

What research is being done?

Recent discoveries show that most individuals (approximately 90 percent) with Alexander disease have a mutation in the gene that makes glial fibrillary acidic protein (GFAP). GFAP is found in Rosenthal fibers; however it is still unclear how the mutation causes the disease. Most of the mutations occur without any known cause and are not inherited from parents. However, there are some people with Alexander disease who do not have the GFAP mutation, which leads researchers to believe that there may be other genetic or perhaps even nongenetic causes of Alexander disease. Current research is aimed at identifying additional mutations in GFAP that may be responsible for Alexander disease, understanding the mechanisms by which the mutations cause disease, and developing better mouse models for the disorder that could ultimately be used for testing treatments. At present, there is no exact animal model for the disease; however, mice have been engineered to produce the same mutant forms of GFAP found in individuals with Alexander disease. These mice form Rosenthal fibers and have a predisposition for seizures, but do not yet mimic all features of the human disease.

Canavan Disease

What is Canavan disease?

Canavan disease, one of the most common cerebral degenerative diseases of infancy, is a gene-linked, neurological birth disorder in which the white matter of the brain degenerates into spongy tissue riddled with microscopic fluid-filled spaces. Canavan disease is one of a group of genetic disorders known as the leukodystrophies. These diseases cause imperfect growth or development of the myelin sheath, the fatty covering that acts as an insulator around nerve fibers in the brain. Myelin, which lends its color to the "white matter" of the brain, is a complex substance made up of at least ten different chemicals. Each of the leukodystrophies affects one (and only one) of these substances. Canavan disease is caused by mutations in the gene for an enzyme called aspartoacylase. Symptoms of Canavan disease, which appear in early infancy and progress rapidly, may include mental retardation, loss of previously acquired motor skills, feeding difficulties, abnormal muscle tone (floppiness or stiffness), and an abnormally large, poorly controlled head. Paralysis, blindness, or hearing loss may also occur. Children are characteristically quiet and apathetic. Although Canavan disease may occur in any ethnic group, it is more frequent among Ashkenazi Jews from eastern Poland, Lithuania, and western Russia, and among Saudi Arabians. Canavan disease can be identified by a simple prenatal blood test that screens for the missing enzyme or for mutations in the gene that controls aspartoacylase. Both parents must be carriers of the defective gene in order to have an affected child. When both parents are found to carry the Canavan gene mutation, there is a one in four (25 percent) chance with each pregnancy that the child will be affected with Canavan disease.

Is there any treatment?

Canavan disease causes progressive brain atrophy. There is no cure, nor is there a standard course of treatment. Treatment is symptomatic and supportive.

What is the prognosis?

The prognosis for Canavan disease is poor. Death usually occurs before age four, although some children may survive into their teens and twenties.

What research is being done?

The gene for Canavan disease has been located. Many laboratories offer prenatal screening for this disorder to populations at risk. Scientists have developed animal models for this disease and are using the models to test potential therapeutic strategies. Research supported by the NINDS includes studies to understand how the brain and nervous system normally develop and function and how they are affected by genetic mutations. These studies contribute to a greater understanding of gene-linked disorders such as Canavan disease, and have the potential to open promising new avenues of treatment.

Infantile Refsum Disease

What is infantile Refsum disease?

Infantile Refsum disease (IRD) is one of a small group of genetic diseases called peroxisome biogenesis disorders (PBD), which are part of a larger group of diseases called the leukodystrophies. These are inherited conditions that damage the white matter of the brain and affect motor movements. IRD is the mildest of the PBDs; Zellweger syndrome, neonatal adrenoleukodystrophy, and rhizomelic chondrodysplasia have similar, but more severe, symptoms. The PBDs are caused by defects in the genes that are associated with the breakdown of phytanic acid, a substance commonly found in foods. As a result, toxic levels of phytanic acid build up in the brain, blood, and other tissues. Symptoms of IRD begin in infancy with a visual impairment called retinitis pigmentosa, which often leads to blindness, and hearing problems that usually progress to deafness by early childhood. Other symptoms may include rapid, jerky eye movements (nystagmus); floppy muscle tone (hypotonia) and lack of muscle coordination (ataxia); mental and growth retardation; mild abnormalities in the form and structure of the face (dysmorphia); enlargement of the liver (hepatomegaly); and low cholesterol (hypocholesterolemia). Although adult Refsum disease and IRD have similar names, they are separate disorders caused by different biomechanisms involved in the breakdown of phytanic acid.

Is there any treatment?

The primary treatment for IRD is to avoid foods that contain phytanic acid, including dairy products; beef and lamb; and fatty fish such as tuna, cod, and haddock. Some infants and children may also require plasma exchange (plasmapheresis) in which blood is drawn, filtered, and reinfused back into the body, to control the buildup of phytanic acid.

What is the prognosis?

IRD is a fatal disease, but some children will survive into their teens and twenties, and possibly even beyond.

What research is being done?

The National Institute of Neurological Disorders and Stroke (NINDS) conducts research related to IRD in its laboratories at the National Institutes of Health (NIH), and also supports additional research through grants to major medical institutions across the country. Research is focused on finding better ways to prevent, treat, and ultimately cure disorders such as the PBDs.

Krabbe Disease

What is Krabbe disease?

Krabbe disease is a rare, inherited degenerative disorder of the central and peripheral nervous systems. It is characterized by the presence of globoid cells (cells that have more than one nucleus), the breakdown of the nerve's protective myelin coating, and destruction of brain cells. Krabbe disease is one of a group of genetic disorders called the leukodystrophies. These disorders impair the growth or development of the myelin sheath, the fatty covering that acts as an insulator around nerve fibers, and cause severe degeneration of mental and motor skills. Myelin, which lends its color to the "white matter" of the brain, is a complex substance made up of at least ten different enzymes. Each of the leukodystrophies affects one (and only one) of these substances. Krabbe disease is caused by a deficiency of galactocerebrosidase, an essential enzyme for myelin metabolism. The disease most often affects infants, with onset before age six months, but can occur in adolescence or adulthood. Symptoms include irritability, unexplained fever, limb stiffness, seizures, feeding difficulties, vomiting, and slowing of mental and motor development. Other symptoms include muscle weakness, spasticity, deafness, and blindness.

Is there any treatment?

There is no cure for Krabbe disease. Results of a very small clinical trial of patients with infantile Krabbe disease found that children who received umbilical cord blood stem cells from unrelated donors prior to symptom onset developed with little neurological impairment. Results also showed that disease progression stabilized faster in patients who receive cord blood compared to those who receive adult bone marrow. Bone marrow transplantation has been shown to benefit mild cases early in the course of the disease. Generally, treatment for the disorder is symptomatic and supportive. Physical therapy may help maintain or increase muscle tone and circulation.

What is the prognosis?

Infantile Krabbe disease is generally fatal before age two. Prognosis may be significantly better for children who receive umbilical cord blood stem cells prior to disease onset or early bone marrow transplantation. Persons with juvenile- or adult-onset cases of Krabbe disease generally have a milder course of the disease and live significantly longer.

What research is being done?

The National Institute of Neurological Disorders and Stroke (NINDS), a part of the National Institutes of Health (NIH), conducts research on the lipid storage diseases in laboratories at the NIH and also supports additional research through grants to major medical institutions across the country.

Metachromatic Leukodystrophy

What is metachromatic leukodystrophy?

Metachromatic leukodystrophy (MLD) is one of a group of genetic disorders called the leukodystrophies. These diseases impair the growth or development of the myelin sheath, the fatty covering that acts as an insulator around nerve fibers. Myelin, which lends its color to the white matter of the brain, is a complex substance made up of at least ten different enzymes. The leukodystrophies are caused by genetic defects in how myelin produces or metabolizes these enzymes. Each of the leukodystrophies is the result of a defect in the gene that controls one (and only one) of the enzymes. MLD is caused by a deficiency of the enzyme arylsulfatase A. MLD is one of several lipid storage diseases, which result in the toxic buildup of fatty materials (lipids) in cells in the nervous system, liver, and kidneys. There are three forms of MLD: late infantile, juvenile, and adult. In the late infantile form, which is the most common MLD, affected children have difficulty walking after the first year of life. Symptoms include muscle wasting and weakness, muscle rigidity, developmental delays, progressive loss of vision leading to blindness, convulsions, impaired swallowing, paralysis, and dementia. Children may become comatose. Most children with this form of MLD die by age five. Children with the juvenile form of MLD (between three and ten years of age) usually begin with impaired school performance, mental deterioration, and dementia and then develop symptoms similar to the infantile form but with slower progression. The adult form commonly begins after age sixteen as a psychiatric disorder or progressive dementia. Adult-onset MLD progresses more slowly than the infantile form.

Is there any treatment?

There is no cure for MLD. Bone marrow transplantation may delay progression of the disease in some cases. Other treatment is symptomatic and supportive.

What is the prognosis?

The prognosis for MLD is poor. Most children with the infantile form die by age five. The progression of symptoms in the juvenile and adult forms is slower and those affected may live a decade or more following diagnosis.

What research is being done?

The National Institute of Neurological Disorders and Stroke (NINDS), a part of the National Institutes of Health (NIH), conducts research on the lipid storage diseases in laboratories at the NIH and also supports additional research through grants to major medical institutions across the country.

Pelizaeus-Merzbacher Disease

What is Pelizaeus-Merzbacher disease?

Pelizaeus-Merzbacher disease (PMD) is a rare, progressive, degenerative central nervous system disorder in which coordination, motor abilities, and intellectual function deteriorate. The disease is one of a group of gene-linked disorders known as the leukodystrophies, which affect growth of the myelin sheath—the fatty covering that wraps around and protects nerve fibers in the brain. The disease is caused by a mutation in the gene that controls the production of a myelin protein called proteolipid protein-1 (PLP1). PMD is inherited as an X-linked recessive trait; the affected individuals are male and the mothers are carriers of the PLP1 mutation. Severity and onset of the disease ranges widely, depending on the type of PLP1 mutation. PMD is one of a spectrum of diseases associated with PLP1, which also includes spastic paraplegia type 2 (SPG2). The PLP1-related disorders span a continuum of neurologic symptoms that range from severe central nervous system involvement (PMD) to progressive weakness and stiffness of the legs (SPG2).

There are four general classifications within this spectrum of diseases. In order of severity, they are:

- connatal PMD, which is the most severe type and involves delayed mental and physical development and severe neurological symptoms;

- classic PMD, in which the early symptoms include muscle weakness, involuntary movements of the eyes (nystagmus), and delays in motor development within the first year of life;

- complicated SPG2, which features motor development issues and brain involvement; and

- pure SPG2, which includes cases of PMD that do not have neurologic complications.

Noticeable changes in the extent of myelination can be detected by magnetic resonance imaging (MRI) analyses of the brain. Additional symptoms of PMD may include slow growth, tremor, failure to develop normal control of head movement, and deteriorating speech and mental function.

Is there any treatment?

There is no cure for Pelizaeus-Merzbacher disease, nor is there a standard course of treatment. Treatment is symptomatic and supportive and may include medication for movement disorders.

What is the prognosis?

The prognosis for those with the severe forms of Pelizaeus-Merzbacher disease is poor, with progressive deterioration until death. On the other end of the disease spectrum, individuals with the mild form, in which spastic paraplegia is the chief symptom, may have nearly normal activity and life span.

What research is being done?

NINDS supports research on gene-linked disorders, including the leukodystrophies. The goals of this research are to increase scientific understanding of these disorders and to find ways to prevent, treat, and ultimately cure them.

Zellweger Syndrome

What is Zellweger syndrome?

Zellweger syndrome is one of a group of four related diseases called peroxisome biogenesis disorders (PBD), which are part of a larger group of diseases known as the leukodystrophies. These are inherited conditions that damage the white matter of the brain and also affect how the body metabolizes particular substances in the blood and organ tissues. Zellweger syndrome is the most severe of the PBDs. Infantile Refsum disease (IRD) is the mildest, and neonatal adrenoleukodystrophy and rhizomelic chondrodysplasia have similar but less severe symptoms. The PBDs are caused by defects in genes that are active in brain development and the formation of myelin, the whitish substance found in the cerebral cortex area of the brain. After birth, defects in the same genes reduce or eliminate the presence of peroxisomes—cell structures that break down toxic substances in the cells of the liver, kidneys, and brain. As a result, in Zellweger syndrome, high levels of iron and copper build up in blood and tissue and cause the characteristic symptoms of the disease. These symptoms include an enlarged liver; facial deformities such as a high forehead, underdeveloped eyebrow ridges, and deformed ear lobes; and neurological abnormalities, such as mental retardation and seizures. Infants with Zellweger syndrome also lack muscle tone, sometimes to the point of being unable to move, and may not be able to suck or swallow. Some babies will be born with glaucoma, retinal degeneration, and impaired hearing. Jaundice and gastrointestinal bleeding may also occur.

Is there any treatment?

There is no cure for Zellweger syndrome, nor is there a standard course of treatment. Since the metabolic and neurological abnormalities that cause the symptoms of Zellweger syndrome are caused during fetal development, treatments to correct these abnormalities after birth are limited. Most treatments are symptomatic and supportive.

What is the prognosis?

The prognosis for infants with Zellweger syndrome is poor. Most infants do not survive past the first six months, and usually succumb to respiratory distress, gastrointestinal bleeding, or liver failure.

What research is being done?

The National Institute of Neurological Disorders and Stroke (NINDS), and other institutes of the National Institutes of Health (NIH), conduct research exploring the molecular and genetic basis of Zellweger syndrome and the other PBDs in laboratories at the NIH, and also support additional research through grants to major medical institutions across the country. Much of this research focuses on finding better ways to prevent, treat, and ultimately cure disorders such as Zellweger syndrome.

Chapter 24

Lipid Storage Diseases

Chapter Contents

Section 24.1

Batten Disease

Excerpted from "Batten Disease Fact Sheet," National Institute
of Neurological Disorders and Stroke, National Institutes of Health,
NIH Publication No. 05-2790, July 15, 2008.

What is Batten disease?

Batten disease is a fatal, inherited disorder of the nervous system that begins in childhood. Early symptoms of this disorder usually appear between the ages of five and ten, when parents or physicians may notice a previously normal child has begun to develop vision problems or seizures. In some cases the early signs are subtle, taking the form of personality and behavior changes, slow learning, clumsiness, or stumbling. Over time, affected children suffer mental impairment, worsening seizures, and progressive loss of sight and motor skills. Eventually, children with Batten disease become blind, bedridden, and demented. Batten disease is often fatal by the late teens or twenties.

Batten disease is named after the British pediatrician who first described it in 1903. Also known as Spielmeyer-Vogt-Sjögren-Batten disease, it is the most common form of a group of disorders called neuronal ceroid lipofuscinoses (or NCLs). Although Batten disease is usually regarded as the juvenile form of NCL, some physicians use the term Batten disease to describe all forms of NCL.

What are the other forms of NCL?

There are three other main types of NCL, including two forms that begin earlier in childhood and a very rare form that strikes adults. The symptoms of these three types are similar to those caused by Batten disease, but they become apparent at different ages and progress at different rates.

Infantile NCL (Santavuori-Haltia disease) begins between about six months and two years of age and progresses rapidly. Affected children fail to thrive and have abnormally small heads (microcephaly). Also typical are short, sharp muscle contractions called myoclonic jerks. Patients usually die before age five, although some have survived in a vegetative state a few years longer.

Late infantile NCL (Jansky-Bielschowsky disease) begins between ages two and four. The typical early signs are loss of muscle coordination (ataxia) and seizures that do not respond to drugs. This form progresses rapidly and ends in death between ages eight and twelve.

Adult NCL (Kufs disease or Parry disease) generally begins before the age of forty, causes milder symptoms that progress slowly, and does not cause blindness. Although age of death is variable among affected individuals, this form does shorten life expectancy.

How many people have these disorders?

Batten disease and other forms of NCL are relatively rare, occurring in an estimated two to four of every hundred thousand live births in the United States. These disorders appear to be more common in Finland, Sweden, other parts of northern Europe, and Newfoundland, Canada. Although NCLs are classified as rare diseases, they often strike more than one person in families that carry the defective genes.

How are NCLs inherited?

Childhood NCLs are autosomal recessive disorders; that is, they occur only when a child inherits two copies of the defective gene, one from each parent. When both parents carry one defective gene, each of their children faces a one in four chance of developing NCL. At the same time, each child also faces a one in two chance of inheriting just one copy of the defective gene. Individuals who have only one defective gene are known as carriers, meaning they do not develop the disease, but they can pass the gene on to their own children. Because the mutated genes that are involved in certain forms of Batten disease are known, carrier detection is possible in some instances.

Adult NCL may be inherited as an autosomal recessive or, less often, as an autosomal dominant disorder. In autosomal dominant inheritance, all people who inherit a single copy of the disease gene develop the disease. As a result, there are no unaffected carriers of the gene.

What causes these diseases?

Symptoms of Batten disease and other NCLs are linked to a buildup of substances called lipofuscins (lipopigments) in the body's tissues. These lipopigments are made up of fats and proteins. Their name comes from the technical word *lipo*, which is short for "lipid" or fat, and from the term *pigment*, used because they take on a greenish-yellow color when viewed under an ultraviolet light microscope. The lipopigments build up in cells of the brain and the eye as well as in skin, muscle, and many other tissues. Inside the cells, these pigments form deposits with distinctive shapes that can be seen under an electron microscope. Some look like half-moons, others like fingerprints. These deposits are what doctors look for when they examine a skin sample to diagnose Batten disease.

The biochemical defects that underlie several NCLs have recently been discovered. An enzyme called palmitoyl-protein thioesterase has been shown to be insufficiently active in the infantile form of Batten disease (this condition is now referred to as CLN1). In the late infantile form (CLN2), a deficiency of an acid protease, an enzyme that hydrolyzes proteins, has been found as the cause of this condition. A mutated gene has been identified in juvenile Batten disease (CLN3), but the protein for which this gene codes has not been identified.

How are these disorders diagnosed?

Because vision loss is often an early sign, Batten disease may be first suspected during an eye exam. An eye doctor can detect a loss of cells within the eye that occurs in the three childhood forms of NCL. However, because such cell loss occurs in other eye diseases, the disorder cannot be diagnosed by this sign alone. Often an eye specialist or other physician who suspects NCL may refer the child to a neurologist, a doctor who specializes in diseases of the brain and nervous system.

In order to diagnose NCL, the neurologist needs the patient's medical history and information from various laboratory tests. Diagnostic tests used for NCLs include the following: blood or urine tests, skin or tissue sampling, electroencephalogram (EEG), electrical studies of the eyes, brain scans, measurement of enzyme activity, and deoxyribonucleic acid (DNA) analysis.

Is there any treatment?

As yet, no specific treatment is known that can halt or reverse the symptoms of Batten disease or other NCLs. However, seizures can sometimes be reduced or controlled with anticonvulsant drugs, and other medical problems can be treated appropriately as they arise.

At the same time, physical and occupational therapy may help patients retain function as long as possible.

Some reports have described a slowing of the disease in children with Batten disease who were treated with vitamins C and E and with diets low in vitamin A. However, these treatments did not prevent the fatal outcome of the disease.

Support and encouragement can help patients and families cope with the profound disability and dementia caused by NCLs. Often, support groups enable affected children, adults, and families to share common concerns and experiences.

Meanwhile, scientists pursue medical research that could someday yield an effective treatment.

What research is being done?

Within the federal government, the focal point for research on Batten disease and other neurogenetic disorders is the National Institute of Neurological Disorders and Stroke (NINDS). The NINDS, a part of the National Institutes of Health, is responsible for supporting and conducting research on the brain and central nervous system. Through the work of several scientific teams, the search for the genetic cause of NCLs is gathering speed.

Other investigators are also working to identify what substances the lipopigments contain. Although scientists know lipopigment deposits contain fats and proteins, the exact identity of the many molecules inside the deposits has been elusive for many years. Scientists have unearthed potentially important clues. For example one NINDS-supported scientist, using animal models of NCL, has found that a large portion of this built-up material is a protein called subunit c. This protein is normally found inside the cell's mitochondria, small structures that produce the energy cells need to do their jobs. Scientists are now working to understand what role this protein may play in NCL, including how this protein winds up in the wrong location and accumulates inside diseased cells. Other investigators are also examining deposits to identify the other molecules they contain.

In addition, research scientists are working with NCL animal models to improve understanding and treatment of these disorders. One research team, for example, is testing the usefulness of bone marrow transplantation in a sheep model, while other investigators are working to develop mouse models. Mouse models will make it easier for scientists to study the genetics of these diseases, since mice breed quickly and frequently.

Section 24.2

Fabry Disease

Reprinted from "NINDS Fabry Disease Information Page,"
National Institute of Neurological Disorders and Stroke (NINDS),
National Institutes of Health, February 13, 2008.

What is Fabry disease?

Fabry disease is caused by the lack of or faulty enzyme needed to metabolize lipids, fatlike substances that include oils, waxes, and fatty acids. The enzyme is known as ceramide trihexosidase, also called alpha-galactosidase-A. A mutation in the gene that controls this enzyme causes insufficient breakdown of lipids, which build up to harmful levels in the eyes, kidneys, autonomic nervous system, and cardiovascular system. Since the gene that is altered is carried on a mother's X chromosome, her sons have a 50 percent chance of inheriting the disorder and her daughters have a 50 percent chance of being a carrier. Some women who carry the genetic mutation may have symptoms of the disease. Symptoms usually begin during childhood or adolescence and include burning sensations in the hands that get worse with exercise and hot weather and small, raised reddish-purple blemishes on the skin. Some boys will also have eye manifestations, especially cloudiness of the cornea. Lipid storage may lead to impaired arterial circulation and increased risk of heart attack or stroke. The heart may also become enlarged and the kidneys may become progressively involved. Other symptoms include decreased sweating, fever, and gastrointestinal difficulties, particularly after eating. Fabry disease is one of several lipid storage disorders.

Is there any treatment?

Enzyme replacement may be effective in slowing the progression of the disease. The pain in the hands and feet usually responds to anticonvulsants such as phenytoin and carbamazepine. Gastrointestinal hyperactivity may be treated with metoclopramide. Some individuals may require dialysis or kidney transplantation.

What is the prognosis?

Patients with Fabry disease often survive into adulthood but are at increased risk of strokes, heart attack and heart disease, and renal failure.

What research is being done?

The National Institute of Neurological Disorders and Stroke (NINDS), a component of the National Institutes of Health, conducts and supports research to find ways to treat and prevent lipid storage diseases such as Fabry disease.

Section 24.3

Gaucher Disease

Excerpted from "Learning about Gaucher Disease,"
National Human Genome Research Institute, National
Institutes of Health, November 7, 2008.

What is Gaucher disease?

Gaucher disease is an autosomal recessive inherited disorder of metabolism where a type of fat (lipid) called glucocerebroside cannot be adequately degraded. Normally, the body makes an enzyme called glucocerebrosidase that breaks down and recycles glucocerebroside—a normal part of the cell membrane. People who have Gaucher disease do not make enough glucocerebrosidase. This causes the specific lipid to build up in the liver, spleen, bone marrow, and nervous system, interfering with normal functioning.

There are three recognized types of Gaucher disease and each has a wide range of symptoms. Type 1 is the most common, does not affect the nervous system, and may appear early in life or adulthood. Many people with type 1 Gaucher disease have findings that are so mild that they never have any problems from the disorder. Type 2 and 3 do affect the nervous system. Type 2 causes serious medical problems beginning in infancy, while type 3 progresses more slowly than type 2. There are also other more unusual forms that are hard to categorize within the three types.

Gaucher disease is caused by changes (mutations) in a single gene called GBA. Mutations in the GBA gene cause very low levels of glucocerebrosidase. A person who has Gaucher disease inherits a mutated copy of the GBA gene from each of his or her parents.

Gaucher disease occurs in about 1 in 50,000 to 1 in 100,000 individuals in the general population. Type 1 is found more frequently among individuals who are of Ashkenazi Jewish ancestry. Type 1 Gaucher disease is present 1 in 500 to 1 in 1,000 people of Ashkenazi Jewish ancestry, and approximately 1 in 14 Ashkenazi Jews is a carrier. Type 2 and type 3 Gaucher disease are not as common and do not occur more often in people of Ashkenazi Jewish ancestry.

What are the symptoms of Gaucher disease?

Symptoms of Gaucher disease vary greatly among those who have the disorder. The major clinical symptoms are as follows:

- Enlargement of the liver and spleen (hepatosplenomegaly)
- A low number of red blood cells (anemia)
- Easy bruising caused by a low level of platelets (thrombocytopenia)
- Bone disease (bone pain and fractures)

Other symptoms depending on the type of Gaucher disease include heart, lung, and nervous system problems.

The symptoms of type 1 Gaucher disease include bone disease, hepatosplenomegaly, anemia and thrombocytopenia, and lung disease.

The symptoms in type 2 and type 3 Gaucher disease include those of type 1 and other problems involving the nervous system such as eye problems, seizures, and brain damage. In type 2 Gaucher disease, severe medical problems begin in infancy. These individuals usually do not live beyond age two. There are also some patients with type 2 Gaucher disease that die in the newborn period, often with severe skin problems or excessive fluid accumulation (hydrops). Individuals with type 3 Gaucher disease may have symptoms before they are two years old, but often have a more slowly progressive disease process and the extent of brain involvement is quite variable. They usually have slowing of their horizontal eye movements.

How is Gaucher disease diagnosed?

The diagnosis of Gaucher disease is based on clinical symptoms and laboratory testing. A diagnosis of Gaucher disease is suspected in individuals who have bone problems, enlarged liver and spleen (hepatosplenomegaly), changes in red blood cell levels, easy bleeding and bruising from low platelets, or signs of nervous system problems.

Laboratory testing involves a blood test to measure the activity level of the enzyme glucocerebrosidase. Individuals who have Gaucher disease have very low levels of this enzyme activity. This type of testing is 90 percent accurate. A second type of laboratory test involves deoxyribonucleic acid (DNA) analysis of the GBA gene for the four most common GBA mutations as well as several more rare mutations. Both enzyme and DNA testing can be done prenatally. A bone marrow or liver biopsy is not necessary to establish the diagnosis.

When the specific gene mutation causing Gaucher disease is known in a family, DNA testing can be used to accurately identify carriers. However it is often not possible to predict the patient's clinical course based upon DNA testing.

What is the treatment for Gaucher disease?

Enzyme replacement therapy is now available as an effective treatment of individuals who have Gaucher disease. The treatment involves giving a modified form of the enzyme, glucocerebrosidase, by intravenous infusion every two weeks. Enzyme replacement therapy helps to stop progression and often reverse the symptoms of Gaucher disease, but does not affect the nervous system involvement.

A type of oral therapy that blocks the enzyme that makes the lipid is also available and clinical trials are still being conducted on this treatment.

Other treatments that may be required include: removal of the spleen (splenectomy); blood transfusions; pain medications; and joint replacement surgery.

Is Gaucher disease inherited?

Gaucher disease is inherited in families in an autosomal recessive manner. Normally, a person has two copies of the genes that provide instructions for making the enzyme glucocerebrosidase. For most individuals, both genes work properly. When one of the two genes is not functioning properly, the person is a carrier. Carriers do not have

Gaucher disease because they have one normally functioning gene that makes enough of the enzyme to carry out normal body functions. When an individual inherits an altered gene from each carrier parent, he or she has Gaucher disease.

Carrier parents have, with each pregnancy, a one in four (25 percent) chance to have a baby born with Gaucher disease; a one in two (50 percent) chance to have a child who is a carrier like themselves; and a one in four (25 percent) chance to have a child who inherits the normally functioning gene from each parent and is neither affected nor a carrier.

Section 24.4

Niemann-Pick Disease

Excerpted from "Niemann-Pick Disease," *Genetics Home Reference*, a service of the U.S. National Library of Medicine, January 2008.

What is Niemann-Pick disease?

Niemann-Pick disease is an inherited condition involving lipid metabolism, which is the breakdown, transport, and use of fats and cholesterol in the body. In people with this condition, abnormal lipid metabolism causes harmful amounts of lipids to accumulate in the spleen, liver, lungs, bone marrow, and brain.

This disorder is divided into four main types based on the genetic cause and the signs and symptoms. Niemann-Pick disease type A appears during infancy and is characterized by an enlarged liver and spleen (hepatosplenomegaly), failure to gain weight and grow at the expected rate (failure to thrive), and progressive deterioration of the nervous system. Due to the involvement of the nervous system, Niemann-Pick disease type A is also known as the neurological type. Children affected by this condition generally do not survive past early childhood.

Niemann-Pick disease type B has a range of features that may include hepatosplenomegaly, growth retardation, and problems with lung function including frequent lung infections. Other signs include blood abnormalities such as elevated levels of cholesterol and other lipids (fats), and decreased numbers of blood cells involved in clotting (platelets). Niemann-Pick disease type B is also known as the non-neurological type because the nervous system is not usually affected. People with Niemann-Pick disease type B usually survive into adulthood.

Niemann-Pick disease type C usually appears in childhood, although infant and adult onsets are possible. Signs of Niemann-Pick disease type C include severe liver disease, breathing difficulties, developmental delay, seizures, poor muscle tone (dystonia), lack of coordination, problems with feeding, and an inability to move the eyes vertically. People with this disorder can survive into adulthood. Niemann-Pick disease type C is further subdivided into types C1 and C2, each caused by a different gene mutation.

How common is Niemann-Pick disease?

Niemann-Pick disease type A occurs more frequently among individuals of Ashkenazi (eastern and central European) Jewish descent than in the general population. The incidence within the Ashkenazi population is approximately 1 in 40,000.

The incidence of both Niemann-Pick disease types A and B in all other populations is estimated to be 1 in 250,000.

The incidence of Niemann-Pick disease type C is estimated to be 1 in 150,000. The disease occurs more frequently in people of French-Acadian descent in Nova Scotia. The French-Acadians were previously designated as having Niemann-Pick disease type D. This term is no longer used since it was shown that affected people have mutations in the gene associated with Niemann-Pick disease type C1.

What genes are related to Niemann-Pick disease?

Mutations in the NPC1, NPC2, and SMPD1 genes cause Niemann-Pick disease.

Mutations in the SMPD1 gene cause Niemann-Pick disease types A and B. This gene provides instructions for producing an enzyme called acid sphingomyelinase. This enzyme is found in the lysosomes (compartments that digest and recycle materials in the cell), where it processes lipids such as sphingomyelin. Mutations in this gene lead to a deficiency of acid sphingomyelinase and the accumulation of sphingomyelin, cholesterol, and other kinds of lipids within the cells and tissues of affected individuals.

Mutations in either the NPC1 or NPC2 gene cause Niemann-Pick disease type C. The NPC1 gene provides instructions for producing a protein that is involved in the movement of cholesterol and lipids within cells. A deficiency of this protein leads to the abnormal storage of lipids within cells as seen in people with Niemann-Pick disease type C1. The NPC2 gene provides instructions to produce a protein that binds and transports cholesterol. Reduced or absent levels of this protein lead to the abnormal accumulation of lipids and cholesterol in the cells as seen in people with Niemann-Pick disease type C2. The exact functions of the NPC1 and NPC2 proteins are not fully understood.

How do people inherit Niemann-Pick disease?

This condition is inherited in an autosomal recessive pattern, which means both copies of the gene in each cell have mutations. The parents of an individual with an autosomal recessive condition each carry one copy of the mutated gene, but they typically do not show signs and symptoms of the condition.

Section 24.5

Sandhoff Disease

Excerpted from "Sandhoff Disease," *Genetics Home Reference*,
a service of the U.S. National Library of Medicine, September 2008.

What is Sandhoff disease?

Sandhoff disease is a rare inherited disorder that progressively destroys nerve cells (neurons) in the brain and spinal cord.

The most common and severe form of Sandhoff disease becomes apparent in infancy. Infants with this disorder typically appear normal until the age of three to six months, when their development slows and muscles used for movement weaken. Affected infants lose motor skills such as turning over, sitting, and crawling. They also develop an exaggerated startle reaction to loud noises. As the disease progresses, children with Sandhoff disease experience seizures, vision and hearing loss, mental retardation, and paralysis. An eye abnormality called a cherry-red spot, which can be identified with an eye examination, is characteristic of this disorder. Some affected children also have enlarged organs (organomegaly) or bone abnormalities. Children with the severe infantile form of Sandhoff disease usually live only into early childhood.

Other forms of Sandhoff disease are very rare. Signs and symptoms can begin in childhood, adolescence, or adulthood and are usually milder than those seen with the infantile form. Characteristic features include muscle weakness, loss of muscle coordination (ataxia) and other problems with movement, speech problems, and mental illness. These signs and symptoms vary widely among people with late-onset forms of Sandhoff disease.

How common is Sandhoff disease?

Sandhoff disease is a rare disorder; its frequency varies among populations. This condition appears to be more common in the Creole population of northern Argentina; the Metis Indians in Saskatchewan, Canada; and people from Lebanon.

265

What genes are related to Sandhoff disease?

Mutations in the HEXB gene cause Sandhoff disease. The HEXB gene provides instructions for making a protein that is part of two critical enzymes in the nervous system, beta-hexosaminidase A and beta-hexosaminidase B. These enzymes are located in lysosomes, which are structures in cells that break down toxic substances and act as recycling centers. Within lysosomes, these enzymes break down fatty substances, complex sugars, and molecules that are linked to sugars. In particular, beta-hexosaminidase A helps break down a fatty substance called GM2 ganglioside.

Mutations in the HEXB gene disrupt the activity of beta-hexosaminidase A and beta-hexosaminidase B, which prevents these enzymes from breaking down GM2 ganglioside and other molecules. As a result, these compounds can accumulate to toxic levels, particularly in neurons of the brain and spinal cord. A buildup of GM2 ganglioside leads to the progressive destruction of these neurons, which causes many of the signs and symptoms of Sandhoff disease.

Because Sandhoff disease impairs the function of lysosomal enzymes and involves the buildup of GM2 ganglioside, this condition is sometimes referred to as a lysosomal storage disorder or a GM2-gangliosidosis.

How do people inherit Sandhoff disease?

This condition is inherited in an autosomal recessive pattern, which means both copies of the gene in each cell have mutations. The parents of an individual with an autosomal recessive condition each carry one copy of the mutated gene, but they typically do not show signs and symptoms of the condition.

Section 24.6

Tay-Sachs Disease

Excerpted from "Learning about Tay-Sachs Disease," National
Human Genome Research Institute, National Institutes of Health,
May 30, 2008.

What do we know about heredity and Tay-Sachs disease?

Tay-Sachs disease (TSD) is a fatal genetic disorder, most commonly occurring in children, that results in progressive destruction of the nervous system. Tay-Sachs is caused by the absence of a vital enzyme called hexosaminidase-A (Hex-A). Without Hex-A, a fatty substance, or lipid, called GM2 ganglioside accumulates abnormally in cells, especially in the nerve cells of the brain. This ongoing accumulation causes progressive damage to the cells.

In children, the destructive process begins in the fetus early in pregnancy. However, a baby with Tay-Sachs disease appears normal until about six months of age when its development slows. By about two years of age, most children experience recurrent seizures and diminishing mental function. The infant gradually regresses, and is eventually unable to crawl, turn over, sit, or reach out. Eventually, the child becomes blind, cognitively impaired, paralyzed, and nonresponsive. By the time a child with Tay-Sachs is three or four years old, the nervous system is so badly affected that death usually results by age five.

A much rarer form of Tay-Sachs, late-onset Tay-Sachs disease, affects adults and causes neurological and intellectual impairment. Only recently identified, the disease has not been extensively described. As for the childhood form of Tay-Sachs, there is no cure. Treatment involves managing the symptoms of the disease.

Defect in Hex-A gene causes Tay-Sachs: Tay-Sachs disease results from defects in a gene on chromosome 15 that codes for production of the enzyme Hex-A. We all have two copies of this gene. If either or both Hex-A genes are active, the body produces enough of the enzyme to prevent the abnormal buildup of the GM2 ganglioside lipid. Carriers of Tay-Sachs—people who have one copy of the inactive gene along with one copy of the active gene—are healthy. They do not have Tay-Sachs disease but they may pass on the faulty gene to their children.

Carriers have a 50 percent chance of passing on the defective gene to their children. A child who inherits one inactive gene is a Tay-Sachs carrier like the parent. If both parents are carriers and their child inherits the defective Hex-A gene from each of them, the child will have Tay-Sachs disease. When both parents are carriers of the defective Tay-Sachs gene, each child has a 25 percent chance of having Tay-Sachs disease and a 50 percent chance of being a carrier.

Eastern European (Ashkenazi) Jews at greater risk for Tay-Sachs disease: While anyone can be a carrier of Tay-Sachs, the incidence of the disease is significantly higher among people of eastern European (Ashkenazi) Jewish descent. Approximately 1 in every 27 Jews in the United States is a carrier of the Tay-Sachs disease gene. Non-Jewish French Canadians living near the St. Lawrence River and in the Cajun community of Louisiana also have a higher incidence of Tay-Sachs. For the general population, about 1 in 250 people are carriers.

There is no cure or effective treatment for Tay-Sachs disease. However, researchers are pursuing several approaches to finding a cure. Scientists are exploring enzyme replacement therapy to provide the Hex-A that is lacking in babies with Tay-Sachs. Bone marrow transplantation has been attempted also, but to date has not been successful in reversing or slowing damage to the central nervous system in babies with Tay-Sachs. Another avenue of research is gene therapy in which scientists transfer a normal gene into cells to replace an abnormal gene. This approach holds great promise for future Tay-Sachs patients.

Is there a test for Tay-Sachs disease?

A simple blood test can identify Tay-Sachs carriers. Blood samples can be analyzed by either enzyme assay or deoxyribonucleic acid (DNA) studies. The enzyme assay is a biochemical test that measures the level of Hex-A in a person's blood. Carriers have less Hex-A in their body fluid and cells than noncarriers.

DNA-based carrier testing looks for specific mutations or changes in the gene that codes for Hex-A. Since 1985, when the Hex-A gene was isolated, more than fifty different mutations in this gene have been identified. Nevertheless, some mutations are not yet known. The current tests detect about 95 percent of carriers of Ashkenazi Jewish background and about 60 percent of carriers in the general population.

If both parents are carriers, they may want to consult with a genetic counselor for help in deciding whether to conceive or whether to have a fetus tested for Tay-Sachs. Extensive carrier testing of Ashkenazi Jews has significantly reduced the number of Tay-Sachs children in this population group. Today most cases of Tay-Sachs disease occur in populations thought not to be at high risk.

Prenatal testing for Tay-Sachs can be performed around the eleventh week of pregnancy using chorionic villi sampling (CVS). This involves removing a tiny piece of the placenta. Alternatively, the fetus can be tested with amniocentesis around the sixteenth week of pregnancy. In this procedure, a needle is used to remove and test a sample of the fluid surrounding the baby.

Assisted reproductive therapy is an option for carrier couples who don't want to risk giving birth to a child with Tay-Sachs. This new technique used in conjunction with in-vitro fertilization enables parents who are Tay-Sachs carriers to give birth to healthy babies. Embryos created in-vitro are tested for Tay-Sachs genetic mutations before being implanted into the mother, allowing only healthy embryos to be selected.

Chapter 25

Mitochondrial Disease

About Mitochondrial Disease

Mitochondrial diseases result from failures of the mitochondria, specialized compartments present in every cell of the body except red blood cells. Mitochondria are responsible for creating more than 90 percent of the energy needed by the body to sustain life and support growth. When they fail, less and less energy is generated within the cell. Cell injury and even cell death follow. If this process is repeated throughout the body, whole systems begin to fail, and the life of the person in whom this is happening is severely compromised. The disease primarily affects children, but adult onset is becoming more and more common.

Diseases of the mitochondria appear to cause the most damage to cells of the brain, heart, liver, skeletal muscles, kidneys, and the endocrine and respiratory systems.

Depending on which cells are affected, symptoms may include loss of motor control, muscle weakness and pain, gastrointestinal disorders and swallowing difficulties, poor growth, cardiac disease, liver disease, diabetes, respiratory complications, seizures, visual/hearing problems, lactic acidosis, developmental delays, and susceptibility to infection.

Diagnosing Mitochondrial Disease

Mitochondrial diseases are difficult to diagnose. Referral to an appropriate research center is critical. If experienced physicians are involved, however, diagnoses can be made through a combination of clinical observations, laboratory evaluation, cerebral imaging, and muscle biopsies. Despite these advances, many cases do not receive a specific diagnosis.

Most hospitals do not have a metabolic laboratory and therefore can run only the most basic tests. However, most hospitals will send specimens to any laboratory in the country. Not all laboratory tests are required for all patients, and your physician may decide that some of these tests are not necessary. In addition, a single blood or urine lab test with normal results does not rule out a mitochondrial disease. This is true for organic acids, lactic acid, carnitine analysis, and amino acid analysis. Even muscle biopsies are not 100 percent accurate.

Initial Evaluation

Metabolic screening in blood and urine (all patients):

- Basic chemistries
- Complete blood count
- Blood lactate, pyruvate, L:P ratio
- Quantitative plasma amino acids
- Liver enzymes and ammonia
- Creatinine kinase (CPK)
- Plasma acylcarnitine analysis
- Quantitative urine organic acids

Characterize systemic involvement (all patients):

- Echocardiogram
- Ophthalmologic exam
- Brain magnetic resonance imaging (MRI)
- Electrocardiogram (EKG)
- Audiology testing

Metabolic screening in spinal fluid (patients with neurological symptoms):

- Lactate and pyruvate
- Routine studies including cell count, glucose and protein measurement
- Quantitative amino acids

Clinical neurogenetics evaluation (patients with developmental delays):

- Karyotype
- Child neurology consultation
- Fragile X test
- Genetics consultation

Treatments and Therapies

At this time, there are no cures for these disorders.

Goals of Treatment

- Alleviate symptoms
- Slow down the progression of the disease

(Note: Goals may never be met.)

Effectiveness of Treatment

- Varies from patient to patient, depending on the exact disorder and the severity of the disorder.
- As a general rule, those with mild disorders tend to respond to treatment better than those with severe disorders.
- In some circumstances, the treatment can be tailored specifically to the patient, and that treatment is effective, whereas in other circumstance, the treatment is "empiric," meaning that the treatment makes sense, but that the benefit of treatment is not obvious or proven to be effective.
- Treatment will not reverse the damage already sustained, such as brain malformations.

Benefits of Treatment and Effectiveness of Therapies Vary

- Treatment may be beneficial and noted immediately in some disorders.

- Benefit of treatment may take a few months to notice.

- Benefit of treatment may never be noticed, but the treatment may be effective in delaying or stopping the progression of the disease.

- Some patients may not benefit from therapy.

Key Points to Treatment

- Never forget there is standard treatment for some symptoms (anticonvulsant medication for epilepsy, physical therapy for motor problems, etc.).

- Dietary.

- Vitamins and supplements.

- Avoidance of stressful factors.

- Treatment must be tailored by the patient's physician to meet that patient's need. Many of these therapies are totally ineffective in some mitochondrial disorders and would be a waste of time, money, and effort. In some cases, the treatment could be dangerous.

Specific Therapies and Things to Avoid

Dietary therapy: Many patients, including young children or mentally impaired persons, have already "self-adjusted" their diet, because they know what foods their body seems to tolerate. The points below are not meant to be suggested therapies for all patients with oxidative phosphorylation (OXPHOS) disorders, and some of the points are dangerous for patients with other disorders (option 2 [below] could be lethal in pyruvate dehydrogenase deficiency, for example). Do not make any of these dietary changes without consulting a physician. A dietitian experienced in metabolic disorders may be helpful.

Avoid fasting. This is perhaps the most important part of the treatment for most people with metabolic disorders. Fasting means "not eating" and avoiding fasting means avoiding prolonged periods without a meal (even an overnight "fast" from 8 p.m. to 8 a.m. may be dangerous in some patients). This also means that some patients should not intentionally try to lose weight by decreasing their food intake. Some patients experiencing an unintended fast resulting from an illness that causes vomiting or loss of appetite (like the flu) should be hospitalized to ensure continuous nutrition (intravenous glucose, for example). In order to ensure adequate frequent nutrition, sometimes a feeding tube needs to be placed in order for the person to receive feeding at night. In some patients, awakening them in the middle of the night for a snack can also be helpful.

Small frequent meals may be better than a typical three-meal-a-day routine for some patients.

A snack before bedtime may be helpful in some patients. This snack should not be mainly "sugar," like a candy bar, JELL-O®, or sweetened cereal. It is usually best if the snack consists of a complex carbohydrate. Cornstarch is the best complex carbohydrate, but this is not very tasty. Theoretically, the best snack would be a homemade low-sugar rice pudding thickened with a lot of cornstarch. If you come up with a tasty recipe, let the United Mitochondrial Disease Foundation know. Pasta, a peanut butter sandwich, bread and butter, unsweetened cereal (oatmeal), or a sandwich are acceptable. Many patients benefit by being woken up in the middle of the night for a small meal and others clearly improve when a gastrostomy tube is placed for continuous feeds. These final two suggestions are a small price to pay for health.

There are conflicting lines of evidence regarding the use of high fat meals in patients with electron transport chain disorders:

1. In patients that seem to gain weight and thrive on a high-fat diet, it makes sense to continue the treatment. The extra fat can also be in the form of MCT (medium chain triglyceride oil), which is easier to metabolize (see point 3 below).

2. In other patients with OXPHOS disorders, reducing fat may be helpful. This includes reducing added oil, butter, and margarine, and cutting down on cheese and fatty meats. This recommendation is not meant to avoid fats altogether. A defect in OXPHOS can create an "energy backup," as the respiratory chain cannot handle the flow of electrons coming into it. This backup may result in the formation of excess free fatty acids (fats waiting to be burned), which can poison the enzyme (adenosine nucleotide translocase) that exchanges the low-energy adenosine diphosphate (ADP) located outside the mitochondria for the high-energy adenosine triphosphate (ATP) formed at complex v. If you take the approach of limiting fats, extra effort

needs to be made to increase the total carbohydrate (in the form of complex carbohydrates) in the diet.

3. In some patients (see points 1 and 2 above), adding fat in the form of medium chain triglycerides (MCT) may be helpful. Medium chain triglycerides of eight to ten carbons long are easier to metabolize (turn into energy) than the longer chain triglycerides (those with twelve to eighteen carbons) because they do not require carnitine to be transported into the mitochondria. "MCT Oil" is mainly made of eight- and ten-carbon triglycerides and this type of oil does not occur in nature, but is made from coconut oil. "MCT Oil" is made by the baby formula company Mead-Johnson. It comes in quart bottles, available by prescription and runs about $70 a quart. It can be added like oil over pasta and rice. You can cook with it, but this is a light oil and burns easily. The special rules are explained in a recipe book that you can request from the pharmacist. Depending on the situation, a patient may benefit from a few teaspoons to a few tablespoons a day. There are oils sold in health food stores called "MCT Oil" or "medium chain triglyceride oil." These are much less expensive ($25 per quart), but make sure there is a certified analysis on the label, stating that the vast majority of the oil is C-8 and C-10 (and not C-12 or higher).

Iron generates free radicals under certain conditions, which is especially bad in mitochondrial diseases because the free radicals injure mitochondrial deoxyribonucleic acid (DNA) and "poke holes" in the mitochondria, making a bad problem worse. Therefore, excess iron is theoretically harmful. In people with mitochondrial disease, there is no routine need to give supplemental iron, nor is there a reason to eat foods rich in iron, such as extra red meat, for the purpose of eating foods rich in iron. This does not mean that the person should not eat red meat, especially if they enjoy it. There is no reason to take vitamins with added iron. There is the rare instance when iron is needed, but this is not common. In addition, vitamin C enhances the absorption of iron from the intestines, and vitamin C should not be given around a meal rich in iron. This is important to remember because some experts feel that vitamin C is a good antioxidant, and also may be helpful in some disorders of OXPHOS.

Supportive therapies: Some mitochondrial disease patients may need additional supportive therapies such as physical therapy, speech therapy, or respiratory therapy. While these therapies will not reverse the disease process, they may preserve or even improve the patient's existing functioning, mobility, and strength.

Avoidance of toxins: Alcohol has been know to hasten the progression of some mitochondrial disorders. Cigarette smoke, probably due to the carbon monoxide, is known to hasten the progression of some conditions. Remember that carbon monoxide kills by inhibiting complex IV of OXPHOS—why make it worse? Cigarette smoke will make it worse.

Monosodium glutamate (MSG) has for years been known to cause migraine headaches in otherwise healthy individuals, and may trigger these events in susceptible people with mitochondrial disease. MSG is frequently added to Chinese (and other Asian) foods, and is also found in high levels in dried and canned soup. Read the label and avoid MSG if there is any sensitivity.

Vitamins and cofactors: Vitamins and cofactors are compounds that are required in order for the chemical reactions, which make energy, to run efficiently. By definition, a cofactor can be made by the body, whereas a vitamin cannot, and therefore must be eaten. For most people, a regular diet contains all the vitamins one could possibly need and their bodies can make as much of any specific cofactor that it needs. For those with mitochondrial disorders, added vitamins and cofactors may be useful. The use of supplemental vitamins and cofactors is largely unproven and their use is therefore controversial in patients with mitochondrial diseases. For disorders of OXPHOS, coenzyme Q10 is considered as a generally accepted effective therapy, although it may not ultimately be effective for an individual patient. Other treatments may be effective in one disorder but not in others. Because of the varied nature of mitochondrial diseases some therapies may be helpful in many but not in all patients and therefore cannot be considered as "proven and effective." Some treatments should only be undertaken under the specific guidance of your physician. For specific information about the controversy, as it relates to your or your child's situation, ask your physician. Most of these vitamins can be purchased from many sources, including the drugstore.

These supplemental compounds can serve two functions:

- Possibly enhance enzyme function and result in improved efficiency of energy generation

- Serve as antioxidants, which may slow the progression of the disease

Avoidance of physiologic "stress": Physiologic stress is triggered by external factors that may result in worsening the metabolic situation, which may result in temporary or sometimes permanent worsening of the condition. It is impossible to avoid all physiologic stressful conditions, so one should not attempt to do so. However, recognizing what may be stressful for patients allows one to adjust the lifestyle. Many patients and their parents have already identified these stresses, despite not knowing why the stresses were important, and avoid them.

Cold stress is extremely important. Thermal regulation (temperature control) is not always normal in people with mitochondrial diseases and exposure to cold can result in severe heat loss and trigger an energy crisis. When going out into the cold, all exposed body parts should be covered, and exposure to extreme cold should be avoided for anything more than a short period. Overbundling can be a problem too (see below).

Heat stress can be a problem in some people. This is especially true of those with an inability to sweat normally. Heat exhaustion and heat stroke may occur on hot days. It is typical for parents to describe that their child seems to "wilt" in situations like hot classrooms or direct sunlight, whereas the other children function normally. Light clothing is important. Patients should avoid direct sunlight on hot days and stay indoors if it is too warm outside. An air-conditioned environment may be needed.

Starvation—avoid fasting.

Lack of sleep may possibly be harmful.

Chapter 26

Neurofibromatosis

Learning about Neurofibromatosis

What is neurofibromatosis?

Neurofibromatosis (NF) is a genetic neurological disorder that can affect the brain, spinal cord, nerves, and skin. Tumors, or neurofibromas, grow along the body's nerves or on or underneath the skin. Scientists have classified NF into two distinct types: neurofibromatosis type 1 (NF1) and neurofibromatosis type 2 (NF2). NF1, formerly known as von Recklinghausen NF, is the more common of the types. It occurs in approximately one in four thousand births. NF2, also referred to as bilateral acoustic NF, central NF, or vestibular NF, occurs less frequently, in one in forty thousand births. Occurrences of NF1 and NF2 are present among all racial groups and affect both sexes equally. The tumors arise from changes in the nerve cells and skin cells. Tumors also may press on the body's vital areas as their size increases. NF may lead to developmental abnormalities and/or increased chances of having learning disabilities. Other forms of NF, where the symptoms are not consistent with that of NF1 or NF2, have

The first part of this chapter is reprinted from "Learning about Neurofibromatosis," National Human Genome Research Institute, National Institutes of Health, November 27, 2007. "Research in Neurofibromatosis" is reprinted from "Researchers Identify Mechanism and Possible Drug Treatment for Growth of Nerve Tumors in Neurofibromatosis," NIH News, National Institutes of Health, October 30, 2008.

been observed. A rare form of NF is schwannomatosis. However, the genetic cause of this form of NF has not been found.

What are the symptoms of neurofibromatosis?

Symptoms for neurofibromatosis type 1 include the following:

- Presence of light brown spots (café au lait) on the skin.

- Appearance of two or more neurofibromas (pea-sized bumps) that can grow either on the nerve tissue, under the skin, or on many nerve tissues

- Manifestation of freckles under the armpits or in the groin areas

- Appearance of tiny tan clumps of pigment in the iris of the eyes (Lisch nodules)

- Tumors along the optic nerve of the eye (optic glioma)

- Severe curvature of the spine (scoliosis)

- Enlargement or malformation of other bones in the skeletal system

Symptoms for NF1 vary for each individual. Those that are skin-related are often present at birth, during infancy, and by a child's tenth birthday. From ages ten to fifteen, neurofibromas may become apparent. Symptoms such as café au lait spots, freckling, and Lisch nodules pose minimal or no health risk to a person. Though neurofibromas are generally a cosmetic concern for those with NF1, they can sometimes be psychologically distressing. For 15 percent of individuals with NF1, the symptoms can be severely debilitating. Neurofibromas can grow inside the body and may affect organ systems. Hormonal changes at puberty and/or even pregnancy may increase the size of neurofibromas. Nearly 50 percent of children with NF1 have speech problems, learning disabilities, seizures, and hyperactivity. Less than 1 percent of those affected with NF1 may have malignant tumors and may require treatment.

Symptoms for neurofibromatosis type 2 include the following:

- Tumors along the eighth cranial nerve (schwannomas)

- Meningiomas and other brain tumors

- Ringing noises inside the ear (tinnitus), hearing loss, and/or deafness

- Cataracts at a young age
- Spinal tumors
- Balance problems
- Wasting of muscles (atrophy)

Individuals with NF2 develop tumors that grow on the eighth cranial nerves and on the vestibular nerves. These tumors often cause pressure on the acoustic nerves, which result in hearing loss. Hearing loss may begin as early as an individual's teenage years. Tinnitus, dizziness, facial numbness, balance problems, and chronic headaches may also surface during the teenage years. Numbness may also occur in other parts of the body, due to spinal cord tumors.

The rare form of NF, schwannomatosis, which was recently identified, does not develop on the eighth cranial nerves, and does not cause hearing loss. It causes pain primarily, and in any part of the body. Though schwannomatosis may also lead to numbness, weakness, or balance problems like NF1 or NF2, the symptoms are less severe.

How is neurofibromatosis diagnosed?

Neurofibromatosis is diagnosed from a combination of findings. For children to be diagnosed with NF1, they must show at least two of the aforementioned symptoms associated with NF1. A physical examination by a doctor familiar with the disorder is usually performed. Doctors may use special lamps to examine the skin for café au lait spots. Doctors may also rely on magnetic resonance imaging (MRI), x-rays, computed tomography (CT scan), and blood tests to detect defects in the NF1 gene.

For NF2, doctors will pay close attention to hearing loss. Hearing tests as well as imaging tests are used to look for tumors in and around the auditory nerves, the spinal cord, or the brain. Audiometry and brainstem auditory evoked response tests can help determine whether the eighth cranial nerve is functioning properly. Family history of NF2 is also a key focal area for diagnosis.

Genetic testing is also used to diagnose NF1 and NF2. Testing conducted before birth (prenatal) is helpful to identify individuals who have a family history of the disorder, but do not yet have the symptoms. Still, gene tests have no way of predicting the severity of NF1 or NF2. Genetic testing is performed by either direct gene mutation analysis and/or linkage analysis. Mutation analysis looks to identify the particular gene changes that cause NF. A linkage analysis is useful if the mutation analysis does not provide enough conclusive information. With a linkage analysis, blood tests from multiple family members are taken to track the chromosome that carry the disease-causing gene through two or more generations. Linkage testing is around 90 percent accurate in determining whether individuals have NF. Mutation analysis is 95 percent accurate in finding a mutation for NF1, and 65 percent accurate for NF2.

How is neurofibromatosis treated?

Though there is no cure for either NF1 or NF2, there are ways to treat the effects the disease. Surgery may be helpful in removing tumors, though there is a risk of the tumors regenerating. For optic gliomas, treatment may include surgery and/or radiation. For scoliosis, treatment may include surgery or back braces. For symptoms associated with NF2, surgery may be a viable option, however not without complications that could result in additional loss of hearing or deafness. Hearing aids are ineffective when parts of the auditory nerve are removed. A breakthrough in treatment became available recently to NF2 patients, when the Food and Drug Administration approved an auditory brainstem implant for those who have parts of their auditory nerve removed and have suffered from subsequent hearing loss. The implant transmits sound signals to the brain directly and allows people to hear certain sounds and speech. Radiation treatment may also help relieve symptoms associated with NF2.

What do we know about heredity and neurofibromatosis?

Neurofibromatosis can either be an inherited disorder or the product of a gene mutation. Both NF1 and NF2 are caused by two separate abnormal genes and may be inherited from parents who have NF or may be the result of a mutation in the sperm or egg cells. NF is considered an autosomal dominant disorder because the gene is located on one of the twenty-two chromosome pairs, called autosomes. The gene for NF1 is located on chromosome 17. The gene for NF2 is located on chromosome 22. Children have a 50 percent chance of inheriting the genes that cause NF if the parent has NF. The type of NF the child inherits will be the same as that of the parent. Therefore, if the parent has NF1, there will be a 50 percent chance the child will have NF1. If the parent has NF2, there will be a 50 percent chance the child will have NF2. The only difference between the child and the parent in these circumstances is the severity of NF and the appearance of symptoms. The presence of only one changed or affected gene can cause the disorder to appear. However, the action of the unaffected gene that is paired with the dominant gene does not prevent the disorder from appearing. People with NF can make two different kinds of reproductive cells: one that can cause a child to have NF and the other that will produce an unaffected child, if that is the gene that happens to be used. When an unaffected individual conceives a child with a person with NF, there are four possible cell combinations—two combinations that will yield a child with NF and the other two that will yield an unaffected child.

Research in Neurofibromatosis

Researchers studying neurofibromatosis type 1—a rare disease in which tumors grow within nerves—have found that the tumors are triggered by crosstalk between cells in the nerves and cells in the blood. The researchers, who were funded by the National Institutes of Health (NIH) and the Department of Defense (DOD), also found that a drug on the market for treating certain kinds of blood cancer curbs tumor growth in a mouse model of neurofibromatosis type 1. A clinical trial of the drug is underway in people with the disease.

The results of the study on mice were published in the October 31, 2008, issue of *Cell*.

The study's senior investigators were Luis F. Parada, Ph.D., a neuroscientist at the University of Texas Southwestern Medical Center in Dallas, and D. Wade Clapp, M.D., a hematologist at the Indiana University School of Medicine in Indianapolis. Their research was supported by NIH's National Institute of Neurological Disorders and Stroke (NINDS), NIH's National Cancer Institute (NCI), and the Neurofibromatosis Research Program of the U.S. Army Medical Research and Material Command.

"By taking a team approach and combining their unique areas of expertise, Drs. Parada and Clapp were able to shed light on a complicated disease mechanism and to develop a potential treatment," says Jane Fountain, Ph.D., a program director with NINDS.

Neurofibromatosis type 1 is a genetic disease that affects about 1 in 3,500 Americans. The nerve-associated tumors, or neurofibromas, that occur in the disease tend to grow just under the skin or at the nerve root. The latter type of tumor, called a plexiform neurofibroma, can cause disabling symptoms by compressing the nerve, the spinal cord, bones, muscles, and internal organs.

The tumor forming cells within a neurofibroma may become malignant and spread to other parts of the body. There is currently no treatment to prevent neurofibroma growth.

In 1990, NIH-funded investigators discovered that neurofibromatosis type 1 is caused by loss-of-function mutations in a tumor suppressor gene, now known as NF1. People with the disease have the genetic makeup NF1+/-, meaning they have one functional copy of the gene and one nonfunctional or mutant copy.

Still, for many years the trigger for neurofibroma growth has been a mystery. Schwann cells, which form a protective sheath around nerve fibers, were a prime suspect. However, neurofibromas also contain nerve fibers themselves, connective tissue, and mast cells, the latter of which circulate in the blood and contribute to inflammation.

Combined with previous findings, the new study suggests that the formation of plexiform neurofibromas requires two steps: complete loss of NF1 in Schwann cells (rendering them NF1 -/-) and an interaction between NF1 -/- Schwann cells and NF1+/- mast cells. While Schwann cells appear to be the primary tumor-causing cell, mast cells appear to stimulate tumor growth by recruiting other cell types and blood vessels to the tumor.

"The mast cell inflammatory response appears to be co-opted by the tumor to enhance tumor growth," says Dr. Parada.

The researchers uncovered the role of mast cells in tumor growth through a series of technically challenging experiments. Previously, Dr. Parada had shown that mice with a targeted deletion of the NF1 gene in their Schwann cells and an NF1+/- genetic background develop plexiform neurofibromas, while mice with the same targeted deletion and an NF1+/+ genetic background do not develop the tumors. Drs. Parada and Clapp now show that in these non-tumorigenic mice, it is possible to induce plexiform neurofibromas by transplantation of NF1+/- bone marrow (which contains mast cells and other blood cells).

The researchers also examined the role of c-kit, a molecule that is expressed by mast cells and other cell types, and is known to become overactive in some kinds of cancer. When c-kit was genetically deleted in NF1+/- bone marrow cells prior to transplantation, the transplanted cells failed to induce neurofibromas. Meanwhile, in mice that were prone to develop neurofibromas, the cancer drug Gleevec®—an inhibitor of c-kit—reduced the metabolic activity and size of the tumors.

Because Gleevec is already prescribed for chronic myelogenous leukemia and other cancers, the researchers were able to secure fast regulatory approval for a phase 2 clinical trial of the drug in children and adults with neurofibromatosis type 1.

In their report, the researchers also discuss the compassionate use of Gleevec in one young neurofibromatosis patient with an airway-compressing plexiform neurofibroma. This patient was not considered an ideal candidate for surgery given the location of the tumor and its vascular nature. A three-month administration of the drug was effective in significantly shrinking the tumor without any observed side effects.

"The results in this one patient are encouraging, but future research is critical to determine any long-term benefits and risks in the majority of patients," Dr. Fountain says.

The researchers say that the complex origin of tumors in neurofibromatosis—which has thwarted therapeutic development until now—could be the chink in the disease's armor. In patients with leukemia, Gleevec directly targets the cancer-causing cells, which can become genetically resistant to the drug over time and render it ineffective.

"In patients with neurofibromatosis type 1, we are using the drug to target a non-tumorigenic cell, so we believe we are less likely to see drug resistance," Dr. Clapp says.

Chapter 27

Neuromuscular Disorders

Chapter Contents

Section 27.1

Charcot-Marie-Tooth Disease

Reprinted from "Charcot-Marie-Tooth Disease Fact Sheet,"
National Institute of Neurological Disorders and Stroke, National
Institutes of Health, NIH Publication No. 07-4897, December 11, 2007.

What is Charcot-Marie-Tooth disease?

Charcot-Marie-Tooth disease (CMT) is one of the most common inherited neurological disorders, affecting approximately 1 in 2,500 people in the United States. The disease is named for the three physicians who first identified it in 1886—Jean-Martin Charcot and Pierre Marie in Paris, France, and Howard Henry Tooth in Cambridge, England. CMT, also known as hereditary motor and sensory neuropathy (HMSN) or peroneal muscular atrophy, comprises a group of disorders that affect peripheral nerves. The peripheral nerves lie outside the brain and spinal cord and supply the muscles and sensory organs in the limbs. Disorders that affect the peripheral nerves are called peripheral neuropathies.

What are the symptoms of Charcot-Marie-Tooth disease?

The neuropathy of CMT affects both motor and sensory nerves. A typical feature includes weakness of the foot and lower leg muscles, which may result in foot drop and a high-stepped gait with frequent tripping or falls. Foot deformities, such as high arches and hammertoes (a condition in which the middle joint of a toe bends upwards) are also characteristic due to weakness of the small muscles in the feet. In addition, the lower legs may take on an "inverted champagne bottle" appearance due to the loss of muscle bulk. Later in the disease, weakness and muscle atrophy may occur in the hands, resulting in difficulty with fine motor skills.

Onset of symptoms is most often in adolescence or early adulthood, however presentation may be delayed until mid-adulthood. The severity of symptoms is quite variable in different patients and even among family members with the disease. Progression of symptoms is gradual. Pain can range from mild to severe, and some patients may need to rely on foot or leg braces or other orthopedic devices to maintain mobility. Although in rare cases patients may have respiratory muscle weakness, CMT is not considered a fatal disease and people with most forms of CMT have a normal life expectancy.

What are the types of Charcot-Marie-Tooth disease?

There are many forms of CMT disease, including CMT1, CMT2, CMT3, CMT4, and CMTX.

CMT1, caused by abnormalities in the myelin sheath, has three main types. CMT1A is an autosomal dominant disease resulting from a duplication of the gene on chromosome 17 that carries the instructions for producing the peripheral myelin protein-22 (PMP-22). The PMP-22 protein is a critical component of the myelin sheath. An overabundance of this gene causes the structure and function of the myelin sheath to be abnormal. Patients experience weakness and atrophy of the muscles of the lower legs beginning in adolescence; later they experience hand weakness and sensory loss. Interestingly, a different neuropathy distinct from CMT1A called hereditary neuropathy with predisposition to pressure palsy (HNPP) is caused by a deletion of one of the PMP-22 genes. In this case, abnormally low levels of the PMP-22 gene result in episodic, recurrent demyelinating neuropathy. CMT1B is an autosomal dominant disease caused by mutations in the gene that carries the instructions for manufacturing the myelin protein zero (P0), which is another critical component of the myelin sheath. Most of these mutations are point mutations, meaning a mistake occurs in only one letter of the DNA genetic code. To date, scientists have identified more than 30 different point mutations in the P0 gene. As a result of abnormalities in P0, CMT1B produces symptoms similar to those found in CMT1A. The gene defect that causes CMT1C, which also has symptoms similar to those found in CMT1A, has not yet been identified.

CMT2 results from abnormalities in the axon of the peripheral nerve cell rather than the myelin sheath. There are many subtypes of CMT2, designated by the letters from A to L. Each subtype is characterized by the mode of inheritance and associated clinical features. The genetic loci have been identified for some subtypes. Recently, a mutation was identified in the gene that codes for the kinesin family member 1B-beta protein in families with CMT2A. Kinesins are proteins that act as motors to help power the transport of materials along the train tracks (microtubules) of the cell. Another recent finding is a mutation in the neurofilament-light gene, identified in a Russian family with CMT2E. Neurofilaments are structural proteins that help maintain the normal shape of a cell.

CMT3 or Dejerine-Sottas disease is a severe demyelinating neuropathy that begins in infancy. Infants have severe muscle atrophy, weakness, and sensory problems. This rare disorder can be caused by a specific point mutation in the P0 gene or a point mutation in the PMP-22 gene.

CMT4 comprises several different subtypes of autosomal recessive demyelinating motor and sensory neuropathies. Each neuropathy subtype is caused by a different genetic mutation, may affect a particular ethnic population, and produces distinct physiologic or clinical characteristics. Patients with CMT4 generally develop symptoms of leg weakness in childhood and by adolescence they may not be able to walk. The gene abnormalities responsible for CMT4 have yet to be identified.

CMTX is an X-linked dominant disease and is caused by a point mutation in the connexin-32 gene on the X chromosome. The connexin-32 protein is expressed in Schwann cells—cells that wrap around nerve axons, making up a single segment of the myelin sheath. This protein may be involved in Schwann cell communication with the axon. Males who inherit one mutated gene from their mothers show moderate to severe symptoms of the disease beginning in late childhood or adolescence (the Y chromosome that males inherit from their fathers does not have the connexin-32 gene). Females who inherit one mutated gene from one parent and one normal gene from the other parent may develop mild symptoms in adolescence or later or may not develop symptoms of the disease at all.

What causes Charcot-Marie-Tooth disease?

A nerve cell communicates information to distant targets by sending electrical signals down a long, thin part of the cell called the axon. In order to increase the speed at which these electrical signals travel, the axon is insulated by myelin, which is produced by another type of cell called the Schwann cell. Myelin twists around the axon like a jellyroll cake and prevents dissipation of the electrical signals. Without an intact axon and myelin sheath, peripheral nerve cells are unable to activate target muscles or relay sensory information from the limbs back to the brain.

CMT is caused by mutations in genes that produce proteins involved in the structure and function of either the peripheral nerve axon or the myelin sheath. Although different proteins are abnormal in different forms of CMT disease, all of the mutations affect the normal function of the peripheral nerves. Consequently, these nerves slowly degenerate and lose the ability to communicate with their distant targets. The degeneration of motor nerves results in muscle weakness and atrophy in the extremities (arms, legs, hands, or feet), and in some cases the degeneration of sensory nerves results in a reduced ability to feel heat, cold, and pain.

The gene mutations in CMT disease are usually inherited. Each of us normally possesses two copies of every gene, one inherited from each parent. Some forms of CMT are inherited in an autosomal dominant fashion, which means that only one copy of the abnormal gene is needed to cause the disease. Other forms of CMT are inherited in an autosomal recessive fashion, which means that both copies of the abnormal gene must be present to cause the disease. Still other forms of CMT are inherited in an X-linked fashion, which means that the abnormal gene is located on the X chromosome. The X and Y chromosomes determine an individual's sex. Individuals with two X chromosomes are female and individuals with one X and one Y chromosome are male. In rare cases the gene mutation causing CMT disease is a new mutation which occurs spontaneously in the patient's genetic material and has not been passed down through the family.

How is Charcot-Marie-Tooth disease diagnosed?

Diagnosis of CMT begins with a standard patient history, family history, and neurological examination. Patients will be asked about the nature and duration of their symptoms and whether other family members have the disease. During the neurological examination a physician will look for evidence of muscle weakness in the arms, legs, hands, and feet, decreased muscle bulk, reduced tendon reflexes, and sensory loss. Doctors look for evidence of foot deformities, such as high arches, hammertoes, inverted heel, or flat feet. Other orthopedic problems, such as mild scoliosis or hip dysplasia, may also be present. A specific sign that may be found in patients with CMT1 is nerve enlargement that may be felt or even seen through the skin. These enlarged nerves, called hypertrophic nerves, are caused by abnormally thickened myelin sheaths.

If CMT is suspected, the physician may order electrodiagnostic tests for the patient. This testing consists of two parts: nerve conduction studies and electromyography (EMG). During nerve conduction studies, electrodes are placed on the skin over a peripheral motor or sensory nerve. These electrodes produce a small electric shock that may cause mild discomfort. This electrical impulse stimulates sensory and motor nerves and provides quantifiable information that the doctor can use to arrive at a diagnosis. EMG involves inserting a needle electrode through the skin to measure the bioelectrical activity of muscles. Specific abnormalities in the readings signify axon degeneration. EMG may be useful in further characterizing the distribution and severity of peripheral nerve involvement.

If all other tests seem to suggest that a patient has CMT, a neurologist may perform a nerve biopsy to confirm the diagnosis. A nerve biopsy involves removing a small piece of peripheral nerve through an incision in the skin. This is most often done by removing a piece of the nerve that runs down the calf of the leg. The nerve is then examined under a microscope. Patients with CMT1 typically show signs of abnormal myelination. Specifically, "onion bulb" formations may be seen which represent axons surrounded by layers of demyelinating and remyelinating Schwann cells. Patients with CMT2 usually show signs of axon degeneration.

Genetic testing is available for some types of CMT and may soon be available for other types; such testing can be used to confirm a diagnosis. In addition, genetic counseling is available to parents who fear that they may pass mutant genes to their children.

How is Charcot-Marie-Tooth disease treated?

There is no cure for CMT, but physical therapy, occupational therapy, braces and other orthopedic devices, and even orthopedic surgery can help patients cope with the disabling symptoms of the disease. In addition, pain-killing drugs can be prescribed for patients who have severe pain.

Physical and occupational therapy, the preferred treatment for CMT, involves muscle strength training, muscle and ligament stretching, stamina training, and moderate aerobic exercise. Most therapists recommend a specialized treatment program designed with the approval of the patient's physician to fit individual abilities and needs. Therapists also suggest entering into a treatment program early; muscle strengthening may delay or reduce muscle atrophy, so strength training is most useful if it begins before nerve degeneration and muscle weakness progress to the point of disability.

Stretching may prevent or reduce joint deformities that result from uneven muscle pull on bones. Exercises to help build stamina or increase endurance will help prevent the fatigue that results from performing everyday activities that require strength and mobility. Moderate aerobic activity can help to maintain cardiovascular fitness and overall health. Most therapists recommend low-impact or no-impact exercises, such as biking or swimming, rather than activities such as walking or jogging, which may put stress on fragile muscles and joints.

Many CMT patients require ankle braces and other orthopedic devices to maintain everyday mobility and prevent injury. Ankle braces can help prevent ankle sprains by providing support and stability during activities such as walking or climbing stairs. High-top shoes or boots can also give the patient support for weak ankles. Thumb splints can help with hand weakness and loss of fine motor skills. Assistive devices should be used before disability sets in because the devices may prevent muscle strain and reduce muscle weakening. Some CMT patients may decide to have orthopedic surgery to reverse foot and joint deformities.

What research is being done?

The National Institute of Neurological Disorders and Stroke (NINDS) supports research on CMT and other peripheral neuropathies in an effort to learn how to better treat, prevent, and even cure these disorders. Ongoing research includes efforts to identify more of the mutant genes and proteins that cause the various disease subtypes, efforts to discover the mechanisms of nerve degeneration and muscle atrophy with the hope of developing interventions to stop or slow down these debilitating processes, and efforts to find therapies to reverse nerve degeneration and muscle atrophy.

One promising area of research involves gene therapy experiments. Research with cell cultures and animal models has shown that it is possible to deliver genes to Schwann cells and muscle. Another area of research involves the use of trophic factors or nerve growth factors, such as the hormone androgen, to prevent nerve degeneration.

Section 27.2

Early-Onset Primary Dystonia

Excerpted from "Early-Onset Primary Dystonia,"
Genetics Home Reference, a service of the U.S. National
Library of Medicine, January 2, 2009.

What is early-onset primary dystonia?

Early-onset primary dystonia is a condition characterized by progressive problems with movement, typically beginning in childhood. Dystonia is a movement disorder that involves involuntary tensing of the muscles (muscle contractions), twisting of specific body parts such as an arm or a leg, rhythmic shaking (tremors), and other uncontrolled movements. A primary dystonia is one that occurs without other neurological symptoms, such as seizures or a loss of intellectual function (dementia). Early-onset primary dystonia does not affect a person's intelligence.

On average, the signs and symptoms of early-onset primary dystonia appear around age twelve. Abnormal muscle spasms in an arm or a leg are usually the first sign. These unusual movements initially occur while a person is doing a specific action, such as writing or walking. In some affected people, dystonia later spreads to other parts of the body and may occur at rest. The abnormal movements persist throughout life, but they do not usually cause pain.

The signs and symptoms of early-onset primary dystonia vary from person to person, even among affected members of the same family. The mildest cases affect only a single part of the body, causing isolated problems such as a writer's cramp in the hand. Severe cases involve abnormal movements affecting many regions of the body.

How common is early-onset primary dystonia?

Early-onset primary dystonia is among the most common forms of childhood dystonia. This disorder occurs most frequently in people of Ashkenazi (central and eastern European) Jewish heritage, affecting one in three thousand to nine thousand people in this population.

The condition is less common among people with other backgrounds; it is estimated to affect one in ten thousand to thirty thousand non-Jewish people worldwide.

What genes are related to early-onset primary dystonia?

A particular mutation in the TOR1A gene (also known as DYT1) is responsible for most cases of early-onset primary dystonia. The TOR1A gene provides instructions for making a protein called torsinA. Although little is known about its function, this protein may help process and transport other proteins within cells. It appears to be critical for the normal development and function of nerve cells in the brain.

A mutation in the TOR1A gene alters the structure of torsinA. The altered protein's effect on the function of nerve cells in the brain is unclear. People with early-onset primary dystonia do not have a loss of nerve cells or obvious changes in the structure of the brain that would explain the abnormal muscle contractions. Instead, the altered torsinA protein may have subtle effects on the connections between nerve cells and likely disrupts chemical signaling between nerve cells that control movement. Researchers are working to determine how a change in this protein leads to the characteristic features of this disorder.

How do people inherit early-onset primary dystonia?

Mutations in the TOR1A gene are inherited in an autosomal dominant pattern, which means one of the two copies of the gene is altered in each cell. Many people who have a mutation in this gene are not affected by the disorder and may never know they have the mutation. Only 30 to 40 percent of people who inherit a TOR1A mutation will ever develop signs and symptoms of early-onset primary dystonia.

Everyone who has been diagnosed with early-onset primary dystonia has inherited a TOR1A mutation from one parent. The parent may or may not have signs and symptoms of the condition, and other family members may or may not be affected.

Section 27.3

Friedreich Ataxia

Reprinted from "Friedreich's Ataxia Fact Sheet," National Institute
of Neurological Disorders and Stroke, National Institutes of Health,
NIH Publication No. 06-87, December 11, 2007.

What is Friedreich ataxia?

Friedreich ataxia is an inherited disease that causes progressive
damage to the nervous system resulting in symptoms ranging from
gait disturbance and speech problems to heart disease. It is named
after the physician Nikolaus Friedreich, who first described the condition in the 1860s. "Ataxia," which refers to coordination problems
such as clumsy or awkward movements and unsteadiness, occurs in
many different diseases and conditions. The ataxia of Friedreich
ataxia results from the degeneration of nerve tissue in the spinal cord
and of nerves that control muscle movement in the arms and legs. The
spinal cord becomes thinner and nerve cells lose some of their myelin sheath—the insular covering on all nerve cells that helps conduct nerve impulses.

Friedreich ataxia, although rare, is the most prevalent inherited
ataxia, affecting about one in every fifty thousand people in the United
States. Males and females are affected equally.

What are the signs and symptoms?

Symptoms usually begin between the ages of five and fifteen but
can, on rare occasions, appear as early as eighteen months or as late
as fifty years of age. The first symptom to appear is usually difficulty
in walking, or gait ataxia. The ataxia gradually worsens and slowly
spreads to the arms and then the trunk. Foot deformities such as clubfoot, flexion (involuntary bending) of the toes, hammertoes, or foot
inversion (turning inward) may be early signs. Over time, muscles
begin to weaken and waste away, especially in the feet, lower legs, and
hands, and deformities develop. Other symptoms include loss of tendon reflexes, especially in the knees and ankles. There is often a

gradual loss of sensation in the extremities, which may spread to other parts of the body. Dysarthria (slowness and slurring of speech) develops, and the person is easily fatigued. Rapid, rhythmic, involuntary movements of the eye (nystagmus) are common. Most people with Friedreich ataxia develop scoliosis (a curving of the spine to one side), which, if severe, may impair breathing.

Other symptoms that may occur include chest pain, shortness of breath, and heart palpitations. These symptoms are the result of various forms of heart disease that often accompany Friedreich ataxia, such as cardiomyopathy (enlargement of the heart), myocardial fibrosis (formation of fiber-like material in the muscles of the heart), and cardiac failure. Heart rhythm abnormalities such as tachycardia (fast heart rate) and heart block (impaired conduction of cardiac impulses within the heart) are also common. About 20 percent of people with Friedreich ataxia develop carbohydrate intolerance and 10 percent develop diabetes mellitus. Some people lose hearing or eyesight.

The rate of progression varies from person to person. Generally, within ten to twenty years after the appearance of the first symptoms, the person is confined to a wheelchair, and in later stages of the disease individuals become completely incapacitated. Life expectancy may be affected, and many people with Friedreich ataxia die in adulthood from the associated heart disease, the most common cause of death. However, some people with less severe symptoms of Friedreich ataxia live much longer, sometimes into their sixties or seventies.

How is Friedreich ataxia diagnosed?

Doctors diagnose Friedreich ataxia by performing a careful clinical examination, which includes a medical history and a thorough physical examination. Tests that may be performed include the following:

- Electromyogram (EMG), which measures the electrical activity of muscle cells

- Nerve conduction studies, which measure the speed with which nerves transmit impulses

- Electrocardiogram (EKG), which gives a graphic presentation of the electrical activity or beat pattern of the heart

- Echocardiogram, which records the position and motion of the heart muscle

- Magnetic resonance imaging (MRI) or computed tomography (CT) scan, which provides a picture of the brain and spinal cord
- Spinal tap to evaluate the cerebrospinal fluid
- Blood and urine tests to check for elevated glucose levels
- Genetic testing to identify the affected gene

How is Friedreich ataxia inherited?

Friedreich ataxia is an autosomal recessive disease, which means the patient must inherit two affected genes, one from each parent, for the disease to develop. A person who has only one abnormal copy of a gene for a recessive genetic disease such as Friedreich ataxia is called a carrier. A carrier will not develop the disease but could pass the affected gene on to his or her children. If both parents are carriers of the Friedreich ataxia gene, their children will have a one in four chance of having the disease and a one in two chance of inheriting one abnormal gene that they, in turn, could pass on to their children. About one in ninety Americans of European ancestry carries one affected gene.

Humans have two copies of each gene—one inherited from the mother and one from the father. Genes are located at a specific place on each of an individual's forty-six chromosomes, which are tightly coiled chains of deoxyribonucleic acid (DNA) containing millions of chemicals called bases. These bases—adenine, thymine, cytosine, and guanine—are abbreviated A, T, C, and G. Certain bases always "pair" together (A with T; C with G), and different combinations of base pairs join in sets of three to form coded messages.

These coded messages are "recipes" for making amino acids, the building blocks of proteins. By combining in long sequences, like long phone numbers, the paired bases tell each cell how to assemble different proteins. Proteins make up cells, tissues, and specialized enzymes that our bodies need to function normally. The protein that is altered in Friedreich ataxia is called frataxin.

In 1996, an international group of scientists identified the cause of Friedreich ataxia as a defect in a gene located on chromosome 9. Because of the inherited abnormal code, a particular sequence of bases (GAA) is repeated too many times. Normally, the GAA sequence is repeated seven to twenty-two times, but in people with Friedreich ataxia it can be repeated hundreds or even over a thousand times. This type of abnormality is called a triplet repeat expansion and has been implicated as the cause of several dominantly inherited diseases.

Friedreich ataxia is the first known recessive genetic disease that is caused by a triplet repeat expansion. Although about 98 percent of Friedreich ataxia carriers have this particular genetic triplet repeat expansion, it is not found in all cases of the disease. A very small proportion of affected individuals have other gene coding defects responsible for causing disease.

The triplet repeat expansion apparently disrupts the normal assembly of amino acids into proteins, greatly reducing the amount of frataxin that is produced. Frataxin is found in the energy-producing parts of the cell called mitochondria. Research suggests that without a normal level of frataxin, certain cells in the body (especially brain, spinal cord, and muscle cells) cannot effectively produce energy and have a buildup of toxic byproducts leading to what is called "oxidative stress." This clue to the possible cause of Friedreich ataxia came after scientists conducted studies using a yeast protein with a chemical structure similar to human frataxin. They found that the shortage of this protein in the yeast cell led to a toxic buildup of iron in the cell's mitochondria. When the excess iron reacted with oxygen, free radicals were produced. Although free radicals are essential molecules in the body's metabolism, they can also destroy cells and harm the body. Research continues on this subject.

Can Friedreich ataxia be cured or treated?

As with many degenerative diseases of the nervous system, there is currently no cure or effective treatment for Friedreich ataxia. However, many of the symptoms and accompanying complications can be treated to help patients maintain optimal functioning as long as possible. Diabetes, if present, can be treated with diet and medications such as insulin, and some of the heart problems can be treated with medication as well. Orthopedic problems such as foot deformities and scoliosis can be treated with braces or surgery. Physical therapy may prolong use of the arms and legs. Scientists hope that recent advances in understanding the genetics of Friedreich ataxia may lead to breakthroughs in treatment.

What services are useful to Friedreich ataxia patients and their families?

Genetic testing is available at some specialized laboratories and can assist with clinical diagnosis, prenatal diagnosis, and carrier status determination. Genetic counselors can help explain how Friedreich ataxia is inherited and its effect on the patient and the family. Psychological counseling and support groups for people with genetic diseases may also help patients and their families cope with the disease. A patient's primary care physician can screen for complications like diabetes and scoliosis, and can refer patients to specialists such as cardiologists and physical therapists to help deal with some of the other associated problems.

What research is being done?

Within the federal government the National Institute of Neurological Disorders and Stroke (NINDS), a component of the National Institutes of Health (NIH), has primary responsibility for sponsoring research on neurological disorders. As part of this mission, the NINDS conducts research on Friedreich ataxia and other forms of inherited ataxias at its facilities at the NIH and supports additional studies at medical centers throughout the United States.

Researchers are optimistic that they will soon be closer to understanding the causes of the disease, which eventually will help scientists develop effective treatments and prevention strategies for Friedreich ataxia.

The studies using yeast proteins with a chemical structure similar to human frataxin led to further studies in mice and humans. These studies revealed that frataxin—like the yeast protein—is a mitochondrial protein that should normally be present in the nervous system, the heart, and the pancreas. Yet in patients with the disease, the amount of frataxin in affected cells of these tissues is severely reduced. Further evidence that frataxin may function similarly to the yeast protein was the finding of abnormally high levels of iron in the heart tissue of people with Friedreich ataxia. It is believed that the nervous system, heart, and pancreas may be particularly susceptible to damage from free radicals (produced when the excess iron reacts with oxygen) because once certain cells in these tissues are destroyed by free radicals they cannot be replaced. Nerve and muscle cells also have metabolic needs that may make them particularly vulnerable to free radical damage. Free radicals have been implicated in other degenerative diseases such as Parkinson and Alzheimer diseases.

Based upon this information, scientists and physicians have tried to reduce the levels of free radicals, also called oxidants, using treatment with "antioxidants." Several clinical studies in Europe suggest that antioxidants like coenzyme Q10, vitamin E, and idebenone may offer patients some limited benefit. There are currently clinical trials in the United States and Europe to evaluate the effectiveness of idebenone in patients with Friedreich ataxia. There is also a clinical trial ongoing in France to examine the efficacy of selectively removing excess iron from the mitochondria. Several other compounds may be brought to clinical trials in the near future.

Since the disease is caused by a reduction in frataxin levels, many scientists are exploring ways to increase those levels through drug treatments, genetic engineering, and protein delivery systems.

Armed with what they currently know about frataxin and Friedreich ataxia, scientists are working to better define frataxin's role, clarify how defects in iron metabolism may be involved in the disease process, and explore new therapeutic approaches for the disease. The discovery by NINDS-supported researchers of the genetic mutation that causes Friedreich ataxia has added new impetus to research efforts on this disease.

Section 27.4

Hereditary Spastic Paraplegia

What is hereditary spastic paraplegia?

Hereditary spastic paraplegia (HSP) is a group of rare, inherited neurological disorders. Their primary symptoms are progressive spasticity and weakness of the leg and hip muscles. Researchers estimate that some thirty different types of HSP exist; the genetic causes are known for eleven. The HSP incidence rate in the United States is twenty thousand people.

The condition is characterized by insidiously progressive lower extremity weakness and spasticity. HSP is classified as uncomplicated or pure if neurological impairment is limited to the lower body. HSP is classified as complicated or complex if other systems are involved or if there are other neurological findings such as seizures, dementia, amyotrophy, extrapyramidal disturbance, or peripheral neuropathy in the absence of other disorders such as diabetes mellitus.

Many different names are used for HSP. The most common are hereditary spastic paraplegia (or paraparesis), familial spastic paraparesis (or paraplegia), and Strümpell-Lorrain disease. Others are spastic paraplegia, hereditary Charcot disease, spastic spinal paralysis, diplegia spinalis progressiva, French settlement disease, Troyer syndrome, and Silver syndrome.

The disorder was first identified in the late 1800s by A. Strümpell, a neurologist in Heidelberg, Germany. He observed two brothers and their father, all of whom had gait disorders and spasticity in their legs. After the death of the brothers, Strümpell showed through autopsy the degeneration of the nerve fibers leading through the spinal cord. HSP was originally named after Strümpell, and later after two Frenchmen, Lorrain and Charcot, who provided more information.

What is (apparently sporadic) spastic paraplegia?

Many individuals with all the signs and symptoms of HSP do not appear to have similarly affected family members. Without proof of a hereditary link, some neurologists call the condition spastic paraplegia or apparently sporadic spastic paraplegia. Other clinicians may diagnosis the same condition as primary lateral sclerosis, which mimics HSP in how it affects the lower body. However, current research indicates that PLS eventually affects the arms and speech and swallowing muscles as well as the leg muscles.

There are many reasons why someone with HSP may not have a family history. Recessive and X-linked forms skip generations, which means the disorder may pass silently for generations and then suddenly appear. In addition, the age of onset, progression rate, and severity vary widely so that the disease could have gone undiagnosed in previous generations or an affected individual may have died before symptom onset. Mistaken parentage or new genetic mutations are also possible.

What are the symptoms?

The hallmark of HSP is progressive difficulty walking due to increasingly weak and stiff (spastic) muscles. Symptoms appear in most people between the second and fourth decade of life, but they can start at any age.

Initial symptoms are typically difficulty with balance, stubbing the toe, or stumbling. Changes begin so gradually that other people often notice the change first. As the disease progresses, canes, walkers, and eventually wheelchairs may become needed, although some people never require assistive devices.

Other common symptoms of HSP are urinary urgency and frequency, hyperactive reflexes, difficulty with balance, clonus, Babinski sign, diminished vibration sense in the feet, muscle spasms, and congenital foot problems such as pes cavus (high arched foot). Some people may experience problems with their arms or fine motor control of their fingers but for most people, this is not significant.

Most people with HSP have uncomplicated HSP. There are also rare, complicated forms, which have additional symptoms, such as peripheral neuropathy, ichthyosis (a skin disorder), epilepsy, ataxia, optic neuropathy, retinopathy, dementia, mental retardation, deafness, or problems with speech, swallowing, or breathing. These symptoms may have other causes though, unrelated to HSP. For example, someone with uncomplicated HSP may have peripheral neuropathy caused by diabetes.

Why are my symptoms different from others in my family?

As noted above, the severity of symptoms and age of onset can vary widely, even within the same family. One reason is that HSP is a group of genetically different disorders, not a single disorder. Some differences may be due to genetic mutations. A child may show symptoms before a parent and it's possible for some family members to have very mild symptoms while others have more severe symptoms. This may be due to other genes, environment, nutrition, general health, or factors not yet understood.

In some families, symptoms tend to start at younger ages with each generation. Although rare, HSP sometimes shows "incomplete penetrance." This means that occasionally, an individual may have the gene mutation, but for unknown reasons never develop symptoms of HSP. Such individuals can still pass HSP to their children.

How does HSP cause symptoms?

HSP is caused by degeneration of the upper motor neurons in the brain and spinal cord. Upper motor neurons control voluntary movement.

The cell bodies of these neurons are located in the motor cortex area of the brain. They have long, hair-like processes called axons that travel to the brainstem and down the spinal cord. Axons relay the messages to move to lower motor neurons that are located all along the brainstem and spinal cord. Lower motor neurons then carry the messages out to the muscles.

When upper motor neurons degenerate, the correct messages cannot reach the lower motor neurons, and the lower motor neurons cannot transmit the correct messages to the muscles. As the degeneration continues, spasticity and weakness increase. The legs are affected because degeneration occurs primarily at the ends of the longest nerves in the spinal cord, which control the legs. In some cases, the upper body can be minimally affected as well, leading to problems with the arms or speech and swallowing muscles.

How severe will my symptoms get?

There is no way to predict rate of progression or severity of symptoms. Generally, once symptoms begin, progression continues slowly throughout life. For some childhood-onset forms, symptoms become apparent, gradually worsen during childhood, and then stabilize after adolescence. HSP rarely results in complete loss of lower limb mobility.

How is HSP diagnosed?

HSP is diagnosed via a careful clinical examination, by excluding other disorders that cause spasticity and weakness in the legs, and by an observation period to see if other symptoms develop that indicate another condition, such as PLS. Disorders that can be ruled out with testing are amyotrophic lateral sclerosis (ALS), tropical spastic paraparesis (TSP), vitamin deficiencies (B_{12} or E), thoracic spine herniated disks, and spinal cord tumors or injuries and multiple sclerosis. HSP can resemble cerebral palsy, however, HSP is degenerative and thereby causes increasing spasticity and weakness of the muscles. Two other disorders with spastic paraplegia symptoms termed lathyrism and konzo are caused by toxins in the plants Lathyrus sativus and cassava.

HSP is hereditary, and examining family history is important in diagnosing HSP. However, many individuals with all the signs and symptoms of HSP do not have a family history.

What genetic testing is available?

Athena Diagnostics offers testing for five different types of HSP out of the thirty or more different forms of HSP. As more genes are discovered, it is hopeful that such information will lead to greater availability of testing.

Genetic counselors can be found at many major medical centers or by contacting the National Society of Genetic Counselors. Gene tests can be used for prenatal testing.

What is the treatment?

No treatments are currently available to prevent, stop, or reverse HSP. Treatment is focused on symptom relief, such as medication to reduce spasticity; physical therapy and exercise to help maintain flexibility, strength, and range of motion; assistive devices and communications aids; supportive therapy and other modalities.

What is the life expectancy?

Life expectancy is normal. However, complications arising from falls or immobility caused by the symptoms of HSP may inadvertently shorten a person's life.

What is the risk of getting HSP?

There are some thirty different forms of HSP, with three different modes of inheritance: autosomal dominant, autosomal recessive, and X-linked. Each mode has a different risk factor, which ranges from almost none to 50 percent.

What other conditions cause spasticity and weakness of muscles?

Muscle spasticity and weakness can also be caused by other conditions including (but not limited to) primary lateral sclerosis, spinal cord injury or tumors, cerebral palsy, multiple sclerosis, amyotrophic lateral sclerosis, vitamin absorption, and thoracic spine herniated disks.

There is a virus-caused disease called tropical spastic paraparesis and conditions called lathyrism and konzo caused by toxins in the plants Lathyrus sativus and cassava that also cause muscle spasticity and weakness.

Does stress affect symptoms?

Many people find the tightness in their muscles worsens when they are angry, stressed, or upset. This may make it more difficult to walk and speak. It is unknown exactly how emotions affect muscle tone, but it may involve adrenalin levels. Most people also report increased stiffness in cold weather.

Is depression normal?

Periods of feeling down about having HSP are normal and expected. It is not uncommon for people to also experience periods of clinical depression.

Do people with HSP experience memory loss?

Memory disturbance has been reported in some individuals with HSP due to spastin gene mutations. In general, it was mild.

Before attributing memory disturbance to HSP, it is important to consider other causes: stress, anxiety, depression, lack of sleep, medications (including baclofen), other health conditions including vitamin B_{12} deficiency.

If memory disturbance is significant, a cause of concern, or worsening, it would be important to discuss this with your primary physician and neurologist.

Are foot problems common?

Yes. Here are a few examples:

- High arched feet (pes cavus). High arches occur because there is more weakness in the foot muscles that extend the foot backward and flatten the arch than in the muscles that flex the foot downward.

- Shortened Achilles tendons. Achilles tendons are often short, and generally shorten further as HSP progresses.

- Jumping feet (clonus). Clonus is an uncontrollable, repetitive jerking of muscles that makes the foot jump rapidly up and down. It occurs when the foot is in a position that causes a disruption of the signals from the brain, leading to an automatic stretch reflex.

- Hammertoes or bunions. These may occur due to imbalances in the strength and tone of muscles that maintain proper alignment of joints in the feet.

- Cold feet and/or foot swelling. This is most likely caused by poor circulation. Normally, muscle contractions in the legs help pump blood from the legs back to the heart. If the muscles are weakened, or if the person is relatively inactive, the blood flow from the legs may be decreased, and fluids may accumulate. This can cause swelling, or a sensation of "cold feet."

Can my arms be affected?

Some people may experience problems with their arms or fine motor control of their fingers. The degeneration in nerves that supply the arms is mild compared to that which occurs in the nerves that supply the legs. For most people, this is not significant.

Can HSP affect sexual function?

The short answer appears to be "yes," although it is important to remember that sexual desire and/or function can be affected by many other factors such as age, stress, depression, fatigue, medical disorders, or medications.

Some people report that stiffness, spasms, and cramps that are part of HSP may either inhibit (or intensify) orgasm, or that orgasm may bring on leg stiffness, spasms, or clonus. Stiffness of the legs or arms may cause difficulty using certain positions for intercourse.

Is HSP an ataxia?

No. The group of disorders known as ataxias (such as Friedreich ataxia) are spinocerebellar disorders in which there is a disturbance either in the part of the brain known as the cerebellum or in the connections to it. HSP does not involve the cerebellum. Ataxias can be hereditary or sporadic.

The term "ataxia" means without coordination, and can also refer to a symptom in which there is a lack of muscle control resulting in a jerky or unsteady movement. People with HSP may have incoordination as a symptom. This does not mean they have ataxia.

Can I donate blood?

HSP cannot be passed to others through donation of blood. There is no medical reason why a person with HSP cannot donate blood.

When was HSP identified?

In the late 1800s, A. Strümpell, a neurologist in Heidelberg, Germany, described this disorder. He observed two brothers and their father, who had gait disorders and spasticity in their legs. After the death of the brothers, Strümpell was able to show through autopsy the degeneration of the nerve fibers leading through the spinal cord. The disorder was originally named after Strümpell, and after two Frenchmen who later provided more information about the disorder, Lorrain and Charcot.

Is HSP more prevalent in certain ethnic groups?

There is no evidence that HSP is more prevalent in one ethnic group than another.

Section 27.5

Muscular Dystrophy

"Muscular Dystrophy," January 2007, reprinted with permission from www.kidshealth.org. Copyright © 2007 The Nemours Foundation. This information was provided by KidsHealth, one of the largest resources online for medically reviewed information written for parents, kids, and teens. For more articles like this one, visit www.KidsHealth.org, or www.TeensHealth.org.

Aside from seeing the telethon hosted by Jerry Lewis on Labor Day weekend, many people don't know much about muscular dystrophy. Yet a quarter of a million kids and adults are living with the disease, so chances are you may know someone who has it.

What is muscular dystrophy?

Muscular dystrophy (MD) is a genetic disorder that weakens the muscles that help the body move. People with MD have incorrect or missing information in their genes, which prevents them from making the proteins they need for healthy muscles. Because MD is genetic, people are born with the problem—it's not contagious and you can't catch it from someone who has it.

MD weakens muscles over time, so children, teens, and adults who have the disease can gradually lose the ability to do the things most people take for granted, like walking or sitting up. Someone with MD might start having muscle problems as a baby or their symptoms might start later. Some people even develop MD as adults.

Several major forms of muscular dystrophy can affect people, each of which weakens different muscle groups in various ways:

- Duchenne (pronounced: due-shen) muscular dystrophy (DMD), the most common type of the disease, is caused by a problem with the gene that makes a protein called dystrophin. This protein helps muscle cells keep their shape and strength. Without it, muscles break down and a person gradually becomes weaker. DMD affects boys. Symptoms usually start between ages two and six. By age ten or twelve, kids with DMD often need to use a wheelchair. The heart may also be affected, and people with DMD need to be followed closely by a lung and heart specialist. They can also develop scoliosis (curvature of the spine) and tightness in their joints. Over time, even the muscles that control breathing get weaker, and a person might need a ventilator to breathe. People with DMD usually do not survive beyond their late teens or early adulthood.

- Becker muscular dystrophy (BMD), like DMD, affects boys. The disease is very similar to DMD, but its symptoms may start later and can be less severe. With BMD, symptoms like muscle breakdown and weakness sometimes don't begin until age ten or even in adulthood. People with BMD can also have breathing, heart, bone, muscle, and joint problems. Many people with BMD can live long, active lives without using a wheelchair. How long a person with BMD can live varies depending on the severity of any breathing and heart problems.

- Emery-Dreifuss (pronounced: em-uh-ree dry-fuss) muscular dystrophy (EDMD) typically starts causing symptoms in late childhood to early teens and sometimes as late as age twenty-five. EDMD is another form of muscular dystrophy that affects mostly boys. It involves muscles in the shoulders, upper arms, and shins, and it often causes joint problems (joints can become tighter in people with EDMD). The heart muscle may also be affected.

- Limb-girdle muscular dystrophy (LGMD) affects boys and girls equally, weakening muscles in the shoulders and upper arms and around the hips and thighs. LGMD can begin as early as childhood or as late as mid-adulthood, and it often progresses slowly.

Over time, a wheelchair might be necessary to get around. There are many different types of LGMD, each with its own specific features.

- Facioscapulohumeral (pronounced: fa-she-o-skap-you-lo-hyoo-meh-rul) muscular dystrophy (FSHD) can affect both guys and girls, and it usually begins during the teens or early adulthood. FSHD affects muscles in the face and shoulders and sometimes causes weakness in the lower legs. People with this type of MD might have trouble raising their arms, whistling, or tightly closing their eyes. How much a person with this form of muscular dystrophy is affected by the condition varies from person to person. It can be quite mild in some people.

- Myotonic (pronounced: my-uh-tah-nick) dystrophy (MMD) is a form of muscular dystrophy in which the muscles have difficulty relaxing. In teens, it can cause a number of problems, including muscle weakness and wasting (where the muscles shrink over time), cataracts, and heart problems.

- Congenital muscular dystrophy (CMD) is the term for all types of MD that show signs in babies and young children, although the MD isn't always diagnosed right away. Like other forms of MD, CMD involves muscle weakness and poor muscle tone. Occurring in both girls and boys, it can have different symptoms. It varies in how severely it affects people and how quickly or slowly it worsens. In rare cases, CMD can cause learning disabilities or mental retardation.

The life expectancy (in other words, how long a person may live) for many of these forms of muscular dystrophy depends on the degree to which a person's muscles are weakened as well as how much the heart and lungs are affected.

How do doctors diagnose MD?

In addition to doing a physical examination, the doctor will ask you about any concerns and symptoms you have, your past health, your family's health, any medications you're taking, any allergies you may have, and other issues. This is called the medical history.

Tests can help the doctor determine which type of MD a person has and rule out other diseases that affect the muscles or nerves. Some tests measure how nerves and muscles are working. Others check the blood for levels of certain enzymes, the proteins that cause chemical changes like converting food to energy. Abnormally high blood levels of certain enzymes from muscle cells are present in many people with MD.

Sometimes a muscle biopsy is needed. The doctor removes a small piece of muscle tissue and examines it under a microscope. If a person has MD, the muscle tissue will have some unusually large fibers, and some of the other fibers will show signs of breaking down. Finally, genetic testing can show if a person has Duchenne MD.

How is MD treated?

There is no cure for MD, but doctors and scientists are working hard to find one. Some scientists are trying to fix the defective genes that lead to MD so they will make the right proteins. Others are trying to make chemicals that will act like these proteins in the body. They hope that this will help the muscles to work properly in people with MD. Doctors are also dedicated to finding the best ways to treat the symptoms of MD so that kids, teens, and adults with the disease can live as comfortably and happily as possible.

People with MD can do some things to help their muscles. Certain exercises and physical therapy can help them avoid contractures, a stiffening of the muscles near the joints that can make it harder to move and can lock the joints in painful positions. Often, people with MD are fitted with special braces to ensure flexible joints and tendons (the strong, rubber band-like tissues that attach muscles to bones). Surgery is sometimes used to reduce pain and increase movement from contractures.

Because we rely on certain muscles to breathe, some people with MD need respiratory aids, such as a ventilator, to help them breathe. People with MD also might need to be treated for problems like scoliosis, which can be caused by weakened muscles or muscles that are contracting or pulling too tightly.

For some types of MD, medication can help. Guys with Duchenne MD may be helped by a medicine called prednisone, and people with myotonic MD might use phenytoin or quinine to relax muscles.

It's also important that people with heart problems caused by muscular dystrophy be monitored by a heart specialist.

What's it like for teens with MD?

Teens have different experiences depending on the type of MD. One person might have weakened shoulder muscles and not be able to raise a hand in class. Someone might be unable to smile because of weak facial muscles. Another person might have weak muscles in the pelvis or legs, making it hard to walk from class to class. In some cases, you might not even be able to tell that a teen has MD.

For teens with MD, it can be hard to come to terms with the disease, especially because it gradually gets worse. For example, when someone who walks to class must start using a wheelchair in school, it can be a difficult adjustment. Support from doctors, family, and friends can make it easier to deal with MD. Changes like wider doorways at home and school can make it easier for teens with MD to do many of the things they enjoy.

If you know someone who has MD, there's a lot you can do to offer help and support. For example, some people with MD may need help getting books out during class or rides to and from events.

Often, people with illnesses that gradually get worse over time can start to feel cut off from friends, especially as their friends may be going out and doing more things while they feel like they're becoming more housebound. Try planning activities that include a friend, brother, or sister with MD, such as playing video games or watching movies at his or her home. Your friend or sibling will always be the same person—just more limited in movement.

Section 27.6

Spinal Muscular Atrophy

Reprinted from "Learning about Spinal Muscular Atrophy,"
National Human Genome Research Institute, National
Institutes of Health, May 30, 2008.

What is spinal muscular atrophy?

Spinal muscular atrophy is a group of inherited disorders that cause progressive muscle degeneration and weakness. Spinal muscular atrophy (SMA) is the second leading cause of neuromuscular disease. It is usually inherited as an autosomal recessive trait (a person must get the defective gene from both parents to be affected).

There are several types of SMA called subtypes. Each of the subtypes is based on the severity of the disorder and the age at which symptoms begin. There are three types of SMA that affect children before the age of one year. There are two types of SMA, type IV and Finkel type, that occur in adulthood, usually after age thirty. Symptoms of adult-onset spinal muscular atrophy are usually mild to moderate and include muscle weakness, tremor, and twitching.

The prognosis for individuals with SMA varies depending on the type of SMA and the degree of respiratory function. The patient's condition tends to deteriorate over time, depending on the severity of the symptoms.

Spinal muscular atrophy affects one in six thousand to one in ten thousand people.

What are the symptoms of spinal muscular atrophy?

Three types of SMA affect children before age one year. Type 0 is the most severe form of spinal muscular atrophy and begins before birth. Usually, the first symptom of type 0 is reduced movement of the fetus that is first seen between thirty and thirty-six weeks of the pregnancy. After birth, these newborns have little movement and have difficulties with swallowing and breathing.

Type I spinal muscular atrophy (called Werdnig-Hoffmann disease) is another severe form of SMA. Symptoms of type 1 may be present

313

at birth or within the first few months of life. These infants usually have difficulty breathing and swallowing, and they are unable to sit without support.

Children with type II SMA usually develop muscle weakness between ages six and twelve months. They cannot stand or walk without help.

Type III SMA (called Kugelberg-Welander disease or juvenile type) is a milder form of SMA than types 0, I, or II. Symptoms appear between early childhood (older than age one year) and early adulthood. Individuals with type III SMA are able to stand and walk without help. They usually lose their ability to stand and walk later in life. There are two other types of spinal muscular atrophy, type IV and Finkel type, that occur in adulthood, usually after age thirty. Symptoms of adult-onset SMA are usually mild to moderate and include muscle weakness, tremor, and twitching.

How is spinal muscular atrophy diagnosed?

To make a diagnosis of SMA, symptoms need to be present. When symptoms are present, diagnosis can be made by genetic testing. Gene alterations (mutations) in the SMN1 and VAPB genes cause SMA. Having extra copies of the SMN2 gene can modify the course of SMA.

Genetic testing on a blood or tissue sample is done to identify whether there is at least one copy of the SMN1 gene by looking for its special makeup. Mutations in the SMN1 gene cause types 0, I, II, III, and IV. Some people who have SMA type II, III, or IV have three or more copies of the SMN2 gene. Having these extra copies can modify the course of SMA. The more copies of SMN2 gene a person has, the less severe his or her symptoms.

Genetic testing for a mutation in the VAPB gene is done to diagnose the Finkel type SMA.

In some situations other tests such as an electromyography (EMG) or muscle biopsy may be needed because it is not possible to conduct the SMN gene tests or no abnormality is identified.

What is the treatment for spinal muscular atrophy?

There is currently no specific cure for SMA. Infants who have a severe form of SMA frequently die of respiratory failure due to weakness of the muscles that help with breathing. Children who have milder forms of SMA will live much longer but they may need extensive medical support.

The current treatment for SMA involves prevention and management of the secondary effect of muscle weakness and loss.

Today, much can be done for SMA patients in terms of medical and in particular respiratory, nutritional, and rehabilitation care. In addition, several drugs have been identified in laboratory experiments that may help patients. Some of the drugs that are currently being investigated include: Butyrates, valproic acid, hydroxyurea, and riluzole.

At present gene therapy—replacing the altered genes with a normal version—is being tested in animals. Researchers believe that gene replacement for SMA will take many more years of research before it can be used in humans. Other approaches to developing better treatment include searching for drugs that increase SMN levels, enhance residual SMN function, or compensate for its loss.

Is spinal muscular atrophy inherited?

SMA types 0, I, II, III, and IV are inherited in an autosomal recessive pattern in families. In autosomal recessive inheritance, a person who has SMA has inherited two altered (mutated) copies of the SMN1 gene from his or her parents. The parents of an individual with an autosomal recessive inherited disorder such as SMA are carriers of one copy of the altered gene. Since they carry a normal version of the gene they do not have signs or symptoms of the disorder.

Finkel type SMA is inherited in an autosomal dominant pattern. This means that the person has one copy of the altered gene in each cell that causes the disorder.

Chapter 28

Noonan Syndrome

What is Noonan syndrome?

Noonan syndrome is a disorder that involves unusual facial characteristics, short stature, heart defects present at birth, bleeding problems, developmental delays, and malformations of the bones of the rib cage.

Noonan syndrome is caused by changes in one of several autosomal dominant genes. A person who has Noonan syndrome may have inherited an altered (mutated) gene from one of his or her parents, or the gene change may be a new change due to an error carried by the egg or sperm or occurring at conception. Alterations in three genes—PTPN11, SOS1, and KRAS—have been identified to date.

Noonan syndrome is present in about 1 in 1,000 to 1 in 2,500 people.

What are the symptoms of Noonan syndrome?

Symptoms of Noonan syndrome may include the following:

- A characteristic facial appearance

- Short stature

- Heart defect present at birth (congenital heart defect)

- A broad or webbed neck

Reprinted from "Learning about Noonan Syndrome," National Human Genome Research Institute, National Institutes of Health, November 7, 2008.

- Minor eye problems such as strabismus in up to 95 percent of individuals

- Bleeding problems such as a history of abnormal bleeding or bruising

- An unusual chest shape with widely spaced and low-set nipples

- Developmental delay of varying degrees, but usually mild

- In males, undescended testes (cryptorchidism)

How is Noonan syndrome diagnosed?

The diagnosis of Noonan syndrome is based on the person's clinical symptoms and signs. The specialist examines the person, looking for the specific features of Noonan syndrome.

Individuals who have Noonan syndrome have normal chromosome studies. Three genes—PTPN11, SOS1, and KRAS—are the only genes that are known to be associated with Noonan syndrome. About 50 percent of individuals who have Noonan syndrome are found to have gene alterations (mutations) in the PTPN11 gene. About 10 percent of individuals who have Noonan syndrome have mutations in the SOS1 gene while less than 5 percent of affected individuals have mutations in the KRAS gene. Genetic testing of all three genes is available clinically.

What is the treatment for Noonan syndrome?

Treatment for individuals who have Noonan syndrome is based on their particular symptoms. Heart problems are treated in the same way as they are for individuals in the general population. Early intervention programs are used to help with developmental disabilities, when present. Bleeding problems that can be present in Noonan syndrome may have a variety of causes and are treated according to their cause. Growth problems may be caused by lack of growth hormone and may be treated with growth hormone treatment. Symptoms such as heart problems are followed on a regular basis.

Is Noonan syndrome inherited?

Noonan syndrome is inherited in families in an autosomal dominant pattern. This means that a person who has Noonan syndrome has one copy of an altered gene that causes the disorder. In about one-third to two-thirds of families one of the parents also has Noonan syndrome. The parent who has Noonan syndrome has a one in two (50 percent) chance to pass on the altered gene to a child who will be affected; and a one in two (50 percent) chance to pass on the normal version of the gene to a child who will not have Noonan syndrome. In many individuals who have Noonan syndrome, the altered gene happens for the first time in them, and neither of the parents has Noonan syndrome. This is called a de novo mutation. The chance for these parents to have another child with Noonan syndrome is very small (less than 1 percent).

Chapter 29

Porphyria

What is porphyria?

The porphyrias are a group of different diseases, each caused by a specific abnormality in the heme production process. Heme is a chemical compound that contains iron and gives blood its red color. The essential functions of heme depend on its ability to bind oxygen. Heme is incorporated into hemoglobin, a protein that enables red blood cells to carry oxygen from the lungs to all parts of the body. Heme also plays a role in the liver where it assists in breaking down chemicals (including some drugs and hormones) so that they are easily removed from the body.

Heme is produced in the bone marrow and liver through a complex process controlled by eight different enzymes. As this production process of heme progresses, several different intermediate compounds (heme precursors) are created and modified. If one of the essential enzymes in heme production is deficient, certain precursors may accumulate in tissues (especially in the bone marrow or liver), appear in excess in the blood, and get excreted in the urine or stool. The specific precursors that accumulate depend on which enzyme is deficient. Porphyria results in a deficiency or inactivity of a specific enzyme in the heme production process, with resulting accumulation of heme precursors.

Reprinted from "Learning about Porphyria," National Human Genome Research Institute, National Institutes of Health, May 19, 2008.

What are the signs and symptoms of porphyria?

The signs and symptoms of porphyria vary among types. Some types of porphyria (called cutaneous porphyria) cause the skin to become overly sensitive to sunlight. Areas of the skin exposed to the sun develop redness, blistering, and often scarring.

The symptoms of other types of porphyria (called acute porphyrias) affect the nervous system. These symptoms include chest and abdominal pain, emotional and mental disorders, seizures, and muscle weakness. These symptoms often appear quickly and last from days to weeks. Some porphyrias have a combination of acute symptoms and symptoms that affect the skin.

Environmental factors can trigger the signs and symptoms of porphyria. These include the following:

- Alcohol
- Smoking
- Certain drugs, hormones
- Exposure to sunlight
- Stress
- Dieting and fasting

How is porphyria diagnosed?

Porphyria is diagnosed through blood, urine, and stool tests, especially at or near the time of symptoms. Diagnosis may be difficult because the range of symptoms is common to many disorders and interpretation of the tests may be complex. A large number of tests are available, however, but results among laboratories are not always reliable.

How is porphyria treated?

Each form of porphyria is treated differently. Treatment may involve treating with heme, giving medicines to relieve the symptoms, or drawing blood. People who have severe attacks may need to be hospitalized.

What do we know about porphyria and heredity?

Most of the porphyrias are inherited conditions. The genes for all the enzymes in the heme pathway have been identified. Some forms of porphyria result from inheriting one altered gene from one parent (autosomal dominant). Other forms result from inheriting two altered genes, one from each parent (autosomal recessive). Each type of porphyria carries a different risk that individuals in an affected family will have the disease or transmit it to their children.

Porphyria cutanea tarda (PCT) is a type of porphyria that is most often not inherited. Eighty percent of individuals with PCT have an acquired disease that becomes active when factors such as iron, alcohol, hepatitis C virus (HCV), human immunodeficiency virus (HIV), estrogens (such as those used in oral contraceptives and prostate cancer treatment), and possibly smoking, combine to cause an enzyme deficiency in the liver. Hemochromatosis, an iron overload disorder, can also predispose individuals to PCT. Twenty percent of individuals with PCT have an inherited form of the disease. Many individuals with the inherited form of PCT never develop symptoms.

If you or someone you know has porphyria, we recommend that you contact a genetics clinic to discuss this information with a genetics professional. To find a genetics clinic near you, contact your primary doctor for a referral.

What triggers a porphyria attack?

Porphyria can be triggered by drugs (barbiturates, tranquilizers, birth control pills, sedatives), chemicals, fasting, smoking, drinking alcohol, infections, emotional and physical stress, menstrual hormones, and exposure to the sun. Attacks of porphyria can develop over hours or days and last for days or weeks.

How is porphyria classified?

The porphyrias have several different classification systems. The most accurate classification is by the specific enzyme deficiency. Another classification system distinguishes porphyrias that cause neurologic symptoms (acute porphyrias) from those that cause photosensitivity (cutaneous porphyrias). A third classification system is based on whether the excess precursors originate primarily in the liver (hepatic porphyrias) or primarily in the bone marrow (erythropoietic porphyrias). Some porphyrias are classified as more than one of these categories.

What are the cutaneous porphyrias?

The cutaneous porphyrias affect the skin. People with cutaneous porphyria develop blisters, itching, and swelling of their skin when it is exposed to sunlight. The cutaneous porphyrias include the following types:

- **Congenital erythropoietic porphyria:** Also called congenital porphyria. This is a rare disorder that mainly affects the skin. It results from low levels of the enzyme responsible for the fourth step in heme production. It is inherited in an autosomal recessive pattern.

- **Erythropoietic protoporphyria:** An uncommon disorder that mainly affects the skin. It results from reduced levels of the enzyme responsible for the eighth and final step in heme production. The inheritance of this condition is not fully understood. Most cases are probably inherited in an autosomal dominant pattern, however, it shows autosomal recessive inheritance in a small number of families.

- **Hepatoerythropoietic porphyria:** A rare disorder that mainly affects the skin. It results from very low levels of the enzyme responsible for the fifth step in heme production. It is inherited in an autosomal recessive pattern.

- **Hereditary coproporphyria:** A rare disorder that can have symptoms of acute porphyria and symptoms that affect the skin. It results from low levels of the enzyme responsible for the sixth step in heme production. It is inherited in an autosomal dominant pattern.

- **Porphyria cutanea tarda:** The most common type of porphyria. It occurs in an estimated one in twenty-five thousand people, including both inherited and sporadic (noninherited) cases. An estimated 80 percent of porphyria cutanea tarda cases are sporadic. It results from low levels of the enzyme responsible for the fifth step in heme production. When this condition is inherited, it occurs in an autosomal dominant pattern.

- **Variegate porphyria:** A disorder that can have symptoms of acute porphyria and symptoms that affect the skin. It results from low levels of the enzyme responsible for the seventh step in heme production. It is inherited in an autosomal dominant pattern.

What are the acute porphyrias?

The acute porphyrias affect the nervous system. Symptoms of acute porphyria include pain in the chest, abdomen, limbs, or back; muscle numbness, tingling, paralysis, or cramping; vomiting; constipation; and personality changes or mental disorders. These symptoms appear intermittently. The acute porphyrias include the following types:

- **Acute intermittent porphyria:** This is probably the most common porphyria with acute (severe but usually not long-lasting) symptoms. It results from low levels of the enzyme responsible for the third step in heme production. It is inherited in an autosomal dominant pattern.

- **Delta-aminolevulinate dehydratase (ALAD) deficiency porphyria:** A very rare disorder that results from low levels of the enzyme responsible for the second step in heme production. It is inherited in an autosomal recessive pattern.

Chapter 30

Retinoblastoma

Retinoblastoma is a disease in which malignant (cancer) cells form in the tissues of the retina.

The retina is the nerve tissue that lines the inside of the back of the eye. The retina senses light and sends images to the brain by way of the optic nerve.

Although retinoblastoma may occur at any age, it usually occurs in children younger than five years of age. The tumor may be in one eye or in both eyes. Retinoblastoma rarely spreads from the eye to nearby tissue or other parts of the body. Retinoblastoma is usually found in only one eye and can usually be cured.

Retinoblastoma is sometimes inherited (passed from the parent to the child). Retinoblastoma that is caused by an inherited gene mutation is called hereditary retinoblastoma. It usually occurs at a younger age than retinoblastoma that is not inherited. Retinoblastoma that occurs in only one eye is usually not inherited. Retinoblastoma that occurs in both eyes is always inherited. When hereditary retinoblastoma first occurs in only one eye, there is a chance it will develop later in the other eye. After diagnosis of retinoblastoma in one eye, regular follow-up exams of the healthy eye should be done every two to four months for at least twenty-eight months. After treatment for

Excerpted from PDQ® Cancer Information Summary. National Cancer Institute; Bethesda, MD. "Retinoblastoma Treatment (PDQ®): Patient Version." Updated November 2008. Available at: http://cancer.gov. Accessed January 12, 2009.

retinoblastoma is finished, it is important that follow-up exams continue until the child is five years of age.

Treatment for both types of retinoblastoma should include genetic counseling (a discussion with a trained professional about inherited diseases). Brothers and sisters of a child who has retinoblastoma should also have regular exams by an ophthalmologist (a doctor with special training in diseases of the eye) and genetic counseling about the risk of developing the cancer.

These and other symptoms may be caused by retinoblastoma. Other conditions may cause the same symptoms. A doctor should be consulted if any of the following problems occur:

- Pupil of the eye appears white instead of red when light shines into it. This may be seen in flash photographs of the child.

- Eyes appear to be looking in different directions.

- Pain or redness in the eye.

The following tests and procedures may be used:

- Physical exam and history

- Eye exam with dilated pupil

- Ultrasound exam

- Computed tomography (CT or CAT) scan

- Magnetic resonance imaging (MRI)

Retinoblastoma is usually diagnosed without a biopsy (removal of cells or tissues so they can be viewed under a microscope to check for signs of cancer).

Treatment Option Overview

Different types of treatment are available for patients with retinoblastoma. Some treatments are standard (the currently used treatment), and some are being tested in clinical trials. A treatment clinical trial is a research study meant to help improve current treatments or obtain information on new treatments for patients with cancer. When clinical trials show that a new treatment is better than the standard treatment, the new treatment may become the standard treatment.

Because cancer in children is rare, taking part in a clinical trial should be considered. Some clinical trials are open only to patients who have not started treatment.

Six types of standard treatment are used.

Enucleation: This is surgery to remove the eye and part of the optic nerve. The eye will be checked with a microscope to see if there are any signs that the cancer is likely to spread to other parts of the body. This is done if the tumor is large and there is little or no chance that vision can be saved. The patient will be fitted for an artificial eye after this surgery.

Radiation therapy: Radiation therapy is a cancer treatment that uses high-energy x-rays or other types of radiation to kill cancer cells or keep them from growing. There are two types of radiation therapy. External radiation therapy uses a machine outside the body to send radiation toward the cancer. Internal radiation therapy uses a radioactive substance sealed in needles, seeds, wires, plaques, or catheters that are placed directly into or near the cancer. The way the radiation therapy is given depends on the type and stage of the cancer being treated.

Cryotherapy: This is a treatment that uses an instrument to freeze and destroy abnormal tissue, such as carcinoma in situ. This type of treatment is also called cryosurgery.

Photocoagulation: This is a procedure that uses laser light to destroy blood vessels to the tumor, causing the tumor cells to die. Photocoagulation may be used to treat small tumors. This is also called light coagulation.

Thermotherapy: This is the use of heat to destroy cancer cells. Thermotherapy may be given using a laser beam aimed through the dilated pupil or onto the outside of the eyeball, or using ultrasound, microwaves, or infrared radiation (light that cannot be seen but can be felt as heat).

Chemotherapy: This is a cancer treatment that uses drugs to stop the growth of cancer cells, either by killing the cells or by stopping them from dividing. When chemotherapy is taken by mouth or injected into a vein or muscle, the drugs enter the bloodstream and can reach cancer cells throughout the body (systemic chemotherapy). When chemotherapy is placed directly into the spinal column, an organ (such as the eye), or a body cavity such as the abdomen, the drugs mainly affect cancer cells in those areas (regional chemotherapy). The way the chemotherapy is given depends on the type and stage of the cancer being treated.

A form of chemotherapy called chemoreduction is used to treat retinoblastoma. Chemoreduction reduces the size of the tumor so it may be treated with local treatment (such as radiation therapy, cryotherapy, photocoagulation, or thermotherapy).

New types of treatment are being tested in clinical trials.

Subtenon chemotherapy: This is the use of drugs injected through the membrane covering the muscles and nerves at the back of the eyeball. This is a type of regional chemotherapy. It is usually combined with systemic chemotherapy and local treatment (such as radiation therapy, cryotherapy, photocoagulation, or thermotherapy).

High-dose chemotherapy with stem cell transplant: This is a way of giving high doses of chemotherapy and replacing blood-forming cells destroyed by the cancer treatment. Stem cells (immature blood cells) are removed from the blood or bone marrow of the patient or a donor and are frozen and stored. After the chemotherapy is completed, the stored stem cells are thawed and given back to the patient through an infusion. These reinfused stem cells grow into (and restore) the body's blood cells.

Biologic therapy: This is a treatment that uses the patient's immune system to fight cancer. Substances made by the body or made in a laboratory are used to boost, direct, or restore the body's natural defenses against cancer. This type of cancer treatment is also called biotherapy or immunotherapy. Clinical trials for retinoblastoma are studying a biologic therapy called gene therapy. This is a treatment that changes a gene to improve the body's ability to fight the disease.

Chapter 31

Rett Syndrome

What is Rett syndrome?

Rett syndrome is a childhood neurodevelopmental disorder characterized by normal early development followed by loss of purposeful use of the hands, distinctive hand movements, slowed brain and head growth, gait abnormalities, seizures, and mental retardation. It affects females almost exclusively.

The disorder was identified by Dr. Andreas Rett, an Austrian physician who first described it in a journal article in 1966. It was not until after a second article about the disorder was published in 1983 that the disorder was generally recognized.

The course of Rett syndrome, including the age of onset and the severity of symptoms, varies from child to child. Before the symptoms begin, however, the child appears to grow and develop normally. Then, gradually, mental and physical symptoms appear. Hypotonia (loss of muscle tone) is usually the first symptom. As the syndrome progresses, the child loses purposeful use of her hands and the ability to speak. Other early symptoms may include problems crawling or walking and diminished eye contact. The loss of functional use of the hands is followed by compulsive hand movements such as wringing and washing. The onset of this period of regression is sometimes sudden.

Reprinted from "Rett Syndrome Fact Sheet," National Institute of Neurological Disorders and Stroke, National Institutes of Health, NIH Publication No. 04-4863, June 6, 2008.

Another symptom, apraxia—the inability to perform motor functions—is perhaps the most severely disabling feature of Rett syndrome, interfering with every body movement, including eye gaze and speech.

Individuals with Rett syndrome often exhibit autistic-like behaviors in the early stages. Other symptoms may include toe walking; sleep problems; wide-based gait; teeth grinding and difficulty chewing; slowed growth; seizures; cognitive disabilities; and breathing difficulties while awake such as hyperventilation, apnea (breath holding), and air swallowing.

What are the stages of the disorder?

There are four stages of Rett syndrome. Stage I, called early onset, generally begins between six and eighteen months of age. Quite frequently, this stage is overlooked because symptoms of the disorder may be somewhat vague, and parents and doctors may not notice the subtle slowing of development at first. The infant may begin to show less eye contact and have reduced interest in toys. There may be delays in gross motor skills such as sitting or crawling. Hand-wringing and decreasing head growth may occur, but not enough to draw attention. This stage usually lasts for a few months but can persist for more than a year.

Stage II, or the rapid destructive stage, usually begins between ages one and four and may last for weeks or months. This stage may have either a rapid or a gradual onset as purposeful hand skills and spoken language are lost. The characteristic hand movements begin to emerge during this stage and often include wringing, washing, clapping, or tapping, as well as repeatedly moving the hands to the mouth. Hands are sometimes clasped behind the back or held at the sides, with random touching, grasping, and releasing. The movements persist while the child is awake but disappear during sleep. Breathing irregularities such as episodes of apnea and hyperventilation may occur, although breathing is usually normal during sleep. Some girls also display autistic-like symptoms such as loss of social interaction and communication. General irritability and sleep irregularities may be seen. Gait patterns are unsteady and initiating motor movements can be difficult. Slowing of head growth is usually noticed during this stage.

Stage III, also called the plateau or pseudo-stationary stage, usually begins between ages two and ten and can last for years. Apraxia, motor problems, and seizures are prominent during this stage. However, there may be improvement in behavior, with less irritability, crying, and autistic-like features. An individual in stage III may show more interest in her surroundings, and her alertness, attention span, and communication skills may improve. Many girls remain in this stage for most of their lives.

The last stage, stage IV—called the late motor deterioration stage—can last for years or decades and is characterized by reduced mobility. Muscle weakness, rigidity (stiffness), spasticity, dystonia (increased muscle tone with abnormal posturing of extremity or trunk), and scoliosis (curvature of the spine) are other prominent features. Girls who were previously able to walk may stop walking. Generally, there is no decline in cognition, communication, or hand skills in stage IV. Repetitive hand movements may decrease, and eye gaze usually improves.

What causes Rett syndrome?

Rett syndrome is caused by mutations (structural alterations or defects) in the MECP2 (pronounced meck-pea-two) gene, which is found on the X chromosome. Scientists identified the gene—which is believed to control the functions of several other genes—in 1999. The MECP2 gene contains instructions for the synthesis of a protein called methyl cytosine binding protein 2 (MeCP2), which acts as one of the many biochemical switches that tell other genes when to turn off and stop producing their own unique proteins. Because the MECP2 gene does not function properly in those with Rett syndrome, insufficient amounts or structurally abnormal forms of the protein are formed. The absence or malfunction of the protein is thought to cause other genes to be abnormally expressed, but this hypothesis has not yet been confirmed.

Seventy to 80 percent of girls given a diagnosis of Rett syndrome have the MECP2 genetic mutation detected by current diagnostic techniques. Scientists believe the remaining 20 to 30 percent of cases may be caused by partial gene deletions, by mutations in other parts of the gene, or by genes that have not yet been identified; thus, they continue to search for other mutations.

Is Rett syndrome inherited?

Although Rett syndrome is a genetic disorder—resulting from a faulty gene or genes—less than 1 percent of recorded cases are inherited or passed from one generation to the next. Most cases are sporadic, which means the mutation occurs randomly, mostly during spermatogenesis, and is not inherited.

Who gets Rett syndrome?

Rett syndrome affects one in every ten thousand to fifteen thousand live female births. It occurs in all racial and ethnic groups worldwide. Prenatal testing is available for families with an affected daughter who has an identified MECP2 mutation. Since the disorder occurs spontaneously in most affected individuals, however, the risk of a family having a second child with the disorder is less than 1 percent.

Genetic testing is also available for sisters of girls with Rett syndrome and an identified MECP2 mutation to determine if they are asymptomatic carriers of the disorder, which is an extremely rare possibility.

Girls have two X chromosomes, but only one is active in any given cell. This means that in a child with Rett syndrome only about half the cells in the nervous system will use the defective gene. Some of the child's brain cells use the healthy gene and express normal amounts of the proteins.

The story is different for boys who have an MECP2 mutation known to cause Rett syndrome in girls. Because boys have only one X chromosome they lack a back-up copy that could compensate for the defective one, and they have no protection from the harmful effects of the disorder. Boys with such a defect die shortly after birth.

Different types of mutations in the MECP2 gene can cause mental retardation in boys.

How is Rett syndrome diagnosed?

Doctors diagnose Rett syndrome by observing signs and symptoms during the child's early growth and development, and conducting ongoing evaluations of the child's physical and neurological status. Recently, scientists developed a genetic test to confirm the clinical diagnosis of this disorder; the test involves searching for the MECP2 mutation on the child's X chromosome. Given what we know about the genes involved in Rett syndrome, such tests are able to confirm a clinical diagnosis in up to 80 percent of all cases.

Some children who have Rett syndrome–like characteristics or MECP2 genetic mutations do not fulfill the diagnostic criteria for the syndrome as defined below. These persons are described as having "atypical" or "variant" Rett syndrome. Atypical cases account for about 15 percent of the total number of diagnosed cases.

A pediatric neurologist or developmental pediatrician should be consulted to confirm the clinical diagnosis of Rett syndrome. The physician will use a highly specific set of guidelines that are divided into three types of clinical criteria: essential, supportive, and exclusion. The presence of any of the exclusion criteria negates a diagnosis of "classic" or "typical" Rett syndrome.

Examples of essential diagnostic criteria or symptoms include having apparently normal development until between the ages of six and eighteen months and having normal head circumference at birth followed by a slowing of the rate of head growth with age (between three months and four years). Other essential diagnostic criteria include severely impaired expressive language, repetitive hand movements, shaking of the torso, and toe-walking or an unsteady, wide-based, stiff-legged gait.

Supportive criteria are not required for a diagnosis of Rett syndrome but may occur in some patients. In addition, these symptoms—which vary in severity from child to child—may not be observed in very young girls but may develop with age. A child with supportive criteria but none of the essential criteria does not have Rett syndrome. Supportive criteria include breathing difficulties; electroencephalogram (EEG) abnormalities; seizures; muscle rigidity, spasticity, and/or joint contracture which worsen with age; scoliosis; teeth-grinding; small feet in relation to height; growth retardation; decreased body fat and muscle mass (although there may be a tendency toward obesity in some affected adults); abnormal sleep patterns, irritability, or agitation; chewing and/or swallowing difficulties; poor circulation of the lower extremities with cold and bluish-red feet and legs; decreased mobility with age; and constipation.

In addition to the essential diagnostic criteria, a number of specific conditions enable physicians to rule out a diagnosis of Rett syndrome. These are referred to as exclusion criteria. Children with any one of the following criteria do not have Rett syndrome: enlargement of body organs or other signs of storage disease, vision loss due to retinal disorder or optic atrophy, microcephaly at birth, an identifiable metabolic disorder or other inherited degenerative disorder, an acquired neurological disorder resulting from severe infection or head trauma, evidence of growth retardation in utero, or evidence of brain damage acquired after birth.

Why are some cases more severe than others?

The course and severity of Rett syndrome vary from individual to individual. Some girls have symptoms from birth onward, while others may have late regression or milder symptoms.

Because females have two copies of the X chromosome and need only one working copy for genetic information, they turn off the extra X chromosome in a process called X inactivation. This process occurs randomly so that each cell is left with one active X chromosome. The severity of Rett syndrome in girls is in part a function of the percentage of cells with a normal copy of the MECP2 gene after X inactivation takes place: if X inactivation turns off the X chromosome that is carrying the defective gene in a large proportion of cells, the symptoms will be mild, but if a larger percentage of cells have the X chromosome with the normal MECP2 gene turned off, onset of the disorder may occur earlier and the symptoms may be more severe.

Is treatment available?

There is no cure for Rett syndrome. Treatment for the disorder is symptomatic—focusing on the management of symptoms—and supportive, requiring a multidisciplinary approach. Medication may be needed for breathing irregularities and motor difficulties, and antiepileptic drugs may be used to control seizures. There should be regular monitoring for scoliosis and possible heart abnormalities. Occupational therapy (in which therapists help children develop skills needed for performing self-directed activities—occupations—such as dressing, feeding, and practicing arts and crafts), physiotherapy, and hydrotherapy may prolong mobility. Some children may require special equipment and aids such as braces to arrest scoliosis, splints to modify hand movements, and nutritional programs to help them maintain adequate weight. Special academic, social, vocational, and support services may also be required in some cases.

What is the outlook for those with Rett syndrome?

Despite the difficulties with symptoms, most individuals with Rett syndrome continue to live well into middle age and beyond. Because the disorder is rare, very little is known about long-term prognosis and life expectancy. While it is estimated that there are many middle-aged women (in their forties and fifties) with the disorder, not enough women have been studied to make reliable estimates about life expectancy beyond age forty.

What research is being done?

Within the federal government, the National Institute of Neurological Disorders and Stroke (NINDS) and the National Institute of

Child Health and Human Development (NICHD), two of the National Institutes of Health (NIH), support clinical and basic research on Rett syndrome. Understanding the cause of this disorder is necessary for developing new therapies to manage specific symptoms, as well as for providing better methods of diagnosis. The discovery of the Rett syndrome gene in 1999 provides a basis for further genetic studies and enables the use of recently developed animal models such as transgenic mice.

One NINDS-supported study is looking for mutations in the MECP2 gene of individuals with Rett syndrome to find out how the MeCP2 protein functions. Information from this study will increase understanding of the disorder and may lead to new therapies.

Scientists know that lack of a properly functioning MeCP2 protein disturbs the function of mature brain cells but they do not know the exact mechanisms by which this happens. Investigators are also trying to find other genetic mutations that can cause Rett syndrome and other genetic switches that operate in a similar way to the MeCP2 protein. Once they discover how the protein works and locate similar switches, they may be able to devise therapies that can substitute for the malfunctioning switch. Another outcome might involve manipulating other biochemical pathways to compensate for the malfunctioning MECP2 gene, thus preventing progression of the disorder.

Chapter 32

Tuberous Sclerosis

What is tuberous sclerosis?

Tuberous sclerosis—also called tuberous sclerosis complex (TSC)[1]—is a rare, multisystem genetic disease that causes benign tumors to grow in the brain and on other vital organs such as the kidneys, heart, eyes, lungs, and skin. It commonly affects the central nervous system and results in a combination of symptoms including seizures, developmental delay, behavioral problems, skin abnormalities, and kidney disease.

The disorder affects as many as twenty-five to forty thousand individuals in the United States and about one to two million individuals worldwide, with an estimated prevalence of one in six thousand newborns. TSC occurs in all races and ethnic groups, and in both genders.

The name tuberous sclerosis comes from the characteristic tuber or potato-like nodules in the brain, which calcify with age and become hard or sclerotic. The disorder—once known as epiloia or Bourneville disease—was first identified by a French physician more than one hundred years ago.

Many TSC patients show evidence of the disorder in the first year of life. However, clinical features can be subtle initially, and many signs and symptoms take years to develop. As a result, TSC can be unrecognized or misdiagnosed for years.

Reprinted from "Tuberous Sclerosis Fact Sheet," National Institute of Neurological Disorders and Stroke, National Institutes of Health, NIH Publication No. 07-1846, September 9, 2008.

What causes tuberous sclerosis?

TSC is caused by defects, or mutations, on two genes—TSC1 and TSC2. Only one of the genes needs to be affected for TSC to be present. The TSC1 gene, discovered in 1997, is on chromosome 9 and produces a protein called hamartin. The TSC2 gene, discovered in 1993, is on chromosome 16 and produces the protein tuberin. Scientists believe these proteins act in a complex as growth suppressors by inhibiting the activation of a master, evolutionarily conserved kinase called mTOR. Loss of regulation of mTOR occurs in cells lacking either hamartin or tuberin, and this leads to abnormal differentiation and development, and to the generation of enlarged cells, as are seen in TSC brain lesions.

Is TSC inherited?

Although some individuals inherit the disorder from a parent with TSC, most cases occur as sporadic cases due to new, spontaneous mutations in TSC1 or TSC2. In this situation, neither parent has the disorder or the faulty gene(s). Instead, a faulty gene first occurs in the affected individual.

In familial cases, TSC is an autosomal dominant disorder, which means that the disorder can be transmitted directly from parent to child. In those cases, only one parent needs to have the faulty gene in order to pass it on to a child. If a parent has TSC, each offspring has a 50 percent chance of developing the disorder. Children who inherit TSC may not have the same symptoms as their parent and they may have either a milder or a more severe form of the disorder.

Rarely, individuals acquire TSC through a process called gonadal mosaicism. These patients have parents with no apparent defects in the two genes that cause the disorder. Yet these parents can have a child with TSC because a portion of one of the parent's reproductive cells (sperm or eggs) can contain the genetic mutation without the other cells of the body being involved. In cases of gonadal mosaicism, genetic testing of a blood sample might not reveal the potential for passing the disease to offspring.

What are the signs and symptoms of TSC?

TSC can affect many different systems of the body, causing a variety of signs and symptoms. Signs of the disorder vary depending on which system and which organs are involved. The natural course of TSC varies from individual to individual, with symptoms ranging from very mild to quite severe. In addition to the benign tumors that frequently occur in TSC, other common symptoms include seizures, mental retardation, behavior problems, and skin abnormalities. Tumors can grow in nearly any organ, but they most commonly occur in the brain, kidneys, heart, lungs, and skin. Malignant tumors are rare in TSC. Those that do occur primarily affect the kidneys.

Kidney problems such as cysts and angiomyolipomas occur in an estimated 70 to 80 percent of individuals with TSC, usually occurring between ages fifteen and thirty. Cysts are usually small, appear in limited numbers, and cause no serious problems. Approximately 2 percent of individuals with TSC develop large numbers of cysts in a pattern similar to polycystic kidney disease[2] during childhood. In these cases, kidney function is compromised and kidney failure occurs. In rare instances, the cysts may bleed, leading to blood loss and anemia.

Angiomyolipomas—benign growths consisting of fatty tissue and muscle cells—are the most common kidney lesions in TSC. These growths are seen in the majority of TSC patients, but are also found in about one of every three hundred people without TSC. Angiomyolipomas caused by TSC are usually found in both kidneys and in most cases they produce no symptoms. However, they can sometimes grow so large that they cause pain or kidney failure. Bleeding from angiomyolipomas may also occur, causing both pain and weakness. If severe bleeding does not stop naturally, there may be severe blood loss, resulting in profound anemia and a life-threatening drop in blood pressure, warranting urgent medical attention.

Other rare kidney problems include renal cell carcinoma, developing from an angiomyolipoma, and oncocytomas, benign tumors unique to individuals with TSC.

Three types of brain tumors are associated with TSC: cortical tubers, for which the disease is named, generally form on the surface of the brain, but may also appear in the deep areas of the brain; subependymal nodules, which form in the walls of the ventricles—the fluid-filled cavities of the brain; and giant-cell tumors (astrocytomas), a type of tumor that can grow and block the flow of fluids within the brain, causing a buildup of fluid and pressure and leading to headaches and blurred vision.

Tumors called cardiac rhabdomyomas are often found in the hearts of infants and young children with TSC. If the tumors are large or there are multiple tumors, they can block circulation and cause death. However, if they do not cause problems at birth—when in most cases they are at their largest size—they usually become smaller with time and do not affect the individual in later life.

Benign tumors called phakomas are sometimes found in the eyes of individuals with TSC, appearing as white patches on the retina. Generally they do not cause vision loss or other vision problems, but they can be used to help diagnose the disease.

Additional tumors and cysts may be found in other areas of the body, including the liver, lung, and pancreas. Bone cysts, rectal polyps, gum fibromas, and dental pits may also occur.

A wide variety of skin abnormalities may occur in individuals with TSC. Most cause no problems but are helpful in diagnosis. Some cases may cause disfigurement, necessitating treatment. The most common skin abnormalities include the following:

- Hypomelanotic macules ("ash leaf spots"), which are white or lighter patches of skin that may appear anywhere on the body and are caused by a lack of skin pigment or melanin—the substance that gives skin its color.

- Reddish spots or bumps called facial angiofibromas (also called adenoma sebaceum), which appear on the face (sometimes resembling acne) and consist of blood vessels and fibrous tissue.

- Raised, discolored areas on the forehead called forehead plaques, which are common and unique to TSC and may help doctors diagnose the disorder.

- Areas of thick leathery, pebbly skin called shagreen patches, usually found on the lower back or nape of the neck.

- Small fleshy tumors called ungual or subungual fibromas that grow around and under the toenails or fingernails and may need to be surgically removed if they enlarge or cause bleeding. These usually appear later in life, ages twenty to fifty.

- Other skin features that are not unique to individuals with TSC, including molluscum fibrosum or skin tags, which typically occur across the back of the neck and shoulders, café au lait spots or flat brown marks, and poliosis, a tuft or patch of white hair that may appear on the scalp or eyelids.

TSC can cause seizures and varying degrees of mental disability. Seizures of all types may occur, including infantile spasms; tonic-clonic seizures (also known as grand mal seizures); or tonic, akinetic, atypical absence, myoclonic, complex partial, or generalized seizures.

Approximately one-half to two-thirds of individuals with TSC have mental disabilities ranging from mild learning disabilities to severe mental retardation. Behavior problems, including aggression, sudden rage, attention deficit hyperactivity disorder, acting out, obsessive-compulsive disorder, and repetitive, destructive, or self-harming behavior, often occur in children with TSC, and can be difficult to manage. Some individuals with TSC may also have a developmental disorder called autism.

How is TSC diagnosed?

In most cases the first clue to recognizing TSC is the presence of seizures or delayed development. In other cases, the first sign may be white patches on the skin (hypomelanotic macules).

Diagnosis of the disorder is based on a careful clinical exam in combination with computed tomography (CT) or magnetic resonance imaging (MRI) of the brain, which may show tubers in the brain, and an ultrasound of the heart, liver, and kidneys, which may show tumors in those organs. Doctors should carefully examine the skin for the wide variety of skin features, the fingernails and toenails for ungual fibromas, the teeth and gums for dental pits and/or gum fibromas, and the eyes for dilated pupils. A Wood's lamp or ultraviolet light may be used to locate the hypomelanotic macules which are sometimes hard to see on infants and individuals with pale or fair skin. Because of the wide variety of signs of TSC, it is best if a doctor experienced in the diagnosis of TSC evaluates a potential patient.

In infants TSC may be suspected if the child has cardiac rhabdomyomas or seizures (infantile spasms) at birth. With a careful examination of the skin and brain, it may be possible to diagnose TSC in a very young infant. However, many children are not diagnosed until later in life when their seizures begin and other symptoms such as facial angiofibromas appear.

How is TSC treated?

There is no cure for TSC, although treatment is available for a number of the symptoms. Antiepileptic drugs may be used to control seizures, and medications may be prescribed for behavior problems. Intervention programs including special schooling and occupational therapy may benefit individuals with special needs and developmental issues. Surgery including dermabrasion and laser treatment may be useful for treatment of skin lesions. Because TSC is a lifelong condition, individuals need to be regularly monitored by a doctor to make sure they are receiving the best possible treatments. Due to the many varied symptoms of TSC, care by a clinician experienced with the disorder is recommended.

Recently much enthusiasm has arisen in regard to the use of rapamycin for treatment of TSC. Rapamycin is a drug that specifically blocks the activity of mTOR. In cell culture experiments and animal models of TSC, rapamycin appears to be very effective. Initial clinical experience with rapamycin and related drugs is also positive, but much additional study is required before these drugs become standard therapy.

What is the prognosis?

The prognosis for individuals with TSC depends on the severity of symptoms, which range from mild skin abnormalities to varying degrees of learning disabilities and epilepsy to severe mental retardation, uncontrollable seizures, and kidney failure. Those individuals with mild symptoms generally do well and live long productive lives, while individuals with the more severe form may have serious disabilities.

In rare cases, seizures, infections, or tumors in vital organs may cause complications in some organs such as the kidneys and brain that can lead to severe difficulties and even death. However, with appropriate medical care, most individuals with the disorder can look forward to normal life expectancy.

What research is being done?

Within the federal government, the leading supporter of research on TSC is the National Institute of Neurological Disorders and Stroke (NINDS). The NINDS, part of the National Institutes of Health (NIH), is responsible for supporting and conducting research on the brain and the central nervous system. NINDS conducts research in its laboratories at NIH and also supports studies through grants to major medical institutions across the country. The National Heart, Lung, and Blood Institute and the National Cancer Institute, also components of the NIH, support and conduct research on TSC.

Scientists who study TSC seek to increase our understanding of the disorder by learning more about the TSC1 and TSC2 genes that can cause the disorder and the function of the proteins—tuberin and hamartin—produced by these genes. Scientists hope knowledge gained from their current research will improve the genetic test for TSC and lead to new avenues of treatment, methods of prevention, and, ultimately, a cure for this disorder.

Research studies run the gamut from very basic scientific investigation to clinical translational research. For example, some investigators are trying to identify all the protein components that are in the same "signaling pathway" in which the TSC1 and TSC2 protein products and the mTOR protein are involved. Other studies are focused on understanding in detail how the disease develops, both in animal models and in patients, to better define new ways of controlling or preventing the development of the disease. Finally, clinical trials of rapamycin are underway (with NINDS and NCI support) to rigorously test the potential benefit of this compound for some of the tumors that are problematic in TSC patients.

Notes

1. Tuberous sclerosis is often referred to as tuberous sclerosis complex (TSC) in medical literature to help distinguish it from Tourette syndrome, an unrelated neurological disorder.

2. Polycystic kidney disease is a genetic disorder characterized by the growth of numerous fluid-filled cysts in the kidneys.

Chapter 33

Vision Disorders

Chapter Contents

Section 33.1

Color Vision Deficiency

Color vision deficiency is the inability to distinguish certain shades of color or in more severe cases, see colors at all. The term "color blindness" is also used to describe this visual condition, but very few people are completely color blind.

Most people with color vision deficiency can see colors, but they have difficulty differentiating between:

- particular shades of reds and greens (most common); or

- blues and yellows (less common).

People who are totally color blind, a condition called achromatopsia, can only see things as black and white or in shades of gray.

The severity of color vision deficiency can range from mild to severe depending on the cause. It will affect both eyes if it is inherited and usually just one if the cause for the deficiency is injury or illness.

Color vision is possible due to photoreceptors in the retina of the eye known as cones. These cones have light-sensitive pigments that enable us to recognize color. Found in the macula, the central portion of the retina, each cone is sensitive to either red, green, or blue light, which the cones recognize based upon light wavelengths.

Normally, the pigments inside the cones register differing colors and send that information through the optic nerve to the brain, enabling you to distinguish countless shades of color. But if the cones lack one or more light-sensitive pigments, you will be unable to see one or more of the three primary colors, thereby causing a deficiency in your color perception.

The most common form of color deficiency is red-green. This does not mean that people with this deficiency cannot see these colors at all; they simply have a harder time differentiating between them. The difficulty they have in correctly identifying them depends on how dark or light the colors are.

Another form of color deficiency is blue-yellow. This is a rarer and more severe form of color vision loss than red-green since persons with blue-yellow deficiency frequently have red-green blindness too. In both cases, it is common for people with color vision deficiency to see neutral or gray areas where a particular color should appear.

What causes color vision deficiency?

Usually, color deficiency is an inherited condition caused by a common X-linked recessive gene, which is passed from a mother to her son. But disease or injury damaging the optic nerve or retina can also result in loss of color recognition. Some specific diseases that can cause color deficits are:

- diabetes;
- glaucoma;
- macular degeneration;
- Alzheimer disease;
- Parkinson disease;
- multiple sclerosis;
- chronic alcoholism;
- leukemia;
- sickle cell anemia.

Other causes for color vision deficiency include:

- **Medications:** Certain medications such as drugs used to treat heart problems, high blood pressure, infections, nervous disorders, and psychological problems can affect color vision.
- **Aging:** The ability to see colors can gradually lessen with age.
- **Chemical exposure:** Contact with certain chemicals such as fertilizers and styrene have been known to cause loss of color vision.

In the majority of cases, genetics is the predominate cause for color deficiency. About 8 percent of Caucasian males are born with some degree of color deficiency. Women are typically just carriers of the color deficient gene, though approximately 0.5 percent of women have color vision deficiency. When the deficiency is hereditary, the severity generally remains constant throughout life. Inherited color vision deficiency does not lead to additional vision loss or blindness.

How is color vision deficiency diagnosed?

Color deficiency can be diagnosed through a comprehensive eye examination. Testing will include the use of a series of specially designed pictures composed of colored dots, called pseudoisochromatic plates, which include hidden numbers or embedded figures that can only be correctly seen by persons with normal color vision:

- **Pseudoisochromatic testing plates:** The patient is asked to look for numbers among the various colored dots, which help distinguish between red, green, and blue color deficiencies. Individuals with normal color vision will see a number, while those with a deficiency do not see it. On some plates, a person with normal color vision may see one number, while a person with a deficiency sees a different number.

Pseudoisochromatic plate testing can be used to determine if a color vision deficiency exists and the type of deficiency. However, additional testing may be needed to determine the exact nature and degree of color deficiency.

It is possible for a person to have poor color vision and not know it. Quite often, people with red-green deficiency aren't even aware of their problem since they've learned to see the "right" color. For example, tree leaves are green, so they call the color they see green.

Also parents may not suspect the condition in their children until a situation causes confusion or misunderstanding. Early detection of color deficiency is vital since many learning materials rely heavily on color perception or color coding. That is one reason that the American Optometric Association recommends a comprehensive optometric examination before a child begins school.

How is color vision deficiency treated?

There is no cure for inherited color deficiency. But if the cause is an illness or eye injury, treating these conditions may improve color vision.

Using special tinted eyeglasses or wearing a red-tinted contact lens on one eye can increase some people's ability to differentiate between colors, though nothing can make you truly see the deficient color.

Most color-deficient persons compensate for their inability to distinguish certain colors with color cues and details that are not consciously evident to people with normal color vision. There are ways to work around the inability to see certain colors by:

- Organizing and labeling clothing, furniture or other colored objects (with the help of friends or family) for ease of recognition.

- Remembering the order of things rather than their color can also increase the chances of correctly identifying colors. For example, a traffic light has red on top, yellow in the middle, and green on the bottom.

Though color vision deficiency can be a frustration and may limit participation in some occupations, in most cases it is not a serious threat to vision and can be adapted to your lifestyle with time, patience, and practice.

Section 33.2

Early-Onset Glaucoma

Excerpted from "Early-Onset Glaucoma," *Genetics Home Reference*, a service of the U.S. National Library of Medicine, February 2009.

What is early-onset glaucoma?

Glaucoma is a group of eye disorders in which the optic nerves connecting the eyes and the brain are progressively damaged. This damage can lead to reduction in side (peripheral) vision and eventual blindness. Other signs and symptoms may include bulging eyes, excessive tearing, and abnormal sensitivity to light (photophobia). The term "early-onset glaucoma" may be used when the disorder appears before the age of forty.

In most people with glaucoma, the damage to the optic nerves is caused by increased pressure within the eyes (intraocular pressure).

Intraocular pressure depends on a balance between fluid entering and leaving the eyes.

Usually glaucoma develops in older adults, in whom the risk of developing the disorder may be affected by a variety of medical conditions including high blood pressure (hypertension) and diabetes mellitus, as well as family history. The risk of early-onset glaucoma depends mainly on heredity.

Structural abnormalities that impede fluid drainage in the eye may be present at birth and usually become apparent during the first year of life. Such abnormalities may be part of a genetic disorder that affects many body systems, called a syndrome. If glaucoma appears before the age of five without other associated abnormalities, it is called primary congenital glaucoma.

Other individuals experience early onset of primary open-angle glaucoma, the most common adult form of glaucoma. If primary open-angle glaucoma develops during childhood or early adulthood, it is called juvenile open-angle glaucoma.

How common is early-onset glaucoma?

Primary congenital glaucoma affects approximately one in ten thousand people. Its frequency is higher in the Middle East. Juvenile open-angle glaucoma affects about one in fifty thousand people. Primary open-angle glaucoma is much more common after the age of forty, affecting about 1 percent of the population worldwide.

What genes are related to early-onset glaucoma?

Approximately 10 to 33 percent of people with juvenile open-angle glaucoma have mutations in the MYOC gene. MYOC mutations have also been detected in some people with primary congenital glaucoma. The MYOC gene provides instructions for producing a protein called myocilin. Myocilin is found in certain structures of the eye, called the trabecular meshwork and the ciliary body, that regulate the intraocular pressure.

Researchers believe that myocilin functions together with other proteins as part of a protein complex. Mutations may alter the protein in such a way that the complex cannot be formed. Defective myocilin that is not incorporated into functional complexes may accumulate in the trabecular meshwork and ciliary body. The excess protein may prevent sufficient flow of fluid from the eye, resulting in increased intraocular pressure and causing the signs and symptoms of early-onset glaucoma.

Between 20 and 40 percent of people with primary congenital glaucoma have mutations in the CYP1B1 gene. CYP1B1 mutations have also been detected in some people with juvenile open-angle glaucoma. The CYP1B1 gene provides instructions for producing a form of the cytochrome P450 protein. Like myocilin, this protein is found in the trabecular meshwork, ciliary body, and other structures of the eye.

It is not well understood how defects in the CYP1B1 protein cause signs and symptoms of glaucoma. Recent studies suggest that the defects may interfere with the early development of the trabecular meshwork. In the clear covering of the eye (the cornea), the CYP1B1 protein may also be involved in a process that regulates the secretion of fluid inside the eye. If this fluid is produced in excess, the high intraocular pressure characteristic of glaucoma may develop.

The CYP1B1 protein may interact with myocilin. Individuals with mutations in both the MYOC and CYP1B1 genes may develop glaucoma at an earlier age and have more severe symptoms than do those with mutations in only one of the genes. Mutations in other genes may also be involved in early-onset glaucoma.

How do people inherit early-onset glaucoma?

Early-onset glaucoma can have different inheritance patterns. Primary congenital glaucoma is usually inherited in an autosomal recessive pattern, which means both copies of the gene in each cell have mutations. Most often, the parents of an individual with an autosomal recessive condition each carry one copy of the mutated gene, but do not show signs and symptoms of the condition.

Juvenile open-angle glaucoma is inherited in an autosomal dominant pattern, which means one copy of the altered gene in each cell is sufficient to cause the disorder. In some families, primary congenital glaucoma may also be inherited in an autosomal dominant pattern.

Section 33.3

X-Linked Juvenile Retinoschisis

Excerpted from "X-Linked Juvenile Retinoschisis,"
Genetics Home Reference, a service of the U.S. National
Library of Medicine, August 2008.

What is X-linked juvenile retinoschisis?

X-linked juvenile retinoschisis is a genetic eye disorder that impairs normal vision. This disorder affects the retina, which is a specialized light-sensitive tissue that lines the back of the eye. Damage to the retina impairs the sharpness of vision (visual acuity). Typically, X-linked juvenile retinoschisis affects cells in the central area of the retina called the macula. The macula is responsible for sharp central vision, which is needed for detailed tasks such as reading, driving, and recognizing faces. X-linked juvenile retinoschisis is one type of a broader disorder called macular degeneration, which involves disruption in the normal functioning of the macula. Occasionally, side (peripheral) vision is affected in people with X-linked juvenile retinoschisis.

X-linked juvenile retinoschisis occurs almost exclusively in males. It is usually diagnosed when affected boys start school and poor vision and difficulty with reading become apparent. In more severe cases, eye squinting and involuntary movement of the eyes (nystagmus) can be seen in infancy. Visual acuity remains unchanged in most people between their teenage years and their forties or fifties, when a significant decline in visual acuity typically occurs. Rarely, severe complications develop, such as separation of the retinal layers (retinal detachment) or leakage of blood vessels in the retina (vitreous hemorrhage). These eye abnormalities can cause impaired vision or blindness.

How common is X-linked juvenile retinoschisis?

The prevalence of X-linked juvenile retinoschisis is estimated to be one in five thousand to twenty-five thousand males worldwide.

What genes are related to X-linked juvenile retinoschisis?

Mutations in the RS1 gene cause most cases of X-linked juvenile retinoschisis. The RS1 gene provides instructions for producing a protein called retinoschisin, which is found in the retina. Studies suggest that retinoschisin plays a role in the development and maintenance of the retina and in specialized cells within the retina that detect light and color (photoreceptor cells).

RS1 gene mutations lead to a reduced amount of retinoschisin, which can cause tiny splits (schisis) or tears to form in the retina. This damage often forms a "spoke-wheel" pattern in the macula, which can be seen during an eye examination. These abnormalities are typically seen in the area of the macula, affecting visual acuity, but can also occur in the sides of the retina, resulting in impaired peripheral vision.

Some individuals with X-linked juvenile retinoschisis do not have a mutation in the RS1 gene. In these individuals, the cause of the disorder is unknown.

How do people inherit X-linked juvenile retinoschisis?

This condition is inherited in an X-linked recessive pattern. The gene associated with this condition is located on the X chromosome, which is one of the two sex chromosomes. In males (who have only one X chromosome), one altered copy of the gene in each cell is sufficient to cause the condition. In females (who have two X chromosomes), a mutation would have to occur in both copies of the gene to cause the disorder. Because it is unlikely that females will have two altered copies of this gene, males are affected by X-linked recessive disorders much more frequently than females. A striking characteristic of X-linked inheritance is that fathers cannot pass X-linked traits to their sons.

Chapter 34

Wilson Disease

What Is Wilson Disease?

Wilson disease is a genetic disorder that prevents the body from getting rid of extra copper. A small amount of copper obtained from food is needed to stay healthy, but too much copper is poisonous. In Wilson disease, copper builds up in the liver, brain, eyes, and other organs. Over time, high copper levels can cause life-threatening organ damage.

Who Gets Wilson Disease?

People who get Wilson disease inherit two abnormal copies of the ATP7B gene, one from each parent. Wilson disease carriers, who have only one copy of the abnormal gene, do not have symptoms. Most people with Wilson disease have no known family history of the disease. A person's chances of having Wilson disease increase if one or both parents have it.

About one in forty thousand people get Wilson disease.[1] It equally affects men and women. Symptoms usually appear between ages five and thirty-five, but new cases have been reported in people aged two to seventy-two years.

Reprinted from "Wilson Disease," National Institute of Diabetes and Digestive and Kidney Diseases, National Institutes of Health, NIH Publication No. 08-4684, July 2008.

What Causes Wilson Disease?

Wilson disease is caused by a buildup of copper in the body. Normally, copper from the diet is filtered out by the liver and released into bile, which flows out of the body through the gastrointestinal tract. People who have Wilson disease cannot release copper from the liver at a normal rate, due to a mutation of the ATP7B gene. When the copper storage capacity of the liver is exceeded, copper is released into the bloodstream and travels to other organs—including the brain, kidneys, and eyes.

What are the Symptoms of Wilson Disease?

Wilson disease first attacks the liver, the central nervous system, or both.

A buildup of copper in the liver may cause ongoing liver disease. Rarely, acute liver failure occurs; most patients develop signs and symptoms that accompany chronic liver disease, including the following:

- Swelling of the liver or spleen
- Jaundice, or yellowing of the skin and whites of the eyes
- Fluid buildup in the legs or abdomen
- A tendency to bruise easily
- Fatigue

A buildup of copper in the central nervous system may result in neurologic symptoms, including the following:

- Problems with speech, swallowing, or physical coordination
- Tremors or uncontrolled movements
- Muscle stiffness
- Behavioral changes

Other signs and symptoms of Wilson disease include the following:

- Anemia
- Low platelet or white blood cell count
- Slower blood clotting, measured by a blood test

- High levels of amino acids, protein, uric acid, and carbohydrates in urine

- Premature osteoporosis and arthritis

Kayser-Fleischer rings result from a buildup of copper in the eyes and are the most unique sign of Wilson disease. They appear in each eye as a rusty-brown ring around the edge of the iris and in the rim of the cornea. The iris is the colored part of the eye surrounding the pupil. The cornea is the transparent outer membrane that covers the eye.

How Is Wilson Disease Diagnosed?

Wilson disease is diagnosed through a physical examination and laboratory tests.

During the physical examination, a doctor will look for visible signs of Wilson disease. A special light called a slit lamp is used to look for Kayser-Fleischer rings in the eyes. Kayser-Fleischer rings are present in almost all people with Wilson disease who show signs of neurologic damage but are present in only 50 percent of those with signs of liver damage alone.

Laboratory tests measure the amount of copper in the blood, urine, and liver tissue. Most people with Wilson disease will have a lower than normal level of copper in the blood and a lower level of corresponding ceruloplasmin, a protein that carries copper in the bloodstream. In cases of acute liver failure caused by Wilson disease, the level of blood copper is often higher than normal. A twenty-four-hour urine collection will show increased copper in the urine in most patients who display symptoms. A liver biopsy—a procedure that removes a small piece of liver tissue—can show if the liver is retaining too much copper. The analysis of biopsied liver tissue with a microscope detects liver damage, which often shows a pattern unique to Wilson disease.

Genetic testing may help diagnose Wilson disease in some people, particularly those with a family history of the disease.

Wilson disease can be misdiagnosed because it is rare and its symptoms are similar to those of other conditions.

Who Should be Screened for Wilson Disease?

Anyone with unexplained liver disease or neurologic symptoms with evidence of liver disease, such as abnormal liver tests and symptoms of liver disease, should be screened for Wilson disease. People with a family history of Wilson disease, especially those with an affected sibling or parent, should also be screened. A doctor can diagnose Wilson disease before the appearance of symptoms. Early treatment can reduce or even prevent illness.

How Is Wilson Disease Treated?

Wilson disease requires lifelong treatment to reduce and control the amount of copper in the body.

Initial therapy includes the removal of excess copper, a reduction of copper intake, and the treatment of any liver or central nervous system damage.

The drugs d-penicillamine (Cuprimine®) and trientine hydrochloride (Syprine®) release copper from organs into the bloodstream. Most of the copper is then filtered out by the kidneys and excreted in urine. A potential major side effect of both drugs is that neurologic symptoms can become worse—a possible result of the newly released copper becoming reabsorbed by the central nervous system. About 20 to 30 percent of patients using d-penicillamine will also initially experience other reactions to the medication, including fever, rash, and other drug-related effects on the kidneys and bone marrow. The risk of drug reaction and neurologic worsening appears to be lower with trientine hydrochloride, which should be the first choice for the treatment of all symptomatic patients.

Pregnant women should take a lower dose of d-penicillamine or trientine hydrochloride during pregnancy to reduce the risk of birth defects. A lower dose will also help reduce the risk of slower wound healing if surgical procedures are performed during childbirth.

Zinc, administered as zinc salts such as zinc acetate (Galzin®), blocks the digestive tract's absorption of copper from food. Zinc removes copper too slowly to be used alone as an initial therapy for people who already have symptoms, but it is often used in combination with d-penicillamine or trientine hydrochloride. Zinc is safe to use at full dosage during pregnancy.

Maintenance therapy begins when symptoms improve and tests show that copper has been reduced to a safe level. Maintenance therapy typically includes taking zinc and low doses of either d-penicillamine or trientine hydrochloride. Blood and urine should be monitored by a health care provider to ensure treatment is keeping copper at a safe level.

People with Wilson disease should reduce their dietary copper intake. They should not eat shellfish or liver, as these foods may contain high levels of copper. Other foods high in copper—including mushrooms, nuts, and chocolate—should be avoided during initial therapy but, in most cases, may be eaten in moderation during maintenance therapy. People with Wilson disease should have their drinking water checked for copper content and should not take multivitamins that contain copper.

If the disorder is detected early and treated effectively, people with Wilson disease can enjoy good health.

Points to Remember

- Wilson disease prevents the body from getting rid of extra copper.

- Wilson disease first attacks the liver, the central nervous system, or both.

- Anyone with unexplained liver disease or neurologic symptoms with evidence of liver disease should be screened for Wilson disease.

- Wilson disease requires lifelong treatment to reduce and control the amount of copper in the body.

- If the disorder is detected early and treated effectively, people with Wilson disease can enjoy good health.

Hope through Research

The National Institute of Diabetes and Digestive and Kidney Diseases conducts and supports Wilson disease research.

The U.S. Food and Drug Administration is evaluating a new anti-copper drug called tetrathiomolybdate (Coprexa®). A National Institutes of Health–supported clinical trial found tetrathiomolybdate to be as effective as trientine hydrochloride in removing copper but with less risk of worsening neurologic symptoms.

Notes

1. Olivarez M, Caggana M, Pass KA, Ferguson P, Brewer GJ. Estimate of the frequency of Wilson's disease in the US Caucasian population: a mutation analysis approach. *Annals of Human Genetics*. 2001;65:459–63.

Part Three

Chromosome Abnormalities

Chapter 35

Angelman Syndrome

Angelman syndrome is a genetic disorder that is characterized by severe learning difficulties, seizures, uncoordinated movements, and a very happy demeanor.

Who

Angelman syndrome occurs in all ethnic groups and equally affects both males and females. The disease occurs in about one in twelve thousand to one in twenty thousand births.

Signs and Symptoms

Angelman syndrome is present at birth but is commonly not recognized right away because the pregnancy and birth are usually normal. The first signs of Angelman syndrome are usually in the first year of life when the child displays developmental delays, low muscle tone, and a slowing of head growth. The most common age of diagnosis is three to seven years old. More than 80 percent of children have onset of seizures before the age of three. The type of seizures varies. Children can experience full body seizures with jerking of the arms and legs, or they can have seizures that just show periods of lack of awareness, or anything in between. The child does not achieve developmental milestones as expected. Language typically does not develop in children with Angelman syndrome. Most can understand simple commands, but are only able to communicate through gestures. Very few children are able to speak more than two or three words. There are physical characteristics that are common in children with Angelman syndrome. For example, they may have crossed eyes, a wide mouth, widely spaced teeth, a protruding tongue, large jaw, and lighter colored skin, eyes, and hair as compared to other family members. When they walk, they have problems with balance, are stiff, and hold their arms and hands flexed. Angelman syndrome can cause a variety of behavioral characteristics. Some of these include frequent laughter and smiling, hyperactivity, short attention span, difficulty sleeping, and hand-flapping movements. There may also be a strong attraction to and fascination with water, reflective surfaces, plastic objects, and balloons. Children typically enjoy being around other people and watching TV, especially slapstick comedy.

Possible Causes

The most common cause of Angelman syndrome is found in about 70 percent of children. This results from a deletion (missing piece) of a part of chromosome 15. We each have two copies of chromosome 15, one from our mother and one from our father. Angelman syndrome occurs if the deletion is on the chromosome that is inherited from the mother. The second most common cause of Angelman syndrome is found in about 11 percent of children. This results from a mutation (change) in a gene called UBE3A. The UBE3A gene is also located in the same region of chromosome 15 that is described above. A third cause of Angelman syndrome is found in about 7 percent of children. This results from inheriting both copies of chromosome 15 from the father. This is called "uniparental disomy" (UPD). A fourth cause of Angelman syndrome is found in about 0.5 percent of children. This results if chromosome 15 does not function properly. This is referred to as an "imprinting" defect. Less than 1 percent of children with Angelman syndrome have another chromosome rearrangement (abnormality). In about 10 percent of cases, the cause of Angelman syndrome is unknown. There are research reports that have found an increased risk of Angelman syndrome associated with artificial reproductive technology.

Diagnosis

When diagnosing Angelman syndrome, chromosome analysis is done to verify that there are no other chromosome abnormalities besides chromosome 15. Several tests can be performed to confirm the diagnosis. Deoxyribonucleic acid (DNA) methylation testing can test for the most common causes of Angelman syndrome, including deletions, uniparental disomy, or imprinting defects. This test will diagnose about 80 percent of individuals. A fluorescent in situ hybridization (FISH) test can be performed to look for a deletion on chromosome 15. Testing of the UBE3A gene will diagnose about 11 percent of individuals.

Treatment

There is no cure for Angelman syndrome. It is important for the child to receive therapy for the physical and behavioral problems associated with the disease. The child's environment should be safe so that the child isn't injured during the hyperactive behaviors. Seizures can often be difficult to treat with anti-seizure medications. Medications may be tried to help with sleep and/or constipation. Programs for the special educational needs of the children are usually helpful. If the individual develops scoliosis or other bone or joint problems, he or she should be treated by an orthopedist. Strabismus (or cross-eyes) may require surgery. Older children have a tendency for obesity and so diet should be monitored.

Prognosis

The facial characteristics of Angelman syndrome become more pronounced in adulthood. The ability to move around often decreases as the individual gets older and they may need a wheelchair. The lifespan of individuals with Angelman syndrome is usually normal but they are unable to live independently. They have relatively good health except for the seizures. They may have problems with constipation, scoliosis (curves in the back or spine), and/or obesity.

Chapter 36

Cri du Chat Syndrome

What is cri du chat syndrome?

Cri du chat syndrome—also known as 5p-syndrome and cat cry syndrome—is a rare genetic condition that is caused by the deletion (a missing piece) of genetic material on the small arm (the p arm) of chromosome 5. The cause of this rare chromosomal deletion is unknown.

What are the symptoms of cri du chat syndrome?

The symptoms of cri du chat syndrome vary among individuals. The variability of the clinical symptoms and developmental delays may be related to the size of the deletion of the 5p arm.

The clinical symptoms of cri du chat syndrome usually include a high-pitched cat-like cry, mental retardation, delayed development, distinctive facial features, small head size (microcephaly), widely spaced eyes (hypertelorism), low birth weight, and weak muscle tone (hypotonia) in infancy. The cat-like cry typically becomes less apparent with time.

Most individuals who have cri du chat syndrome have difficulty with language. Half of children learn sufficient verbal skills to communicate. Some individuals learn to use short sentences, while others express themselves with a few basic words, gestures, or sign language.

Reprinted from "Learning about Cri du Chat Syndrome," National Human Genome Research Institute, National Institutes of Health, March 26, 2007.

Other characteristics may include feeding difficulties, delays in walking, hyperactivity, scoliosis, and significant retardation. A small number of children are born with serious organ defects and other life-threatening medical conditions, although most individuals with cri du chat syndrome have a normal life expectancy.

Both children and adults with this syndrome are usually friendly and happy, and enjoy social interaction.

How is cri du chat syndrome diagnosed?

The diagnosis of cri du chat syndrome is generally made in the hospital at birth. A health care provider may note the clinical symptoms associated with the condition. The cat-like cry is the most prominent clinical feature in newborn children and is usually diagnostic for the cri du chat syndrome.

Additionally, analysis of the individual's chromosomes may be performed. The missing portion (deletion) of the short arm of chromosome 5 may be seen on a chromosome analysis. If not, a more detailed type of genetic test called fluorescence in situ hybridization (FISH) analysis may be needed to reveal the deletion.

What is the treatment for cri du chat syndrome?

No specific treatment is available for this syndrome. Children born with this genetic condition will most likely require ongoing support from a team made up of the parents, therapists, and medical and educational professionals to help the child achieve his or her maximum potential. With early and consistent educational intervention, as well as physical and language therapy, children with cri du chat syndrome are capable of reaching their fullest potential and can lead full and meaningful lives.

Is cri du chat syndrome inherited?

Most cases of cri du chat syndrome are not inherited. The chromosomal deletion usually occurs as a random event during the formation of reproductive cells (eggs or sperm) or in early fetal development. People with cri du chat typically have no history of the condition in their family.

About 10 percent of people with cri du chat syndrome inherit the chromosome with a deleted segment from an unaffected parent. In these cases, the parent carries a chromosomal rearrangement called a balanced translocation, in which no genetic material is gained or lost. Balanced translocations usually do not cause any medical problems; however, they can become unbalanced as they are passed to the next generation. A deletion in the short arm of chromosome 5 is an example of an unbalanced translocation, which is a chromosomal rearrangement with extra or missing genetic material. Unbalanced translocations can cause birth defects and other health problems such as those seen in cri du chat syndrome.

Chapter 37

DiGeorge Syndrome

What

DiGeorge syndrome is a rare disorder whose symptoms generally consist of increased susceptibility to infection (immune deficiency), defects of the heart, and a number of characteristic facial features, although there is great variability from person to person. Often the thymus and parathyroid glands are underdeveloped or dysfunctional. DiGeorge syndrome is actually one of the most common genetic disorders and is known by a variety of names, including velo-cardio-facial syndrome (VCFS). It used to be thought that these were different disorders, but the ability to do specific genetic tests has shown that they all have a similar cause.

Who

DiGeorge syndrome affects male and females with equal frequency and is usually diagnosed shortly after birth because of the obvious abnormalities in facial features, and because the heart problems are often recognized then. Recent data suggests that the incidence of DiGeorge and related syndromes is one in three thousand persons.

Signs and Symptoms

Cardiac defects are among the major physical manifestations associated with DiGeorge syndrome. Such defects may include abnormalities of the blood vessels leaving the heart (the aorta and pulmonary arteries) and ventricular septal defects (VSD), which consist of a hole between the lower chambers of the heart. Facial manifestations include down-slanting eyes, low-set rotated ears, a small round mouth, high-arched palate, and relative smallness of the jaw. Speech impairment is often observed in these individuals when they get older. Low calcium levels are often observed since the parathyroid glands are intimately involved in maintaining normal serum calcium levels, and may be missing in DiGeorge syndrome. If thymus gland development is compromised, then adequate T-cell production is lost and these children will suffer from immune deficiency and thus experience an increased incidence of fungal or viral infections.

Possible Causes

DiGeorge syndrome is a genetic problem caused by the microdeletion of the long arm of chromosome 22. In DiGeorge syndrome, the genetic abnormality consists of a deletion, or missing segment, of chromosome 22. Humans have twenty-three pairs of chromosomes (forty-six total) numbered 1 to 22 in decreasing order of size, plus the two sex chromosomes that determine gender. The deleted chromosomal segment means that several genes are absent, thereby affecting the development of the fetus and causing a number of abnormalities. The variability in symptoms is due to the amount of genetic information that is missing. Sometimes the parents will have a similar deletion, but often not. The parents may or may not have symptoms, even if they have the deletion.

Diagnosis

The observance in an individual of any one or more of the major signs and symptoms associated with DiGeorge syndrome should raise suspicion. In infants, hypocalcemia is often a characteristic feature, although this condition may occur intermittently and even resolve itself at around age one. Blood tests help analyze the function of the immune and endocrine systems. In addition, imaging studies reveal cardiac defects and other developmental anomalies. A standard karyotype, which produces a picture of all the chromosomes, does not usually detect the disease. A special genetic test called a fluorescence in situ hybridization (FISH) probe is needed.

Treatment

Supportive management includes the correction of low calcium with calcium supplements and vitamin D administration. Surgery is often performed to correct cardiac lesions and transplantation surgeries of the thymus and/or bone marrow may also be performed to treat the immunodeficiency associated with DiGeorge syndrome. In addition to a general pediatrician, children with this genetic disorder will consult specialist physicians, such as a cardiologist and an immunologist, to address specific abnormalities associated with DiGeorge syndrome.

Prognosis

The prognosis for patients with DiGeorge syndrome varies significantly according to the degree of involvement of the cardiac and immune systems, respectively. A congenital heart defect is the major cause of morbidity and mortality, with most deaths occurring within six months of age. Opportunistic infections occurring due to severe immune deficiency are the second most common cause of death. However, if the immune problem is not too severe, many children outgrow it with time.

Chapter 38

Down Syndrome and Other Trisomy Disorders

Chapter Contents

Section 38.1

Down Syndrome

What is Down syndrome?

Down syndrome is a chromosomal disorder that includes a combination of birth defects. Affected individuals have some degree of mental retardation, characteristic facial features, and, often, heart defects and other health problems. The severity of these problems varies greatly among affected individuals.

How common is Down syndrome?

Down syndrome is one of the most common genetic birth defects, affecting about one in eight hundred babies.[1] According to the National Down Syndrome Society, there are approximately 350,000 individuals with Down syndrome in the United States.[2]

What causes Down syndrome?

Down syndrome is caused by extra genetic material from chromosome 21. Chromosomes are the structures in cells that contain the genes.

Each person normally has twenty-three pairs of chromosomes, or forty-six in all. An individual inherits one chromosome per pair from the mother's egg and one from the father's sperm. When an egg and sperm cell join together, they normally form a fertilized egg with forty-six chromosomes.

Sometimes something goes wrong before fertilization. A developing egg or sperm cell may divide incorrectly, sometimes resulting in an egg or sperm cell with an extra chromosome number 21. When this cell joins with a normal egg or sperm cell, the resulting embryo has 47 chromosomes instead of 46. Down syndrome also is called trisomy

21 because affected individuals have three number 21 chromosomes, instead of two. This type of error in cell division causes about 95 percent of the cases of Down syndrome.[3]

Occasionally, before fertilization, a part of chromosome 21 breaks off during cell division and becomes attached to another chromosome in the egg or sperm cell. The resulting embryo may have what is called translocation Down syndrome. Affected individuals have two normal copies of chromosome 21 plus extra chromosome 21 material attached to another chromosome. This type of error in cell division causes about 3 to 4 percent of the cases of Down syndrome.[3] In some cases, the parent has a rearrangement of chromosome 21, called a balanced translocation, which does not affect his or her health.

About 1 to 2 percent of individuals with Down syndrome have a form called mosaicism.[3] In this form, the error in cell division occurs after fertilization. Affected individuals have some cells with an extra chromosome 21 and others with the normal number.

What health problems might a child or adult with Down syndrome have?

The outlook for individuals with Down syndrome is far brighter than it once was. Most of the health problems associated with Down syndrome can be treated, and life expectancy is now about fifty-five years.[2] Individuals with Down syndrome are more likely than unaffected individuals to have one or more of the following health conditions:

- **Heart defects:** Almost half of babies with Down syndrome have heart defects.[3] Some defects are minor and may be treated with medications, while others require surgery. All babies with Down syndrome should be examined by a pediatric cardiologist, a doctor who specializes in heart diseases of children, and have an echocardiogram (a special ultrasound examination of the heart) in the first two months of life so that heart defects can be treated.[2,3]

- **Intestinal defects:** About 12 percent of babies with Down syndrome are born with intestinal malformations that require surgery.[3]

- **Vision problems:** More than 60 percent of children with Down syndrome have vision problems, including crossed eyes (esotropia), near- or farsightedness, and cataracts.[3] Glasses, surgery, or other treatments usually can improve vision. A child with Down

379

syndrome should be examined by a pediatric ophthalmologist (eye doctor) within the first six months of life and have regular vision exams.[3]

- **Hearing loss:** About 75 percent of children with Down syndrome have some hearing loss.[3] Hearing loss may be due to fluid in the middle ear (which may be temporary), a nerve, or both. Babies with Down syndrome should be screened for hearing loss at birth or by three months of age. They also should have regular hearing exams so any problems can be treated before they hinder development of language and other skills.[3]

- **Infections:** Children with Down syndrome tend to have many colds and ear infections, as well as bronchitis and pneumonia. Children with Down syndrome should receive all the standard childhood immunizations, which help prevent some of these infections.

- **Thyroid problems, leukemia, and seizures.**[3]

- **Memory loss:** Individuals with Down syndrome are more likely than unaffected individuals to develop Alzheimer disease (characterized by progressive memory loss, personality changes, and other problems). Adults with Down syndrome tend to develop Alzheimer disease at an earlier age than unaffected individuals. Studies suggest that about 25 percent of adults with Down syndrome over age thirty-five have symptoms of Alzheimer disease.[2]

Some individuals with Down syndrome may have a number of these problems, while others may have none. The severity of these conditions varies greatly.

What does a child with Down syndrome look like?

A child with Down syndrome may have eyes that slant upward and small ears that my fold over a little at the top. The child's mouth may be small, making the tongue appear large. The nose also may be small, with a flattened nasal bridge. Some babies with Down syndrome have short necks and small hands with short fingers. Having less muscle tone, they may appear somewhat "floppy."

The child or adult with Down syndrome is often short and has unusual looseness of the joints. Most children with Down syndrome have some, but not all, of these features.

How serious is the mental retardation?

The degree of mental retardation varies widely. Most fall within the mild to moderate range. With proper intervention, few will have severe mental retardation.[3] There is no way to predict the mental development of a child with Down syndrome based upon physical features.

What can a child with Down syndrome do?

Children with Down syndrome usually can do most things that any young child can do, such as walking, talking, dressing, and being toilet-trained. However, they generally start learning these things later than other children.

The exact age that these developmental milestones will be achieved cannot be predicted. However, early intervention programs beginning in infancy can help these children achieve their developmental milestones sooner.

Can a child with Down syndrome go to school?

Yes. There are special programs beginning in the preschool years to help children with Down syndrome develop skills as fully as possible. Along with benefiting from early intervention and special education, many children are integrated into the regular classroom. Many affected children learn to read and write, and some graduate from high school and go on to postsecondary programs or college. Individuals with Down syndrome participate in diverse childhood activities both at school and in their neighborhoods.

While there are special work programs designed for adults with Down syndrome, many people with the disorder hold regular jobs. Today, an increasing number of adults with Down syndrome live semi-independently in community group homes where they take care of themselves, participate in household chores, develop friendships, partake in leisure activities, and work in their communities.

Can Down syndrome be cured or prevented?

There is no cure for Down syndrome, nor is there any way to prevent it. However, some studies suggest that women who have certain variant genes that affect how their bodies metabolize (process) the B vitamin folic acid may be at increased risk for having a baby with Down syndrome.[4,5] If confirmed, this finding may provide yet another reason why all women who might become pregnant should take a daily multivitamin containing 400 micrograms of folic acid (which has been shown to reduce the risk of certain birth defects of the brain and spinal cord).

Does the risk of Down syndrome increase with the mother's age?

Yes. The risk of Down syndrome increases from about 1 in 1,250 at age twenty-five to 1 in 1,000 at age thirty, 1 in 400 at age thirty-five, 1 in 100 at age forty, and 1 in 30 at age forty-five.[6] Women over age thirty-five have been traditionally considered most likely to have a baby with Down syndrome. However, about 80 percent of babies with Down syndrome are born to women who are under age thirty-five, as younger women have far more babies.[2]

What is the risk that parents of a child with Down syndrome will have another affected child?

In general, in each subsequent pregnancy, the chance of having another baby with Down syndrome is 1 percent plus whatever additional risk a mother has, based upon her age.[2, 7] If, however, the first child has translocation Down syndrome, the chance of having another child with Down syndrome may be greatly increased.

After birth, the provider takes a blood sample from a baby suspected of having Down syndrome and sends it to a laboratory. The lab examines the chromosomes (called a karyotype) to determine if the baby has Down syndrome and what genetic form of Down syndrome the baby has. This information is important in determining the risk in future pregnancies. The doctor may refer parents to a genetic counselor who can explain the results of chromosomal tests in detail, including what the recurrence risks may be in another pregnancy.

Can Down syndrome be diagnosed before the child is born?

Yes. The American College of Obstetricians and Gynecologists (ACOG) recommends that all pregnant women be offered a screening test for Down syndrome, regardless of the woman's age. Screening may consist of a maternal blood test done in the first trimester (at eleven to thirteen weeks of pregnancy), along with a special ultrasound examination of the back of the baby's neck (called nuchal translucency), or a maternal blood test done in the second trimester (at fifteen to twenty weeks).[8] A screening test helps identify pregnancies that are at higher-than-average risk of Down syndrome. However, a screening test cannot diagnose Down syndrome or other birth defects.

Women who have an abnormal screening test result are offered a diagnostic test, such as amniocentesis or chorionic villus sampling (CVS). These tests are highly accurate at diagnosing, or more likely, ruling out Down syndrome.

ACOG also recommends that pregnant women of all ages have the option of bypassing the screening test and choosing a diagnostic test for Down syndrome instead.[8] Until recently, only women over age thirty-five and others considered at increased risk for having a baby with Down syndrome were offered diagnostic testing because amniocentesis and CVS pose a very small risk of miscarriage.

Most parents-to-be receive reassuring news from a screening or diagnostic test for Down syndrome. However, if a prenatal diagnostic test shows that the baby has Down syndrome, parents have an opportunity to prepare medically, emotionally, and financially for the birth of a child with special needs, such as arranging for delivery in a medically appropriate setting.

Can people with Down syndrome have children?

Some people with Down syndrome marry. With rare exceptions, men with Down syndrome cannot father a child.[3] In any pregnancy, a woman with Down syndrome has a 50-50 chance of conceiving a child with Down syndrome, but many affected fetuses are miscarried.

Is the March of Dimes conducting research on Down syndrome?

Some March of Dimes grantees are investigating why errors in chromosome division occur, in the hope of someday preventing Down syndrome and other birth defects caused by abnormalities in the number or structure of chromosomes. Other grantees are investigating the role of specific genes in causing the brain abnormalities associated with Down syndrome, with the goal of treating the mental retardation associated with the disorder. An international team of scientists has mapped all the genes of chromosome 21. This information eventually may pave the way for treatment of many features of this disorder.

References

1. Centers for Disease Control and Prevention (CDC). Birth Defects: Frequently Asked Questions. Updated 12/12/06.

2. National Down Syndrome Society. Information Topics. Accessed 1/11/07.

3. American Academy of Pediatrics Committee on Genetics. Health Supervision for Children with Down Syndrome. *Pediatrics*, volume 107, number 2, February 2001, pages 442–49.

4. O'Leary, V.B., et al. MTRR and MTHFR Polymorphism: Link to Down Syndrome? *American Journal of Medical Genetics*, January 15, 2002, volume 107, number 2, pages 151–55.

5. Scala, I., et al. Analysis of Seven Maternal Polymorphisms of Genes Involved in Homocysteine/Folate Metabolism and Risk of Down Syndrome. *Genetics in Medicine*, volume 8, number 7, July 2006, pages 409–16.

6. American College of Obstetricians and Gynecologists (ACOG). *Your Pregnancy and Birth*, 4th Edition. ACOG, Washington, DC, 2005.

7. National Institute of Child Health and Human Development (NICHD). Facts About Down Syndrome. Last updated 8/18/06.

8. American College of Obstetricians and Gynecologists (ACOG). Screening for Fetal Chromosomal Abnormalities. ACOG Practice Bulletin, number 77, January 2007.

Section 38.2

Edwards Syndrome (Trisomy 18)

Excerpted from "Trisomy 18," © 2009 A.D.A.M., Inc.
Reprinted with permission.

Trisomy 18 is a genetic disorder associated with the presence of extra material from chromosome 18.

Causes

Trisomy 18 is a relatively common syndrome affecting approximately one out of three thousand live births. It is three times more common in girls than boys. The syndrome is caused by the presence of an extra material from chromosome 18. The extra material interferes with normal development.

Symptoms

- Clenched hands
- Crossed legs (preferred position)
- Heart disease (congenital)
- Hole, split, or cleft in the iris (coloboma)
- Kidney problems
- Low birth weight
- Low-set ears
- Mental deficiency
- Separation between the left and right side of the rectus abdominis muscle (diastasis recti)
- Small head (microcephaly)
- Small jaw (micrognathia)
- Umbilical hernia or inguinal hernia
- Underdeveloped fingernails

- Undescended testicle
- Unusual shaped chest (pectus carinatum)

Exams and Tests

Examination of the pregnant woman may show an unusually large uterus and extra amniotic fluid. An unusually small placenta may be seen when the baby is born.

Physical examination of the infant may show unusual fingerprint patterns. X-rays may show a short breastbone. Chromosome studies show trisomy 18, partial trisomy, or translocation.

There are often signs of congenital heart disease, such as:

- VSD (ventricular septal defect);
- ASD (atrial septal defect);
- PDA (patent ductus arteriosus).

Tests may also show kidney problems, including:

- horseshoe kidney;
- hydronephrosis;
- polycystic kidney.

Treatment

Medical management of children with trisomy 18 is planned on a case-by-case basis and depends on the individual circumstances of the patient.

Outlook (Prognosis)

Fifty percent of infants with this condition do not survive beyond the first week of life. Some children have survived to teenage years, but with serious medical and developmental problems.

Possible Complications

Complications depend on the specific defects and symptoms.

When to Contact a Medical Professional

Call your health care provider and genetic counselor if you have had a child with trisomy 18 and you plan to have another child.

Prevention

Prenatal diagnosis of trisomy 18 is possible with an amniocentesis or chorionic villus sampling and chromosome studies on amniotic cells. Parents who have a child with translocational trisomy 18 and want additional children should have chromosome studies, because they are at increased risk to have another child with trisomy 18.

Section 38.3

Patau Syndrome (Trisomy 13)

Excerpted from "Trisomy 13," © 2009 A.D.A.M., Inc.
Reprinted with permission.

Trisomy 13, also called Patau syndrome, is a genetic disorder associated with the presence of extra material from chromosome 13.

Causes

Trisomy 13 occurs when extra DNA from chromosome 13 appears in some or all of the body's cells:

- **Trisomy 13:** The presence of an extra (third) chromosome 13 in all of the cells.

- **Trisomy 13 mosaicism:** The presence of an extra chromosome 13 in some of the cells.

- **Partial trisomy:** The presence of a part of an extra chromosome 13 in the cells.

The extra material interferes with normal development.
Trisomy 13 occurs in about one out of every ten thousand newborns. Most cases are not passed down through families (inherited). Instead, the events that lead to trisomy 13 occur in either the sperm or the egg that forms the fetus.

Symptoms

- Cleft lip or palate
- Close-set eyes—eyes may actually fuse together into one
- Decreased muscle tone
- Extra fingers or toes (polydactyly)
- Hernias: umbilical hernia, inguinal hernia
- Hole, split, or cleft in the iris (coloboma)
- Low-set ears
- Mental retardation, severe
- Scalp defects (absent skin)
- Seizures
- Single palmar crease
- Skeletal (limb) abnormalities
- Small eyes
- Small head (microcephaly)
- Small lower jaw (micrognathia)
- Undescended testicle (cryptorchidism)

Exams and Tests

The infant may have a single umbilical artery at birth. There are often signs of congenital heart disease, such as:

- abnormal placement of the heart toward the right side of the chest instead of the left;
- atrial septal defect;
- patent ductus arteriosus;
- ventricular septal defect.

Gastrointestinal x-rays or ultrasound may show rotation of the internal organs.

Magnetic resonance imaging (MRI) or computed tomography (CT) scans of the head may reveal a problem with the structure of the brain. The problem is called holoprosencephaly. It is the joining together of the two sides of the brain.

Chromosome studies show trisomy 13, trisomy 13 mosaicism, or partial trisomy.

Treatment

Medical management of children with trisomy 13 is planned on a case-by-case basis and depends on the individual circumstances of the patient.

Outlook (Prognosis)

The syndrome involves multiple abnormalities, many of which are not compatible with life. More than 80 percent of children with trisomy 13 die in the first month.

Possible Complications

Complications begin almost immediately. Congenital heart disease is present in approximately 80 percent of infants with trisomy 13. Complications may include:

- breathing difficulty or lack of breathing (apnea);
- deafness;
- feeding problems;
- heart failure;
- seizures;
- vision problems.

When to Contact a Medical Professional

Call for an appointment with your health care provider if you have had a child with trisomy 13 and you plan to have another child.

Prevention

Trisomy 13 can be diagnosed prenatally by amniocentesis with chromosome studies of the amniotic cells.

Parents of infants with trisomy 13 caused by a translocation should have genetic testing and counseling, which may help them prevent recurrence.

Section 38.4

Triple X Syndrome

"XXX Syndrome (Trisomy X)," June 2008, compiled by Kyla Boyse, RN, reviewed by Autumn Tansky, MS. Reprinted with permission of the University of Michigan Health System. © 2008 Regents of the University of Michigan.

What is XXX or triple X syndrome?

XXX syndrome (also called trisomy X or triple X) is caused by the presence of an extra "X" chromosome in every cell. Typically, a female has two X chromosomes in every cell of their body, so the extra "X" is unusual. The extra "X" chromosome is typically inherited from the mother, but is a random event—not caused by anything she did or could prevent. Trisomy X is often not diagnosed until later in life, if ever. The risk of having a second child with an extra chromosome is approximately 1 percent, until mom is older than thirty-eight years of age, as it is thought that this random event becomes more common as a woman ages. Prenatal testing is available in future pregnancies.

How common is trisomy X?

The extra "X" chromosome occurs in about one in every one thousand newborn girls.

What are the features of triple X syndrome?

Many girls and women with triple X have no signs or symptoms. Signs and symptoms vary a lot between individuals, but can include the following:

- Physical:
  - Tall stature (height)
  - Possible mild facial characteristics: increased width between eyes, skin fold at inner eyelid (epicanthal fold), proportionately smaller head size

- Developmental:
  - Learning disabilities (70 percent): Normal IQ, but may be 10–15 points below siblings
  - Speech and language delays (50 percent)
  - Delayed motor skills: poor coordination, awkwardness, clumsiness
- Behavioral: introverted, difficulty with interpersonal relationships

How is triple X diagnosed and treated?

XXX syndrome is diagnosed prenatally, through chorionic villus sampling (CVS) or amniocentesis, or after the child is born by a blood test. These tests are all able to look at a person's chromosomes (karyotype.) There is no way to remove the extra X chromosome. Treatment depends on what needs the child has. Girls with XXX syndrome may need to be seen by physical, developmental, occupational, or speech therapists if they have developmental or speech problems. Additionally, a pediatric psychologist or group therapy may be helpful if they have social troubles. Girls with trisomy X are treated as any other child with a developmental or psychological concern would be treated.

What is 46,XX/47,XXX mosaicism?

This describes a chromosome study that shows a mixture of normal cells and cells with an extra X chromosome. A girl with mosaicism will usually have fewer effects of the extra chromosome, because not all of her cells have this extra genetic material. She will probably not be much different than she would be if her chromosome study showed all normal cells.

Chapter 39

Fragile X Syndrome

What is fragile X syndrome?

Fragile X syndrome is the most common form of inherited mental retardation in males and is also a significant cause of mental retardation in females. It affects about one in four thousand males and one in eight thousand females and occurs in all racial and ethnic groups.

Nearly all cases of fragile X syndrome are caused by an alteration (mutation) in the FMR1 gene where a DNA segment, known as the CGG triplet repeat, is expanded. Normally, this DNA segment is repeated from five to about forty times. In people with fragile X syndrome, however, the CGG segment is repeated more than two hundred times. The abnormally expanded CGG segment inactivates (silences) the FMR1 gene, which prevents the gene from producing a protein called fragile X mental retardation protein. Loss of this protein leads to the signs and symptoms of fragile X syndrome. Both boys and girls can be affected, but because boys have only one X chromosome, a single fragile X is likely to affect them more severely.

What are the symptoms of fragile X syndrome?

A boy who has the full FMR1 mutation has fragile X syndrome and will have moderate mental retardation. They have a particular facial appearance, characterized by a large head size, a long face, prominent

Reprinted from "Learning about Fragile X Syndrome," National Human Genome Research Institute, National Institutes of Health, April 10, 2008.

forehead and chin, and protruding ears. In addition males who have fragile X syndrome have loose joints (joint laxity), and large testes (after puberty).

Affected boys may have behavioral problems such as hyperactivity, hand flapping, hand biting, temper tantrums, and autism. Other behaviors in boys after they have reached puberty include poor eye contact, perseverative speech, problems in impulse control, and distractibility. Physical problems that have been seen include eye, orthopedic, heart, and skin problems.

Girls who have the full FMR1 mutation have mild mental retardation.

Family members who have fewer repeats in the FMR1 gene may not have mental retardation, but may have other problems. Women with less severe changes may have premature menopause or difficulty becoming pregnant.

Both men and women may have problems with tremors and poor coordination.

What does it mean to have a fragile X premutation?

People with about fifty-five to two hundred repeats of the CGG segment are said to have an FMR1 premutation (an intermediate variation of the gene). In women, the premutation is liable to expand to more than two hundred repeats in cells that develop into eggs. This means that women with the FMR1 premutation have an increased risk of having a child with fragile X syndrome. By contrast, the premutation CGG repeat in men remains at the same size or shortens as it is passed to the next generation.

Males and females who have a fragile X premutation have normal intellect and appearance. A few individuals with a premutation have subtle intellectual or behavioral symptoms, such as learning difficulties or social anxiety. The difficulties are usually not socially debilitating, and these individuals may still marry and have children.

Males who have a premutation with fifty-nine to two hundred CGG trinucleotide repeats are usually unaffected and are at risk for fragile X–associated tremor/ataxia syndrome (FXTAS). The fragile X–associated tremor/ataxia syndrome (FXTAS) is characterized by late-onset, progressive cerebellar ataxia and intention tremor in males who have a premutation. Other neurologic findings include short-term memory loss, executive function deficits, cognitive decline, parkinsonism, peripheral neuropathy, lower-limb proximal muscle weakness, and autonomic dysfunction.

The degree to which clinical symptoms of fragile X are present (penetrance) is age related; symptoms are seen in 17 percent of males aged fifty to fifty-nine years, in 38 percent of males aged sixty to sixty-nine years, in 47 percent of males aged seventy to seventy-nine years, and in 75 percent or males aged eighty years or older. Some female premutation carriers may also develop tremor and ataxia.

Females who have a premutation usually are unaffected, but may be at risk for premature ovarian failure and FXTAS. Premature ovarian failure (POF) is defined as cessation of menses before age forty years, and has been observed in carriers of premutation alleles. A review by Sherman (2005) concluded that the risk for POF was 21 percent in premutation carriers compared to 1 percent for the general population.

How is fragile X syndrome diagnosed?

There are very few outward signs of fragile X syndrome in babies, but one is a tendency to have a large head circumference. An experienced geneticist may note subtle differences in facial characteristics. Mental retardation is the hallmark of this condition and, in females, this may be the only sign of the problem.

A specific genetic test (polymerase chain reaction [PCR]) can now be performed to diagnose fragile X syndrome. This test looks for an expanded mutation (called a triplet repeat) in the FMR1 gene.

How is fragile X syndrome treated?

There is no specific treatment available for fragile X syndrome. Supportive therapy for children who have fragile X syndrome includes the following:

- Special education and anticipatory management including avoidance of excessive stimulation to decrease behavioral problems.

- Medication to manage behavioral issues, although no specific medication has been shown to be beneficial.

- Early intervention, special education, and vocational training.

- Vision, hearing, connective tissue problems, and heart problems when present are treated in the usual manner.

Is fragile X syndrome inherited?

This condition is inherited in an X-linked dominant pattern. A condition is considered X-linked if the mutated gene that causes the disorder is located on the X chromosome, one of the two sex chromosomes. The inheritance is dominant if one copy of the altered gene in each cell is sufficient to cause the condition. In most cases, males experience more severe symptoms of the disorder than females. A striking characteristic of X-linked inheritance is that fathers cannot pass X-linked traits to their sons.

Chapter 40

Klinefelter Syndrome

What Is Klinefelter Syndrome?

In 1942, Dr. Harry Klinefelter and his coworkers at the Massachusetts General Hospital in Boston published a report about nine men who had enlarged breasts, sparse facial and body hair, small testes, and an inability to produce sperm.

By the late 1950s, researchers discovered that men with Klinefelter syndrome, as this group of symptoms came to be called, had an extra sex chromosome, XXY instead of the usual male arrangement, XY.

In the early 1970s, researchers around the world sought to identify males having the extra chromosome by screening large numbers of newborn babies. One of the largest of these studies, sponsored by the National Institute of Child Health and Human Development (NICHD), checked the chromosomes of more than forty thousand infants.

Based on these studies, the XXY chromosome arrangement appears to be one of the most common genetic abnormalities known, occurring as frequently as one in five hundred to one in one thousand male births. Although the syndrome's cause, an extra sex chromosome, is widespread, the syndrome itself—the set of symptoms and characteristics that may result from having the extra chromosome—is uncommon.

Excerpted from "Understanding Klinefelter Syndrome: A Guide for XXY Males and Their Families," National Institute of Child Health and Human Development, National Institutes of Health, NIH Publication No. 93-3202, August 15, 2006.

Many men live out their lives without ever even suspecting that they have an additional chromosome.

"I never refer to newborn babies as having Klinefelter, because they don't have a syndrome," said Arthur Robinson, M.D., a pediatrician at the University of Colorado Medical School in Denver and the director of the NICHD-sponsored study of XXY males. "Presumably, some of them will grow up to develop the syndrome Dr. Klinefelter described, but a lot of them won't."

For this reason, the term "Klinefelter syndrome" has fallen out of favor with medical researchers. Most prefer to describe men and boys having the extra chromosome as "XXY males."

In addition to occasional breast enlargement, lack of facial and body hair, and a rounded body type, XXY males are more likely than other males to be overweight, and tend to be taller than their fathers and brothers.

For the most part, these symptoms are treatable. Surgery, when necessary, can reduce breast size. Regular injections of the male hormone testosterone, beginning at puberty, can promote strength and facial hair growth—as well as bring about a more muscular body type.

A far more serious symptom, however, is one that is not always readily apparent. Although they are not mentally retarded, most XXY males have some degree of language impairment. As children, they often learn to speak much later than do other children and may have difficulty learning to read and write. And while they eventually do learn to speak and converse normally, the majority tend to have some degree of difficulty with language throughout their lives. If untreated, this language impairment can lead to school failure and its attendant loss of self-esteem.

Fortunately, however, this language disability usually can be compensated for. Chances for success are greatest if begun in early childhood. Sections that follow describe possible strategies for meeting the special educational needs of many XXY males.

Chromosomes and Klinefelter Syndrome

Chromosomes, the spaghetti-like strands of hereditary material found in each cell of the body, determine such characteristics as the color of our eyes and hair, our height, and whether we are male or female.

Women usually inherit two X chromosomes—one from each parent. Men tend to inherit an X chromosome from their mothers, and a Y chromosome from their fathers. Most males with the syndrome Dr.

Klinefelter described, however, have an additional X chromosome for a total of two X chromosomes and one Y chromosome.

Causes

No one knows what puts a couple at risk for conceiving an XXY child. Advanced maternal age increases the risk for the XXY chromosome count, but only slightly. Furthermore, recent studies conducted by NICHD grantee Terry Hassold, a geneticist at Case Western Reserve University in Cleveland, Ohio, show that half the time, the extra chromosome comes from the father.

Dr. Hassold explained that cells destined to become sperm or eggs undergo a process known as meiosis. In this process, the forty-six chromosomes in the cell separate, ultimately producing two new cells having twenty-three chromosomes each. Before meiosis is completed, however, chromosomes pair with their corresponding chromosomes and exchange bits of genetic material. In women, X chromosomes pair; in men, the X and Y chromosome pair. After the exchange, the chromosomes separate, and meiosis continues.

In some cases, the Xs or the X chromosome and Y chromosome fail to pair and fail to exchange genetic material. Occasionally, this results in their moving independently to the same cell, producing either an egg with two Xs, or a sperm having both an X and a Y chromosome. When a sperm having both an X and a Y chromosome fertilizes an egg having a single X chromosome, or a normal Y- bearing sperm fertilizes an egg having two X chromosomes, an XXY male is conceived.

Diagnosis

Because they often don't appear any different from anyone else, many XXY males probably never learn of their extra chromosome. However, if they are to be diagnosed, chances are greatest at one of the following times in life: before or shortly after birth, early childhood, adolescence, and in adulthood (as a result of testing for infertility).

In recent years, many XXY males have been diagnosed before birth, through amniocentesis or chorionic villus sampling (CVS). In amniocentesis, a sample of the fluid surrounding the fetus is withdrawn. Fetal cells in the fluid are then examined for chromosomal abnormalities. CVS is similar to amniocentesis, except that the procedure is done in the first trimester, and the fetal cells needed for examination are taken from the placenta. Neither procedure is used routinely, except when there is a family history of genetic defects, the pregnant woman is older than thirty-five, or other medical indications are present.

"If I were going to say something to parents who have had a prenatal diagnosis, it would be 'You are so lucky that you know,'" said Melissa, the mother of one XXY boy. "Because there are parents who don't know that their sons have this problem. And they will never be able to help them lead a normal life. But you can."

The next most likely opportunity for diagnosis is when the child begins school. A physician may suspect a boy is an XXY male if he is delayed in learning to talk and has difficulty with reading and writing. XXY boys may also be tall and thin and somewhat passive and shy. Again, however, there are no guarantees. Some of the boys who fit this description will have the XXY chromosome count, but many others will not.

A few XXY males are diagnosed at adolescence, when excessive breast development forces them to seek medical attention. Like some chromosomally normal males, many XXY males undergo slight breast enlargement at puberty. Of these, only about a third—10 percent of XXY males in all—will develop breasts large enough to embarrass them.

The final chance for diagnosis is at adulthood, as a result of testing for infertility. At this time, an examining physician may note the undersized testes characteristic of an XXY male. In addition to infertility tests, the physician may order tests to detect increased levels of hormones known as gonadotropins, common in XXY males.

A karyotype is used to confirm the diagnosis. In this procedure, a small blood sample is drawn. White blood cells are then separated from the sample, mixed with tissue culture medium, incubated, and checked for chromosomal abnormalities, such as an extra X chromosome.

What to Tell Families, Friends, and XXY Boys

Expectant parents awaiting the arrival of their XXY baby have difficult choices to make: whom to tell and how much to tell about their son's extra chromosome. Fortunately, however, there are some guidelines that new parents can take into account when making their decisions.

One school of thought holds that the best course is to go on slowly, waiting at least one year before telling anyone—grandparents included—about the child's extra chromosome. Many people are frightened by the diagnosis, and their fears will color their perceptions of the child. For example, some people may confuse the term Klinefelter syndrome with Down syndrome, a condition resulting in mild to moderate mental retardation.

Others may prefer to reveal the diagnosis early. Some parents have found that grandparents, aunts, uncles—and even extended family members—are more supportive when given accurate information. Another important decision parents must make is when to tell their son about his diagnosis. Some experts recommend telling the child early. When the truth is withheld, children often suspect that their parents are hiding something and may imagine a condition that is worse than their actual diagnosis.

This school of thought maintains that by the time he is ten or eleven years old, the child can be told that his cells differ slightly from those of other people. Soon after, he can be filled in on the details: that the cell difference is due to an additional X chromosome, which is responsible for his undersized testes and any reading difficulties he may have. At this time, the child can be reassured that he does not have a disease and will not become sick. The child should also be told that some people may misunderstand this information and that he should exercise discretion in sharing it with others.

By roughly the age of twelve, depending on the child's emotional maturity, he can be told that he will most probably be infertile. Parents should stress that neither the X chromosome nor the infertility associated with it mean that he is in any way less masculine than other males his age. The child's parents or his physician can explain that although he may not be able to make a baby, he can consider adopting one. Parents may also need to reassure an XXY boy that his small testes will in no way interfere with his ability to have a normal sex life.

Adherents of this school of thought believe that learning about possible infertility in such a gradual manner will be less of a shock than finding out about it all at once, late in the teen years.

Conversely, other experts believe that holding back the information does not appear to do any harm. Instead, telling an XXY boy about his extra chromosome too early may have some unpleasant consequences. An eleven- or twelve-year-old, for example, may associate infertility with sexual disorders and other concepts he may not yet understand.

Moreover, children, when making friends, tend to share secrets. But childhood friendships may be fleeting, and early confidences are sometimes betrayed. A malicious or thoughtless child may tell all the neighborhood children that his former companion is a "freak" because he has an extra chromosome.

For this reason, the best time to reveal the information may be mid-to-late adolescence, when an XXY male is old enough to understand his condition and better able to decide with whom he wishes to share this knowledge.

Childhood

According to Dr. Robinson, the director of the NICHD-funded study, XXY babies differ little from other children their age. They tend to start life as what many parents call "good" babies—quiet, undemanding, and perhaps even a little passive. As toddlers, they may be somewhat shy and reserved. They usually learn to walk later than most other children, and may have similar delays in learning to speak.

In some, the language delays may be more severe, with the child not fully learning to talk until about age five. Others may learn to speak at a normal rate, and not meet with any problems until they begin school, where they may experience reading difficulties. A few may not have any problems at all in learning to speak or in learning to read.

XXY males usually have difficulty with expressive language—the ability to put thoughts, ideas, and emotions into words. In contrast, their faculty for receptive language—understanding what is said—is close to normal.

"It's one of the conflicts they have," said Melissa, the mother of an XXY boy. "My son can understand the conversations of other ten-year-olds. But his inability to use the language the way other ten-year-olds use it makes him stand out."

In addition to academic help, XXY boys, like other language-disabled children, may need help with social skills. Language is essential not only for learning the school curriculum, but also for building social relationships. By talking and listening, children make friends—in the process, sharing information, attitudes, and beliefs. Through language, they also learn how to behave—not just in the schoolroom, but also on the playground. If their sons' language disability seems to prevent them from fitting in socially, the parents of XXY boys may want to ask school officials about a social skills training program.

Throughout childhood—perhaps, even, for the rest of their lives—XXY boys retain the same temperament and disposition they first displayed as infants and toddlers. As a group, they tend to be shy, somewhat passive, and unlikely to take a leadership role. Although they do make friends with other children, they tend to have only a few friends at a time. Researchers also describe them as cooperative and eager to please.

Detecting Language Problems Early

The parents of XXY babies can compensate for their children's language disability by providing special help in language development, beginning at an early age. However, there is no easy formula to meet the language needs of all XXY boys. Like everyone else, XXY males are unique individuals. A few may not have any trouble learning to read and write, while the rest may have language impairments ranging from mild to severe.

If their son's speech seems to be lagging behind that of other children, parents should ask their child's pediatrician for a referral to a speech pathologist for further testing. A speech pathologist specializes in the disorders of voice, speech, and language.

Parents should also pay particular attention to their children's hearing. Like other small children, XXY infants and toddlers may suffer from frequent ear infections. With any child, such infections may impair hearing and delay the acquisition of language. Such a hearing impairment may be a further setback for an XXY child who is already having language difficulties.

Guidelines for Detecting Language Problems

Shortly after the first birthday, children should be able to make their wishes known with simple one-word utterances. For example, a child may say "milk" to mean "I want more milk." Gradually, children begin to combine words to produce two-word sentences, such as "More milk." By age three, most children use an average of about four words per sentence.

If a child is not communicating effectively with single words by eighteen to twenty-four months, then parents should seek a consultation with a speech and language pathologist.

The XXY Boy in the Classroom

Although there are exceptions, XXY boys are usually well behaved in the classroom. Most are shy, quiet, and eager to please the teacher. But when faced with material they find difficult, they tend to withdraw into quiet daydreaming. Teachers sometimes fail to realize they have a language problem, and dismiss them as lazy, saying they could do the work if they would only try. Many become so quiet that teachers forget they're even in the room. As a result, they fall farther and farther behind, and eventually may be held back a grade.

Help under the Law

According to Dr. Robinson, XXY boys do best in small, uncrowded classrooms where teachers can give them a lot of individual attention. He suggests that parents who can meet the expense consider sending their sons to a private school offering special educational services.

Parents who cannot afford private schools should become familiar with Public Law 94-142, the Education of the Handicapped Act—now called the Individuals with Disabilities Education Act. This law, adopted by Congress in 1975, states that all children with disabilities have a right to a free, appropriate public education. The law cannot ensure that every child who needs special educational services will automatically get them. But the law does allow parents to take action when they suspect their child has a learning disability.

Chances for success are greatest for parents who are well informed and work cooperatively with the schools to plan educational and related service programs for their sons.

Parents may also wish to contact their local and state boards of education for information on how the law has been implemented in their area. In addition, local educational groups may be able to provide useful information on working with school systems. Parents should also consider taking a course in educational advocacy. The local public school system, the state board of education, or local parents groups may be able to tell parents where they can enroll in such a course.

Services for Infants, Toddlers, and Preschoolers

The chances for reducing the impact of a learning disability are greatest in early childhood. Public Law 99-457 is an amendment to Public Law 94-142 that assists states in providing special educational services for infants, toddlers, and preschoolers. Eligibility requirements and entrance procedures vary from state to state.

Adolescence

In general, XXY boys enter puberty normally, without any delay of physical maturity. But as puberty progresses, they fail to keep pace with other males. In chromosomally normal teenaged boys, the testes gradually increase in size, from an initial volume of about 2 ml, to about 15 ml. In XXY males, while the penis is usually of normal size, the testes remain at 2 ml, and cannot produce sufficient quantities of the male hormone testosterone. As a result, many XXY adolescents, although taller than average, may not be as strong as other teenaged boys, and may lack facial or body hair.

As they enter puberty, many boys will undergo slight breast enlargement. For most teenaged males, this condition, known as gynecomastia, tends to disappear in a short time. About one-third of XXY boys develop enlarged breasts in early adolescence slightly more than do chromosomally normal boys. Furthermore, in XXY boys, this condition may be permanent. However, only about 10 percent of XXY males have breast enlargement great enough to require surgery.

Most XXY adolescents benefit from receiving an injection of testosterone every two weeks, beginning at puberty. The hormone increases strength and brings on a more muscular, masculine appearance.

Adolescence and the high school years can be difficult for XXY boys and their families, particularly in neighborhoods and schools where the emphasis is on athletic ability and physical prowess.

"They're usually tall, good-looking kids, but they tend to be awkward," Dr. Robinson said of the XXY teenagers he has met through his study. "They don't necessarily make good football players or good basketball players."

Lack of strength and agility, combined with a history of learning disabilities, may damage self-esteem. Unsympathetic peers, too, sometimes may make matters worse, through teasing or ridicule.

"Lots of kids have a tough time during adolescence," Dr. Robinson said. "But a higher proportion of XXY boys have a tough time. High school is very competitive, and these kids are not very good competitors, in general."

Dr. Robinson again stressed, however, that while XXY males share many characteristics, they cannot be pigeonholed into rigid categories. Several of his patients have played football, and one, in particular, is an excellent tennis player.

Damage to self-esteem may be more severe in XXY teenagers who are diagnosed in early or late adolescence. Teachers—and even parents—may have dismissed their scholastic difficulties as laziness. Lack of athletic prowess and the inability to use language properly in social settings may have helped to isolate them from their peers. Some may react by sliding quietly into depression and withdraw from contact with other people. Others may find acceptance in a dangerous crowd.

For these reasons, XXY males diagnosed as teenagers may need psychological counseling as well as help in overcoming their learning disabilities. Help with learning disabilities is available through public school systems for XXY males high-school age and under. Referrals to qualified mental health specialists may be obtained from family physicians.

Testosterone Treatment

Ideally, XXY males should begin testosterone treatment as they enter puberty. XXY males diagnosed in adulthood are also likely to benefit from the hormone. A regular schedule of testosterone injections will increase strength and muscle size, and promote the growth of facial and body hair.

In addition to these physical changes, testosterone injections often bring on psychological changes as well. As they begin to develop a more masculine appearance, the self-confidence of XXY males tends to increase. Many become more energetic and stop having sudden, angry changes in moods. What is not clear is whether these psychological changes are a direct result of testosterone treatment or are a side benefit of the increased self-confidence that the treatment may bring. As a group, XXY boys tend to suffer from depression, principally because of their scholastic difficulties and problems fitting in with other males their age. Sudden, angry changes in mood are typical of depressed people.

Other benefits of testosterone treatment may include decreased need for sleep, an enhanced ability to concentrate, and improved relations with others. But to obtain these benefits an XXY male must decide, on his own, that he is ready to stick to a regular schedule of injections.

Sometimes, younger adolescents, who may be somewhat immature, seem not quite ready to take the shots. It is an inconvenience, and many don't like needles.

Most physicians do not push the young men to take the injections. Instead, they usually recommend informing XXY adolescents and their parents about the benefits of testosterone injections and letting them take as much time as they need to make their decision.

Individuals may respond to testosterone treatment in different ways. Although the majority of XXY males ultimately will benefit from testosterone, a few will not.

To ensure that the injections will provide the maximum benefit, XXY males who are ready to begin testosterone injections should consult a qualified endocrinologist (a specialist in hormonal interactions) who has experience treating XXY males.

Side effects of the injections are few. Some individuals may develop a minor allergic reaction at the injection site, resulting in an itchy welt resembling a mosquito bite. Applying a nonprescription hydrocortisone cream to the area will reduce swelling and itching.

In addition, testosterone injections may result in a condition known as benign prostatic hyperplasia (BPH). This condition is common in chromosomally normal males as well, affecting more than 50 percent of men in their sixties, and as many as 90 percent in their seventies and eighties. In XXY males receiving testosterone injections, this condition may begin sometime after age forty.

The prostate is a small gland about the size of a walnut, which helps to manufacture semen. The gland is located just beneath the bladder and surrounds the urethra, the tube through which urine passes out of the body.

In BPH, the prostate increases in size, sometimes squeezing the bladder and urethra and causing difficulty urinating, "dribbling" after urination, and the need to urinate frequently.

XXY males receiving testosterone injections should consult their physicians about a regular schedule of prostate examinations. BPH can often be detected early by a rectal exam. If the prostate greatly interferes with the flow of urine, excess prostate tissue can be trimmed away by a surgical instrument that is inserted in the penis, through the urethra.

Chromosomal Variations

Occasionally, variations of the XXY chromosome count may occur, the most common being the XY/XXY mosaic. In this variation, some of the cells in the male's body have an additional X chromosome, and the rest have the normal XY chromosome count. The percentage of cells containing the extra chromosome varies from case to case. In some instances, XY/XXY mosaics may have enough normally functioning cells in the testes to allow them to father children.

A few instances of males having two or even three additional X chromosomes have also been reported in the medical literature. In these individuals, the classic features of Klinefelter syndrome may be exaggerated, with low IQ or moderate to severe mental retardation also occurring.

In rare instances, an individual may possess both an additional X and an additional Y chromosome. The medical literature describes

XXYY males as having slight to moderate mental retardation. They may sometimes be aggressive or even violent. Although they may have a rounded body type and decreased sex drive, experts disagree whether testosterone injections are appropriate for all of them.

One group of researchers reported that after receiving testosterone injections, an XXYY male stopped having violent sexual fantasies and ceased his assaults on teenaged girls. In contrast, Dr. Robinson found that testosterone injections seemed to make an XXYY boy he had been treating more aggressive.

Scientists admit, however, that because these cases are so rare, not much is known about them. Most of the XXYY males who have been studied were referred to treatment because they were violent and got into trouble with the law. It is not known whether XXYY males are inherently aggressive by nature, or whether only a few extreme individuals come to the attention of researchers precisely because they are aggressive.

Sexuality

The parents of XXY boys are sometimes concerned that their sons may grow up to be homosexual. This concern is unfounded, however, as there is no evidence that XXY males are any more inclined toward homosexuality than are other men.

In fact, the only significant sexual difference between XXY men and teenagers and other males their age is that the XXY males may have less interest in sex. However, regular injections of the male sex hormone testosterone can bring sex drive up to normal levels.

In some cases, testosterone injections lead to a false sense of security: After receiving the hormone for a time, XXY males may conclude they've derived as much benefit from it as possible and discontinue the injections. But when they do, their interest in sex almost invariably diminishes until they resume the injections.

Infertility

The vast majority of XXY males do not produce enough sperm to allow them to become fathers. If these men and their wives wish to become parents, they should seek counseling from their family physician regarding adoption and infertility.

However, no XXY male should automatically assume he is infertile without further testing. In a very small number of cases, XXY males have been able to father children.

In addition, a few individuals who believe themselves to be XXY males may actually be XY/XXY mosaics. Along with having cells with the XXY chromosome count, these males may also have cells with the normal XY chromosome count. If the number of XY cells in the testes is great enough, the individual should be able to father children.

Karyotyping, the method traditionally used to identify an individual's chromosome count, may sometimes fail to identify XY/XXY mosaics. For this reason, a karyotype should never be used to predict whether an individual will be infertile or not.

Health Considerations

Compared with other males, XXY males have a slightly increased risk of autoimmune disorders. In this group of diseases, the immune system, for unknown reasons, attacks the body's organs or tissues. The most well known of these diseases are type I (insulin-dependent) diabetes, autoimmune thyroiditis, and lupus erythematosus. Most of these conditions can be treated with medication.

XXY males with enlarged breasts have the same risk of breast cancer as do women—roughly fifty times the risk XY males have. For this reason, these XXY adolescents and men need to practice regular breast self-examination. XXY males may also wish to consult their physicians about the need for more thorough breast examinations by medical professionals.

In addition, XXY males who do not receive testosterone injections may have an increased risk of developing osteoporosis in later life. In this condition, which usually afflicts women after the age of menopause, the bones lose calcium, becoming brittle and more likely to break.

Adulthood

Unfortunately, comparatively little is known about XXY adults. Studies in the United States have focused largely on XXY males identified in infancy from large random samples. Only a few of these individuals have reached adulthood; most are still in adolescence. At this time, researchers simply do not know what kind of adults they will become.

"Some of them have really struggled through adolescence," said Dr. Bruce Bender, the psychologist for the NICHD-sponsored study of XXY males. "But we don't know whether they'll have serious problems in adulthood, or, like many troubled teenagers, overcome their problems and lead productive lives."

Comparatively few studies of XXY males diagnosed in adulthood have been conducted. By and large, the men who took part in these studies were not selected at random but identified by a particular characteristic, such as height. For this reason, it is not known whether these individuals are truly representative of XXY men as a whole or represent a particular extreme.

One study found a group of XXY males diagnosed between the ages of twenty-seven and thirty-seven to have suffered a number of setbacks, in comparison to a similar group of XY males. The XXY men were more likely to have had histories of scholastic failure, depression, and other psychological problems, and to lack energy and enthusiasm.

But by the time the XXY men had reached their forties, most had surmounted their problems. The majority said that their energy and activity levels had increased, that they were more productive on the job, and that their relationships with other people had improved. In fact, the only difference between the XY males and the XXY males was that the latter were less likely to have been married.

That these men eventually overcame their troubled pasts is encouraging for all XXY males and particularly encouraging for those diagnosed in childhood. Had they received counseling, support, and testosterone treatments beginning in childhood, these men might have avoided the difficulties of their twenties and thirties.

Although a supportive environment through childhood and adolescence appears to offer the greatest chance for a well-adjusted adulthood, it is not too late for XXY men diagnosed as adults to seek help.

Research has shown that testosterone injections, begun in adulthood, can be beneficial. Psychological counseling also offers the best hope of overcoming depression and other psychological problems. For referrals to endocrinologists qualified to administer testosterone or to mental health specialists, XXY men should consult their physicians.

Chapter 41

Prader-Willi Syndrome

What is Prader-Willi syndrome (PWS)?

PWS is a complex genetic disorder that typically causes low muscle tone, short stature, incomplete sexual development, cognitive disabilities, problem behaviors, and a chronic feeling of hunger that can lead to excessive eating and life-threatening obesity.

Is PWS inherited?

Most cases of PWS are attributed to a spontaneous genetic error that occurs at or near the time of conception for unknown reasons. In a very small percentage of cases (2 percent or less), a genetic mutation that does not affect the parent is passed on to the child, and in these families more than one child may be affected. A PWS-like disorder can also be acquired after birth if the hypothalamic portion of the brain is damaged through injury or surgery. All families with a child diagnosed with PWS should see a geneticist for genetic counseling in order to fully understand their chances of having another child with PWS.

How common is PWS?

It is estimated that one in twelve thousand to fifteen thousand people has PWS. Although considered a "rare" disorder, Prader-Willi

"Questions and Answers on Prader-Willi Syndrome," © 2008 Prader-Willi Syndrome Association. Reprinted with permission. For additional information and resources for support, visit www.pwsausa.org, or call the toll-free helpline at 800-926-4797.

syndrome is one of the most common conditions seen in genetics clinics and is the most common genetic cause of obesity that has been identified. PWS is found in people of both sexes and all races.

How is PWS diagnosed?

Suspicion of the diagnosis is first assessed clinically, then confirmed by specialized genetic testing on a blood sample. Formal diagnostic criteria for the clinical recognition of PWS have been published (Holm et al, 1993), as have laboratory testing guidelines for PWS (ASHG, 1996).

What is known about the genetic abnormality?

Basically, the occurrence of PWS is due to lack of several genes on one of an individual's two chromosome 15s— the one normally contributed by the father. In the majority of cases, there is a deletion— the critical genes are somehow lost from the chromosome. In most of the remaining cases, the entire chromosome from the father is missing and there are instead two chromosome 15s from the mother (uniparental disomy). The critical paternal genes lacking in people with PWS have a role in the regulation of appetite. This is an area of active research in a number of laboratories around the world, since understanding this defect may be very helpful not only to those with PWS but to understanding obesity in otherwise normal people.

What causes the appetite and obesity problems in PWS?

People with PWS have a flaw in the hypothalamus part of their brain, which normally registers feelings of hunger and satiety. While the problem is not yet fully understood, it is apparent that people with this flaw never feel full; they have a continuous urge to eat that they cannot learn to control. To compound this problem, people with PWS need less food than their peers without the syndrome because their bodies have less muscle and tend to burn fewer calories.

Does the overeating associated with PWS begin at birth?

No. In fact, newborns with PWS often cannot get enough nourishment because low muscle tone impairs their sucking ability. Many require special feeding techniques or tube feeding for several months after birth, until muscle control improves. Sometime in the following years, usually before school age, children with PWS develop an intense interest in food and can quickly gain excess weight if calories are not restricted.

Do diet medications work for the appetite problem in PWS?

Unfortunately, no appetite suppressant has worked consistently for people with PWS. Most require an extremely low-calorie diet all their lives and must have their environment designed so that they have very limited access to food. For example, many families have to lock the kitchen or the cabinets and refrigerator. As adults, most affected individuals can control their weight best in a group home designed specifically for people with PWS, where food access can be restricted without interfering with the rights of those who don't need such restriction.

What kinds of behavior problems do people with PWS have?

In addition to their involuntary focus on food, people with PWS tend to have obsessive/compulsive behaviors that are not related to food, such as repetitive thoughts and verbalizations, collecting and hoarding of possessions, picking at skin irritations, and a strong need for routine and predictability. Frustration or changes in plans can easily set off a loss of emotional control in someone with PWS, ranging from tears to temper tantrums to physical aggression. While psychotropic medications can help some individuals, the essential strategies for minimizing difficult behaviors in PWS are careful structuring of the person's environment and consistent use of positive behavior management and supports.

Does early diagnosis help?

While there is no medical prevention or cure, early diagnosis of Prader-Willi syndrome gives parents time to learn about and prepare for the challenges that lie ahead and to establish family routines that will support their child's diet and behavior needs from the start. Knowing the cause of their child's developmental delays can facilitate a family's access to important early intervention services and may help program staff identify areas of specific need or risk. Additionally, a diagnosis of PWS opens the doors to a network of information and support from professionals and other families who are dealing with the syndrome.

What does the future hold for people with PWS?

With help, people with PWS can expect to accomplish many of the things their "normal" peers do—complete school, achieve in their outside areas of interest, be successfully employed, even move away from their family home. They do, however, need a significant amount of support from their families and from school, work, and residential service providers to both achieve these goals and avoid obesity and the serious health consequences that accompany it. Even those with IQs in the normal range need lifelong diet supervision and protection from food availability.

Although in the past many people with PWS died in adolescence or young adulthood, prevention of obesity can enable those with the syndrome to live a normal lifespan. New medications, including psychotropic drugs and synthetic growth hormone, are already improving the quality of life for some people with PWS. Ongoing research offers the hope of new discoveries that will enable people affected by this unusual condition to live more independent lives.

Chapter 42

Smith-Magenis Syndrome

What is Smith-Magenis syndrome?

Smith-Magenis syndrome is a developmental disorder that affects many parts of the body. The major features of this condition include mild to moderate mental retardation, delayed speech and language skills, distinctive facial features, sleep disturbances, and behavioral problems.

Most people with Smith-Magenis syndrome have a broad, square-shaped face with deep-set eyes, full cheeks, and a prominent lower jaw. The middle of the face and the bridge of the nose often appear flattened. The mouth tends to turn downward with a full, outward-curving upper lip. These facial differences can be subtle in early childhood, but they usually become more distinctive in later childhood and adulthood. Dental abnormalities are also common in affected individuals.

Disrupted sleep patterns are characteristic of Smith-Magenis syndrome, typically beginning early in life. Affected people may be very sleepy during the day, but have trouble falling asleep and awaken several times each night.

People with Smith-Magenis syndrome have affectionate, engaging personalities, but most also have behavioral problems. These include frequent temper tantrums and outbursts, aggression, anxiety, impulsiveness, and difficulty paying attention. Self-injury, including biting,

Excerpted from "Smith-Magenis Syndrome," *Genetics Home Reference*, a service of the U.S. National Library of Medicine, February 2007.

hitting, head banging, and skin picking, is very common. Repetitive self-hugging is a behavioral trait that may be unique to Smith-Magenis syndrome. People with this condition also compulsively lick their fingers and flip pages of books and magazines (a behavior known as "lick and flip").

Other signs and symptoms of Smith-Magenis syndrome include short stature, abnormal curvature of the spine (scoliosis), reduced sensitivity to pain and temperature, and a hoarse voice. Some people with this disorder have ear abnormalities that lead to hearing loss. Affected individuals may have eye abnormalities that cause nearsightedness (myopia) and other vision problems. Although less common, heart and kidney defects also have been reported in people with Smith-Magenis syndrome.

How common is Smith-Magenis syndrome?

Smith-Magenis syndrome affects at least one in twenty-five thousand individuals worldwide. Researchers believe that many people with this condition are not diagnosed, however, so the true prevalence may be closer to one in fifteen thousand individuals.

What are the genetic changes related to Smith-Magenis syndrome?

Smith-Magenis syndrome is related to chromosome 17.
Mutations in the RAI1 gene cause Smith-Magenis syndrome.
Most people with Smith-Magenis syndrome have a deletion of genetic material from a specific region of chromosome 17. Although this region contains multiple genes, researchers believe that the loss of one particular gene, RAI1, in each cell is responsible for most of the characteristic features of this condition. The loss of other genes in the deleted region may help explain why the features of Smith-Magenis syndrome vary among affected individuals.

A small percentage of people with Smith-Magenis syndrome have a mutation in the RAI1 gene instead of a chromosomal deletion. Although these individuals have many of the major features of the condition, they are less likely than people with a chromosomal deletion to have short stature, hearing loss, and heart or kidney abnormalities. The RAI1 gene provides instructions for making a protein whose function is unknown. Mutations in one copy of this gene lead to the production of a nonfunctional version of the RAI1 protein or reduce the amount of this protein that is produced in cells. Researchers are uncertain how changes in this protein result in the physical, mental, and behavioral problems associated with Smith-Magenis syndrome.

Can Smith-Magenis syndrome be inherited?

Smith-Magenis syndrome is typically not inherited. This condition usually results from a genetic change that occurs during the formation of reproductive cells (eggs or sperm) or in early fetal development. Most often, people with Smith-Magenis syndrome have no history of the condition in their family.

Chapter 43

Turner Syndrome

What is Turner syndrome?

Turner syndrome is a chromosomal condition that alters development in females. Women with this condition tend to be shorter than average and are usually unable to conceive a child (infertile) because of an absence of ovarian function. Other features of this condition that can vary among women who have Turner syndrome include: extra skin on the neck (webbed neck), puffiness or swelling (lymphedema) of the hands and feet, skeletal abnormalities, heart defects, and kidney problems.

This condition occurs in about 1 in 2,500 female births worldwide, but is much more common among pregnancies that do not survive to term (miscarriages and stillbirths).

Turner syndrome is a chromosomal condition related to the X chromosome.

Researchers have not yet determined which genes on the X chromosome are responsible for most signs and symptoms of Turner syndrome. They have, however, identified one gene called SHOX that is important for bone development and growth. Missing one copy of this gene likely causes short stature and skeletal abnormalities in women with Turner syndrome.

Reprinted from "Learning about Turner Syndrome," National Human Genome Research Institute, National Institutes of Health, May 29, 2008.

What are the symptoms of Turner syndrome?

Girls who have Turner syndrome are shorter than average. They often have normal height for the first three years of life, but then have a slow growth rate. At puberty they do not have the usual growth spurt.

Nonfunctioning ovaries are another symptom of Turner syndrome. Normally a girl's ovaries begin to produce sex hormones (estrogen and progesterone) at puberty. This does not happen in most girls who have Turner syndrome. They do not start their periods or develop breasts without hormone treatment at the age of puberty.

Even though many women who have Turner have nonfunctioning ovaries and are infertile, their vagina and womb are totally normal.

In early childhood, girls who have Turner syndrome may have frequent middle ear infections. Recurrent infections can lead to hearing loss in some cases.

Girls with Turner syndrome are usually of normal intelligence with good verbal skills and reading skills. Some girls, however, have problems with math, memory skills, and fine-finger movements.

Additional symptoms of Turner syndrome include the following:

- An especially wide neck (webbed neck) and a low or indistinct hairline.

- A broad chest and widely spaced nipples.

- Arms that turn out slightly at the elbow.

- A heart murmur, sometimes associated with narrowing of the aorta (blood vessel exiting the heart).

- A tendency to develop high blood pressure (so this should be checked regularly).

- Minor eye problems that are corrected by glasses.

- Scoliosis (deformity of the spine) occurs in 10 percent of adolescent girls who have Turner syndrome.

- The thyroid gland becomes underactive in about 10 percent of women who have Turner syndrome. Regular blood tests are necessary to detect it early and if necessary treat with thyroid replacement.

- Older or overweight women with Turner syndrome are slightly more at risk of developing diabetes.

- Osteoporosis can develop because of a lack of estrogen, but this can largely be prevented by taking hormone replacement therapy.

How is Turner syndrome diagnosed?

A diagnosis of Turner syndrome may be suspected when there are a number of typical physical features observed such as webbed neck, a broad chest, and widely spaced nipples. Sometimes diagnosis is made at birth because of heart problems, an unusually wide neck, or swelling of the hands and feet.

The two main clinical features of Turner syndrome are short stature and the lack of the development of the ovaries.

Many girls are diagnosed in early childhood when a slow growth rate and other features are identified. Diagnosis sometimes takes place later when puberty does not occur.

Turner syndrome may be suspected in pregnancy during an ultrasound test. This can be confirmed by prenatal testing—chorionic villous sampling or amniocentesis—to obtain cells from the unborn baby for chromosomal analysis. If a diagnosis is confirmed prenatally, the baby may be under the care of a specialist pediatrician immediately after birth.

Diagnosis is confirmed by a blood test, called a karyotype. This is used to analyze the chromosomal composition of the female.

What is the treatment for Turner syndrome?

During childhood and adolescence, girls may be under the care of a pediatric endocrinologist, who is a specialist in childhood conditions of the hormones and metabolism.

Growth hormone injections are beneficial in some individuals with Turner syndrome. Injections often begin in early childhood and may increase final adult height by a few inches.

Estrogen replacement therapy is usually started at the time of normal puberty, around twelve years to start breast development. Estrogen and progesterone are given a little later to begin a monthly "period," which is necessary to keep the womb healthy. Estrogen is also given to prevent osteoporosis.

Babies born with a heart murmur or narrowing of the aorta may need surgery to correct the problem. A heart expert (cardiologist) will assess and follow up any treatment necessary.

Girls who have Turner syndrome are more likely to get middle ear infections. Repeated infections may lead to hearing loss and should be evaluated by the pediatrician. An ear, nose, and throat specialist (ENT) may be involved in caring for this health issue.

High blood pressure is quite common in women who have Turner syndrome. In some cases, the elevated blood pressure is due to narrowing of the aorta or a kidney abnormality. However, most of the time, no specific cause for the elevation is identified. Blood pressure should be checked routinely and, if necessary, treated with medication. Women who have Turner syndrome have a slightly higher risk of having an underactive thyroid or developing diabetes. This should also be monitored during routine health maintenance visits and treated if necessary.

Regular health checks are very important. Special clinics for the care of girls and women who have Turner syndrome are available in some areas, with access to a variety of specialists. Early preventive care and treatment is very important.

Almost all women with Turner syndrome are infertile, but pregnancy with donor embryos may be possible.

Having appropriate medical treatment and support allows a woman with Turner syndrome to lead a normal, healthy, and happy life.

Is Turner syndrome inherited?

Turner syndrome is not usually inherited in families. Turner syndrome occurs when one of the two X chromosomes normally found in women is missing or incomplete. Although the exact cause of Turner syndrome is not known, it appears to occur as a result of a random error during the formation of either the eggs or sperm.

Humans have forty-six chromosomes, which contain all of a person's genes and deoxyribonucleic acid (DNA). Two of these chromosomes, the sex chromosomes, determine a person's gender. Both of the sex chromosomes in females are called X chromosomes. (This is written as XX.) Males have an X and a Y chromosome (written as XY). The two sex chromosomes help a person develop fertility and the sexual characteristics of their gender.

In Turner syndrome, the girl does not have the usual pair of two complete X chromosomes. The most common scenario is that the girl has only one X chromosome in her cells. Some girls with Turner syndrome do have two X chromosomes, but one of the X chromosomes is incomplete. In another scenario, the girl has some cells in her body with two X chromosomes, but other cells have only one. This is called mosaicism.

Chapter 44

Williams Syndrome

Alternative Names

Williams-Beuren syndrome

Definition

Williams syndrome is a rare genetic disorder that can lead to problems with development.

Causes

Williams syndrome is a rare condition caused by missing genes. Parents may not have any family history of the condition. However, a person with Williams syndrome has a 50 percent chance of passing the disorder on to each of his or her children. The cause usually occurs randomly.

Williams syndrome occurs in about one in eight thousand births.

One of the twenty-five missing genes is the gene that produces elastin, a protein that allows blood vessels and other tissues in the body to stretch. It is likely that having only one copy of this gene results in the narrowing of blood vessels seen in this condition.

Symptoms

- Delayed speech that may later turn into strong speaking ability and strong learning by hearing

- Developmental delay

- Easily distracted, attention deficit disorder (ADD)

- Feeding problems including colic, reflux, and vomiting

- Inward bend of the small finger (clinodactyly)

- Learning disorders

- Mild to moderate mental retardation

- Narrowing of the large artery that leaves the heart (aorta)

- Personality traits including being very friendly, trusting strangers, fearing loud sounds or physical contact, and being interested in music

- Short compared to the rest of the person's family

- Slack joints that may change to stiffness as patient gets older

- Sunken chest (pectus excavatum)

- Unusual appearance of the face

- Flattened nasal bridge with small upturned nose

- Long ridges in the skin that run from the nose to the upper lip (philtrum)

- Prominent lips with an open mouth

- Skin that covers the inner corner of the eye (epicanthal folds)

- Partially missing teeth, defective tooth enamel, or small, widely spaced teeth

Exams and Tests

Signs include:

- blood vessel narrowing including supravalvular aortic stenosis, pulmonary stenosis, and pulmonary artery stenosis;

- farsightedness;

- high blood calcium level (hypercalcemia) that may cause seizures and rigid muscles;

- high blood pressure;

- unusual pattern ("stellate" or star-like) in iris of the eye.

Tests for Williams syndrome:

- blood pressure check;

- blood test for missing chromosome (fluorescence in situ hybridization [FISH] test);

- echocardiography combined with Doppler ultrasound;

- kidney ultrasound.

Treatment

There is no cure for Williams syndrome. Avoid taking extra calcium and vitamin D. Treat high levels of blood calcium if present. Blood vessel narrowing can be a significant health problem and is treated based on how severe it is.

Physical therapy is helpful to patients with joint stiffness. Developmental and speech therapy can also help these children; for example, verbal strengths can help make up for other weaknesses. Other treatments are based on a patient's symptoms.

It can help to have treatment coordinated by a geneticist who is experienced with Williams syndrome.

Outlook (Prognosis)

About 75 percent of those with Williams syndrome have some mental retardation.

Most patients will not live as long as normal, due to complications.

Most patients require full-time caregivers and often live in supervised group homes.

Possible Complications

- Calcium deposits in the kidney and other kidney problems

- Death (in rare cases from anesthesia)

- Heart failure due to narrowed blood vessels
- Pain in the abdomen

When to Contact a Medical Professional

Many of the symptoms and signs of Williams syndrome may not be obvious at birth. Call your health care provider if your child has features similar to those of Williams syndrome. Seek genetic counseling if you have a family history of Williams syndrome.

Prevention

There is no known way to prevent the genetic problem that causes Williams syndrome. Prenatal testing is available for couples with a family history of Williams syndrome who wish to conceive.

Part Four

Complex Disorders with Genetic and Environmental Components

Chapter 45

Gene-Environment
Interaction in Human Disease

Virtually all human diseases result from the interaction of genetic susceptibility factors and modifiable environmental factors, broadly defined to include infectious, chemical, physical, nutritional, and behavioral factors.

This is perhaps the most important fact in understanding the role of genetics and environment in the development of disease. Many people tend to classify the cause of disease as either genetic or environmental. Indeed, some rare diseases, such as Huntington or Tay-Sachs disease, may be the result of a deficiency of a single gene product, but these diseases represent a very small proportion of all human disease. Common diseases, such as diabetes or cancer, are a result of the complex interplay of genetic and environmental factors.

Genetic Variations

Variations in genetic makeup are associated with almost all disease. Even so-called single-gene disorders actually develop from the interaction of both genetic and environmental factors. For example, phenylketonuria (PKU) results from a genetic variant that leads to deficient metabolism of the amino acid phenylalanine; in the presence of normal protein intake, phenylalanine accumulates and is neurotoxic. PKU occurs only when both the genetic variant (phenylalanine

Reprinted from "Gene-Environment Interaction Fact Sheet," Centers for Disease Control and Prevention, November 27, 2007.

hydroxylase deficiency) and the environmental exposure (dietary phenylalanine) are present.

Environmental Factors

Genetic variations do not cause disease but rather influence a person's susceptibility to environmental factors. We do not inherit a disease state per se. Instead, we inherit a set of a susceptibility factors to certain effects of environmental factors and therefore inherit a higher risk for certain diseases. This concept also explains why individuals are differently affected by the same environmental factors. For example, some health-conscious individuals with "acceptable" cholesterol levels suffer myocardial infarction at age forty. Other individuals seem immune to heart disease in spite of smoking, poor diet, and obesity. Genetic variations account, at least in part, for this difference in response to the same environmental factors.

Intervention Strategies

Genetic information can be used to target interventions. We all carry genetic variants that increase our susceptibility to some diseases. By identifying and characterizing gene-environment interactions, we have more opportunities to effectively target intervention strategies. Many of the genetic risk factors for diseases have not been identified, and the complex interaction of genes with other genes and genes with environmental factors is not yet understood. Clinical and epidemiological studies are necessary to further describe these factors and their interactions. However, as our understanding of genetic variations increases, so should our knowledge of environmental factors, so that ultimately, genetic information can be used to plan appropriate intervention strategies for high-risk individuals.

Chapter 46

Genetics and Addiction

Chapter Contents

Section 46.1

The Genetics of Alcoholism

Excerpted from "The Genetics of Alcoholism," National Institute on Alcohol Abuse and Alcoholism, National Institutes of Health, July 2003. Reviewed by David A. Cooke, M.D., FACP, July 2009.

Research has shown conclusively that familial transmission of alcoholism risk is at least in part genetic and not just the result of family environment.[1] The task of current science is to identify what a person inherits that increases vulnerability to alcoholism and how inherited factors interact with the environment to cause disease. This information will provide the basis for identifying people at risk and for developing behavioral and pharmacologic approaches to prevent and treat alcohol problems.

A Complex Genetic Disease

Studies in recent years have confirmed that identical twins, who share the same genes, are about twice as likely as fraternal twins, who share on average 50 percent of their genes, to resemble each other in terms of the presence of alcoholism. Recent research also reports that 50 to 60 percent of the risk for alcoholism is genetically determined, for both men and women.[2–5] Genes alone do not preordain that someone will be alcoholic; features in the environment along with gene-environment interactions account for the remainder of the risk.

Research suggests that many genes play a role in shaping alcoholism risk. Like diabetes and heart disease, alcoholism is considered genetically complex, distinguishing it from genetic diseases, such as cystic fibrosis, that result primarily from the action of one or two copies of a single gene and in which the environment plays a much smaller role, if any. The methods used to search for genes in complex diseases have to account for the fact that the effects of any one gene may be subtle and a different array of genes underlies risk in different people.

Scientists have bred lines of mice and rats that manifest specific and separate alcohol-related traits or phenotypes, such as sensitivity to alcohol's intoxicating and sedative effects, the development of tolerance, the susceptibility to withdrawal symptoms, and alcohol-related organ damage.[6,7] Risk for alcoholism in humans reflects the mix and magnitude of these and other phenotypes, shaped by underlying genes, in interaction with an environment in which alcohol is available. Genetic research on alcoholism seeks to tease apart the genetic underpinnings of these phenotypes and how they contribute to risk.

One well-characterized relationship between genes and alcoholism is the result of variation in the liver enzymes that metabolize (break down) alcohol. By speeding up the metabolism of alcohol to a toxic intermediate, acetaldehyde, or slowing down the conversion of acetaldehyde to acetate, genetic variants in the enzymes alcohol dehydrogenase (ADH) or aldehyde dehydrogenase (ALDH) raise the level of acetaldehyde after drinking, causing symptoms that include flushing, nausea, and rapid heartbeat. The genes for these enzymes and the alleles, or gene variants, that alter alcohol metabolism have been identified. Genes associated with flushing are more common among Asian populations than other ethnic groups, and the rates of drinking and alcoholism are correspondingly lower among Asian populations.[8,9]

Genes, Behavior, and the Brain

Addiction is based in the brain. It involves memory, motivation, and emotional state. The processes involved in these aspects of brain function have thus been logical targets for the search for genes that underlie risk for alcoholism. Much of the information on potential alcohol-related genes has come from research on animals. Research has demonstrated a similarity in the mechanisms of many brain functions across species as well as an overlap between the genomes of animals—even invertebrates—and humans.

One approach to identifying alcohol-related genes is to start with an aspect of brain chemistry on which alcohol is thought to have an impact, and work forward, identifying and manipulating the underlying genes and ultimately determining whether the presence or absence of different forms, or alleles, of a gene influence alcoholism risk. For example, genetic technology now permits scientists to delete or inactivate specific genes, or alternatively, to increase the expression of specific genes, and watch the effects in living animals. Because genes act in the context of many other genes, interpretation of these studies can be difficult. If one gene is disabled, for example, others may compensate for the loss of function. Alternatively, the loss of a single gene throughout development may be harmful or lethal. Nonetheless, these techniques can provide important clues to function. These approaches have been used to study how altering the expression of genes encoding the receptors (or their subunits) for neurotransmitters and intracellular messenger molecules alters the response to alcohol.[10]

Scientists also have an increasing array of methods for locating alcohol-related genes and gene locations and only then determining how the genes function, an approach known as reverse genetics. Quantitative trait loci (QTL) analysis seeks to identify stretches of deoxyribonucleic acid (DNA) along chromosomes that influence traits, like alcohol sensitivity, that vary along a spectrum (height is another quantitative trait). QTLs have been identified for alcohol sensitivity, alcohol preference, and withdrawal severity.[11] Ultimately, the goal is to identify and determine which candidate genes within the QTLs are responsible for the observed trait. Among the candidate genes already known to lie near alcohol-related QTLs are several that encode neurotransmitter receptors and neurotransmitters themselves. One of these, neuropeptide Y (NPY), lies within a QTL for alcohol preference in rats. NPY is a small protein molecule that is abundant in the brain and has been shown to influence the response to alcohol.[12]

Scientists also can scan the genome to identify genes whose activity differs among animals that respond differently to alcohol. The methods used are designed to measure the amount of messenger RNA, which, as the first intermediary in the process by which DNA is translated into protein, is a reflection of gene expression. The advantage of this approach is its power to survey the activities of thousands of genes, some of which might not otherwise have been identified as candidates for involvement in alcohol-related behavior. Recent work in rats identified a gene that is differentially expressed in brain regions of alcohol-preferring rats and nonpreferring rats. The gene is within an already identified QTL for alcohol preference and codes for alpha-synuclein, a protein that has been shown to regulate dopamine transmission.[13]

Genetic Studies in Humans

Knowledge gained from animal studies has assisted scientists in identifying the genes underlying brain chemistry in humans. Much research suggests that genes affecting the activity of the neurotransmitters serotonin and GABA (gamma-aminobutyric acid) are likely candidates for involvement in alcoholism risk. A recent preliminary study looked at five genes related to these two neurotransmitters in a group of men who had been followed over a fifteen-year period.[14] The men who had particular variants of genes for a serotonin transporter and for one type of GABA receptor showed lower response to alcohol at age twenty and were more likely to have met the criteria for alcoholism. Another study found that college students with a particular variant of the serotonin transporter gene consumed more alcohol per occasion, more often drank expressly to become inebriated, and engaged more frequently in binge drinking than students with another variant of the gene.[15] The relationships between neurotransmitter genes and alcoholism are complex, however; not all studies have shown a connection between alcoholism risk and these genes.

Individual variation in response to stressors such as pain is genetically influenced and helps shape susceptibility to psychiatric diseases, including alcoholism. Scientists recently found that a common genetic variation in an enzyme (catechol-0-methyltransferase) that metabolizes the neurotransmitters dopamine and norepinephrine results in a less efficient form of the enzyme and increased pain susceptibility.[16] Scientists in another study found that the same genetic variant influences anxiety in women. In this study, women who had the enzyme variant scored higher on measures of anxiety and exhibited an electroencephalogram (EEG) pattern associated with anxiety disorders and alcoholism.[17]

The drug naltrexone has been shown to help some, but not all, alcohol-dependent patients reduce their drinking. Preliminary results from a recent study showed that alcoholic patients with different variations in the gene for a receptor on which naltrexone is known to act (the mu-opioid receptor) responded differently to treatment with the drug.[18] This work demonstrates how genetic typing may in the future be helpful in tailoring treatment for alcoholism to each individual.

The National Institute on Alcohol Abuse and Alcoholism's (NIAAA's) Collaborative Study on the Genetics of Alcoholism (COGA) is searching for alcohol-related genes through studies of families with multiple generations of alcoholism. Using existing markers—known variations in the DNA sequence that serve as signposts along the length of a chromosome—and observing to what extent specific markers are inherited along with alcoholism risk, they have found "hotspots" for alcoholism risk on five chromosomes and a protective area on one chromosome near the location of genes for alcohol dehydrogenase.[19] They have also examined patterns of brain waves measured by electroencephalogram. EEGs measure differences in electrical potential across the brain caused by synchronized firing of many neurons. Brain wave patterns are characteristic to individuals and are shaped genetically—they are quantitative genetic traits, varying along a spectrum among individuals. COGA researchers have found that reduced amplitude of one wave that characteristically occurs after a stimulus correlates with alcohol dependence, and they have identified chromosomal regions that appear to affect this P300 wave amplitude.[20] Recently, COGA researchers found that the shape of a characteristic brain wave measured in the frequency stretch between 13 and 25 cycles per second (the "beta" wave) reflected gene variations at a specific chromosomal site containing genes for one type of GABA receptor.[21] They suggest that this site is in or near a previously identified QTL for alcoholism risk. Thus, brain wave patterns reflect underlying genetic variation in a receptor for a neurotransmitter known to be involved in the brain's response to alcohol. Findings of this type promise to help researchers identify markers of alcoholism risk and ultimately, suggest ways to reduce the risk or to treat the disease pharmacologically.

References

1. National Institute on Alcohol Abuse and Alcoholism (NIAAA). The Genetics of Alcoholism. *Alcohol Alert* No. 18. Rockville, MD: NIAAA, 1992.

2. Heath, A.C.; Bucholz, K.K.; Madden, P.A.F.; et al. Genetic and environmental contributions to alcohol dependence risk in a national twin sample: Consistency of findings in women and men. *Psychological Medicine* 27:1381–96, 1997.

3. Heath, A.C., and Martin, N.G. Genetic influences on alcohol consumption patterns and problem drinking: Results from the Australian NH&MRC twin panel follow–up survey. *Annals of the New York Academy of Sciences* 708:72–85, 1994.

4. Kendler, K.S.; Neale, M.C.; Heath, A.C.; et al. A twin-family study of alcoholism in women. *American Journal of Psychiatry* 151:707–15, 1994.

5. Prescott, C.A., and Kendler, K.S. Genetic and environmental contributions to alcohol abuse and dependence in a population–based sample of male twins. *American Journal of Psychiatry* 156: 34–40, 1999.

6. Crabbe, J.C. Alcohol and genetics: New models. *American Journal of Medical Genetics (Neuropsychiatric Genetics)* 114:969–74, 2002.

7. Tabakoff, B., and Hoffman, P.L. Animal models in alcohol research. *Alcohol Research & Health* 24(2):77–84, 2000.

8. Li, T.K. Pharmacogenetics of responses to alcohol and genes that influence alcohol drinking. *Journal of Studies on Alcohol* 61:5–12, 2000.

9. Makimoto, K. Drinking patterns and drinking problems among Asian–Americans and Pacific Islanders. *Alcohol Health & Research World* 22(4):270–75, 1998.

10. Bowers, B.J. Applications of transgenic and knockout mice in alcohol research. *Alcohol Research & Health* 24(3):175–84, 2000.

11. Crabbe, J.C.; Phillips, T.J.; Buck, K.J.; et al. Identifying genes for alcohol and drug sensitivity: Recent progress and future directions. *Trends in Neurosciences* 22(4):173–79, 1999.

12. Pandey, S.C.; Carr, L.G.; Heilig, M.; et al. Neuropeptide Y and alcoholism: Genetic, molecular, and pharmacological evidence. *Alcoholism: Clinical and Experimental Research* 27:149–54, 2003.

13. Liang, T.; Spence, J.; Liu, L.; et al. α-Synuclein maps to a quantitative trait locus for alcohol preference and is differentially expressed in alcohol-preferring and -nonpreferring rats. *Proceedings of the National Academy of Sciences of the U.S.A.* 100(8): 4690–95, 2003.

14. Schuckit, M.A.; Mazzanti, C.; Smith, T.L.; et al. Selective genotyping for the role of 5-HT2A, 5-HT2C, and GABAα6 receptors and the serotonin transporter in the level of response to alcohol: A pilot study. *Biological Psychiatry* 45: 647–51, 1999.

15. Herman, A.I.; Philbeck, J.W.; Vasilopoulos, N.L.; and Depetrillo, P.B. Serotonin transporter promoter polymorphism and differences in alcohol consumption behaviour in a college student population. *Alcohol and Alcoholism* 38: 446–49, 2003.

16. Zubieta, J.–K.; Heitzeg, M.M.; Smith, Y.R.; et al. COMT val158met genotype affects μ-opioid neurotransmitter responses to a pain stressor. *Science* 299:1240–43, 2003.

17. Enoch, M.A.; Xu, K.; Ferro, E.; et al. Genetic origins of anxiety in women: A role for a functional catechol-O-methyltransferase polymorphism. *Psychiatric Genetics* 13(1):33–41, 2003.

18. Oslin, D.W.; Berrettini, W.; Kranzler, H.R.; et al. A functional polymorphism of the µ-opioid receptor gene is associated with naltrexone response in alcohol-dependent patients. *Neuropsychopharmacology* 28:1546–52, 2003.

19. Edenberg, H.J. The collaborative study on the genetics of alcoholism: An update. *Alcohol Research & Health* 26(3):214–17, 2002.

20. Begleiter, H.; Porjesz, B.; Reich, T.; et al. Quantitative trait loci analysis of human event–related brain potentials: P3 voltage. *Electroencephalography and Clinical Neurophysiology* 103(3):244–50, 1998.

21. Porjesz, B.; Almasy, L.; Edenberg, H.J.; et al. Linkage disequilibrium between the beta frequency of the human EEG and a GABAA receptor gene locus. *Proceedings of the National Academy of Sciences of the U.S.A.* 99:3729–33, 2002.

Section 46.2

Genetic Trait Linked to Alcoholism

Variations in the genetic makeup of alcoholics may affect how much they drink, a new study suggests.

And the key might be the brain's control of serotonin, a mood-influencing neurological chemical.

The research could potentially help doctors understand who might be at highest risk of becoming an alcoholic, and then treat that person, said study co-author Ming D. Li, head of neurobiology at the University of Virginia.

Li added that the research is unique, because it shows that a single gene variation is connected to a kind of behavior—alcoholism.

The genetic blueprint that people inherit from their parents accounts for an estimated 40 percent to 50 percent of a person's risk of becoming alcoholic, said Dr. Robert Philibert, director of the Laboratory of Psychiatric Genetics at the University of Iowa.

The interplay between genetic makeup and environmental factors is responsible for the rest of the risk, said Philibert, who's familiar with the new study's findings.

"This study really takes the next step down the line," he said, in understanding the role that genes play in alcoholism.

For the study, the researchers looked at the deoxyribonucleic acid (DNA) of 275 alcoholics who had sought treatment. Almost 80 percent were men, and all were of European descent. The researchers found that differences in the genes that affect serotonin levels in the brain coincided with the amount of alcohol consumed by the drinkers.

The findings were published online November 20, 2008, and were expected to be in the February 2009 issue of *Alcoholism: Clinical & Experimental Research.*

Scientists think serotonin, a neurotransmitter, is crucial to human moods and emotions as well as things like sleep. Low levels of serotonin can lead to depression; some antidepressants aim to help the brain do a better job of processing serotonin.

"We know that serotonin is critical to maintaining a positive sense of self and for controlling our anxiety," Philibert said. That could explain a possible connection between serotonin levels and alcoholism, he added.

Li cautioned, however, that it's unlikely that a single genetic trait by itself would make someone more susceptible to alcoholism. It's more likely that a genetic variation works with other genes to raise the risk, he said.

Philibert said research might lead to a day when doctors could look at an alcoholic's genetic traits and discover whether antidepressants could help that person.

Doctors, he said, might say, "You have this genotype and you drink a lot, so you may benefit from a drug like Prozac®."

Section 46.3

Genetics of Addiction: A Research Update

Reprinted from "Genetics of Addiction," National Institute of Drug Abuse, National Institutes of Health, April 2008.

Genetics: The Blueprint of Health and Disease

Why do some people become addicted, while others do not? Studies of identical twins indicate that as much as half of an individual's risk of becoming addicted to nicotine, alcohol, or other drugs depends on his or her genes. Pinning down the biological basis for this risk is an important avenue of research for scientists trying to solve the problem of drug abuse.

Genes—functional units that make up our DNA (deoxyribonucleic acid)—provide the information that directs our bodies' basic cellular activities. Research on the human genome has shown that the DNA sequences of any two individuals are 99.9 percent identical. However, that 0.1 percent variation is profoundly important, contributing to visible differences, like height and hair color, and to invisible differences, such as increased risks for, or protection from, heart attack, stroke, diabetes, and addiction.

Some diseases, like sickle cell anemia or cystic fibrosis, are caused by an error in a single gene. Medical research has been strikingly successful at unraveling the mechanisms of these single-gene disorders. However, most diseases, including addiction, are more complicated: variations in many different genes contribute to an individual's overall level of risk or resistance.

Linking Genes to Health: Genome-Wide Association Studies

Recent advances in DNA analysis are enabling researchers to untangle complex genetic interactions by examining a person's entire genome at once. These genome-wide association studies (GWAS) identify subtle variations in DNA sequence called single-nucleotide polymorphisms (SNPs)—places where individuals differ in just a single letter of the genetic code. If a SNP appears more often in individuals with a disease than in those without, it is presumed to be located in or near a gene that influences susceptibility to that disease.

Genome wide association studies are extremely powerful because they are unbiased and comprehensive: they can implicate a known gene in a disorder, and they can identify genes which may have been overlooked or previously unknown. Building on GWAS results, scientists gather additional evidence from affected families, animal models, and biochemical experiments to verify and understand the link between a gene and risk for a disease.

Research Advance: Genetic Variation May Increase Risk of Nicotine Addiction and Lung Cancer

A genome-wide association study sponsored by the National Institute on Drug Abuse (NIDA) recently found that a variant in the gene for a nicotinic receptor subunit doubled the risk for nicotine addiction among smokers (Saccone et al., 2007). A study in Iceland verified this association, finding that this region is also linked to vulnerability to lung cancer and peripheral arterial disease (Thorgeirsson et al., 2008). This is the first evidence of a genetic variation influencing both the likelihood of nicotine addiction and an individual's risk for the severe health consequences of tobacco use.

What Role Does the Environment Play in a Disease Like Addiction?

That old saying "nature or nurture" might be better phrased "nature and nurture," because research shows that individual health is the result of dynamic interactions between genes and environmental conditions. For example, susceptibility to high blood pressure is influenced by both genetics and lifestyle, including diet, stress, and exercise. Environmental influences, such as exposure to drugs or stress, can alter both gene expression and gene function. In some cases, these effects may persist throughout a person's life. Research suggests that genes can also influence how a person responds to his or her environment, placing some individuals at higher risk than others.

Research Advance

A recent study highlights the complex interactions between genetics, drug exposure, and age of use in the risk of developing a mental disorder.

The COMT gene produces an enzyme that regulates dopamine, a brain chemical involved in schizophrenia. COMT comes in two forms: "Met" and "Val." Individuals with one or two copies of the "Val" variant have a higher risk of developing symptoms of psychosis and schizophrenic-type disorders if they use cannabis during adolescence.

The Promise of Personalized Medicine

The emerging science of pharmacogenomics promises to harness the power of genomic information to improve treatments for addiction. Clinicians often find substantial variability in how individual patients respond to treatment. Part of that variability is due to genetics. Genes influence the numbers and types of receptors in our brains, how quickly our bodies metabolize drugs, and how well we respond to different medications.

Armed with an understanding of genetics, health providers will be better equipped to match patients with the most suitable treatments, adjust medication dosages, and avoid or minimize adverse reactions.

Research Advance

A NIDA-sponsored study of alcohol-dependent patients treated with naltrexone found that patients with a specific variant in an opioid receptor gene, Asp40, had a significantly lower rate of relapse (26.1 percent) than patients with the Asn40 variant (47.9 percent).

In the future, identifying which mu-opioid receptor gene variant a patient possesses may help predict the most effective choice of medication for alcohol addiction.

Chapter 47

Genes and Alzheimer Disease

Chapter Contents

Section 47.1

Genetics of Alzheimer Disease

Reprinted from "Alzheimer's Disease Genetics Fact Sheet,"
National Institute on Aging, National Institutes of Health,
NIH Publication No. 08-6424, November 2008.

Scientists don't yet fully understand what causes Alzheimer disease (AD). However, the more they learn about AD, the more they realize that genes play an important role in the development of this devastating disease. Research conducted and funded by the National Institute on Aging (NIA) and others is advancing the field of AD genetics.

The Genetics of Disease

Some diseases are caused by a genetic mutation, or permanent change, in one specific gene. If a person inherits a genetic mutation that is linked to a certain disease from a parent, then he or she will usually get the disease. Cystic fibrosis, muscular dystrophy, and Huntington disease are examples of single-gene disorders.

In other diseases, a genetic variant, or a change in a gene, may occur, but it doesn't necessarily cause the person to develop the disease. More than one gene variant may be necessary to cause the disease, or the variant may increase a person's risk of developing the disease. When this happens, the changed gene is called a genetic risk factor.

The Genetics of Alzheimer Disease

AD is an irreversible, progressive brain disease characterized by the development of amyloid plaques and neurofibrillary tangles, the loss of connections between nerve cells in the brain, and the death of these nerve cells. AD has two types: early-onset and late-onset. Both types have genetic links.

Early-Onset AD

Early-onset AD is a rare form of AD, affecting only about 5 percent of all people who have AD. It develops in people ages thirty to sixty.

Some cases of early-onset AD, called familial AD (FAD), are inherited. FAD is caused by a number of different gene mutations on chromosomes 21, 14, and 1, and each of these mutations causes abnormal proteins to be formed. Mutations on chromosome 21 cause the formation of abnormal amyloid precursor protein (APP). A mutation on chromosome 14 causes abnormal presenilin 1 to be made, and a mutation on chromosome 1 leads to abnormal presenilin 2.

Even if only one of these mutated genes is inherited from a parent, the person will almost always develop early-onset AD. This inheritance pattern is referred to as "autosomal dominant" inheritance. In other words, offspring in the same generation have a 50/50 chance of developing FAD if one of their parents had it.

Scientists know that each of these mutations causes an increased amount of the beta-amyloid protein to be formed. Beta-amyloid, a major component of AD plaques, is formed from APP.

These early-onset findings were critical because they showed that genetics were involved in AD, and they helped identify key players in the AD process. The studies also helped explain some of the variation in the age at which AD develops.

Late-Onset AD

Most cases of Alzheimer are of the late-onset form, developing after age sixty. Scientists studying the genetics of AD have found that the mutations seen in early-onset AD are not involved in this form of the disease.

Although a specific gene has not been identified as the cause of late-onset AD, one predisposing genetic risk factor does appear to increase a person's risk of developing the disease. This increased risk is related to the apolipoprotein E (APOE) gene found on chromosome 19. APOE contains the instructions needed to make a protein that helps carry cholesterol in the bloodstream. APOE comes in several different forms, or alleles. Three forms—APOE epsilon2, APOE epsilon3, and APOE epsilon4—occur most frequently.

APOE epsilon2 is relatively rare and may provide some protection against the disease. If AD does occur in a person with this allele, it develops later in life than it would in someone with the APOE epsilon4 gene.

APOE epsilon3 is the most common allele. Researchers think it plays a neutral role in AD—neither decreasing nor increasing risk.

APOE epsilon4 occurs in about 40 percent of all people who develop late-onset AD and is present in about 25 to 30 percent of the population.

People with AD are more likely to have an APOE epsilon4 allele than people who do not develop AD. However, many people with AD do not have an APOE epsilon4 allele.

Dozens of studies have confirmed that the APOE epsilon4 allele increases the risk of developing AD, but how that happens is not yet understood. These studies also have helped explain some of the variation in the age at which AD develops, as people who inherit one or two APOE epsilon4 alleles tend to develop AD at an earlier age than those who do not have any. APOE epsilon4 is called a risk-factor gene because it increases a person's risk of developing AD. However, inheriting an APOE epsilon4 allele does not mean that a person will definitely develop AD. Some people with one or two APOE epsilon4 alleles never get the disease, and others who develop AD do not have any APOE epsilon4 alleles.

Scientists believe that four to seven other AD risk-factor genes exist and are using a new approach called a genome-wide association study (GWAS) to help speed the discovery process. Another possible risk-factor gene, SORL1, was discovered in 2007. This gene is involved in transporting APP within cells, and its association with AD has been identified and confirmed in three separate studies. Researchers found that when SORL1 is present at low levels or in a variant form, beta-amyloid levels increase and may harm neurons.

DNA, Chromosomes, and Genes

The nucleus of almost every human cell contains a "blueprint" that carries the instructions a cell needs to do its job. The blueprint is made up of deoxyribonucleic acid (DNA), which is present in long strands that would stretch to nearly six feet in length if attached end to end. The DNA is packed tightly together with proteins into compact structures called chromosomes in the nucleus of each cell. Each cell has forty-six chromosomes in twenty-three pairs. The DNA in nearly all cells of an individual is identical.

Each chromosome contains many thousands of segments, called genes. People inherit two copies of each gene from their parents, except for genes on the X and Y chromosomes, which, among other functions, determine a person's sex. The gene tells the cell how to make specific proteins, which determine the different kinds of cells that make up an organism and direct almost every aspect of the cell's construction, operation, and repair. Even slight alterations in a gene can produce an abnormal protein, which may lead to cell malfunction and, eventually, to disease. Other changes in genes may not cause disease but can increase a person's risk of developing a particular disease.

APOE Testing

A blood test is available that can identify which APOE alleles a person has, but it is not yet possible to predict who will or will not develop AD. Because APOE epsilon4 is only a risk factor for AD, this blood test cannot say for sure whether a person will develop AD. Some researchers believe that screening measures may never be able to predict AD with 100 percent accuracy. However, a small battery of tests for other risk-factor genes might eventually be useful.

At present, APOE testing is used in a research setting to identify study participants who may have an increased risk of developing AD. This knowledge helps scientists look for early brain changes in participants and compare the effectiveness of treatments for people with different APOE profiles. Most researchers believe that the APOE test is useful for studying AD risk in large groups of people but not for determining any one person's specific risk. Someday, perhaps, screening in otherwise healthy people may be useful if an accurate and reliable test is developed and effective ways to treat or prevent AD become available.

Research Questions

Learning more about the role of APOE epsilon4 and other risk-factor genes in the development of AD is a vitally important area of AD research. Understanding more about the genetic underpinnings of the disease will help researchers do the following:

- Answer remaining basic questions about mechanisms—What makes the disease process begin, and why do some people who have memory problems go on to develop AD while others do not?

- Determine how AD risk-factor genes may interact with other genes and lifestyle or environmental factors to affect AD risk in any one person.

- Identify people who are at high risk so they can possibly receive early treatment.

- Focus on new prevention or treatment approaches.

Major AD Genetics Research Efforts Underway

As AD genetics research has intensified, it has become clear that scientists need many genetic samples to make further progress. The National Institute on Aging (NIA) has launched two large programs, the Alzheimer's Disease Genetics Study and the Alzheimer's Disease Genetics Consortium, to collect and analyze blood samples and other biological information from thousands of families around the world with members who do and do not have late-onset AD. The National Institute on Aging (NIA) also funds the National Cell Repository for Alzheimer's Disease (NCRAD), a national resource where clinical information and DNA can be stored and accessed by qualified researchers. Through these programs, AD researchers are working together to develop new technologies and methods and to share data.

The AD Genetics Study is gathering genetic and other information from one thousand or more families in the United States that include a pair of living siblings (brothers or sisters) who have late-onset AD. Families who meet this criteria are urged to participate.

The AD Genetics Consortium is a collaborative effort of AD geneticists to collect more than ten thousand samples to do GWAS, the DNA analysis studies needed to identify risk-factor genes.

The participation of volunteer families is a critical part of AD genetics research. The more genetic information that researchers can gather and analyze from a wide range of families, the more clues they will have for finding additional risk-factor genes.

Section 47.2

New Research on the Genetics of Alzheimer Disease

Scientists have new information about the complex genetic signature associated with Alzheimer's disease, the leading cause of cognitive decline and dementia in the elderly.

The new research uses a powerful, high-resolution analysis to look for genes associated with this devastating neurodegenerative disorder.

Previous research linked late-onset Alzheimer's disease, the most common form, with the apolipoprotein E gene. However, the genetics of the disease are complex and are not well understood.

"Though apolipoprotein E has been universally confirmed as a risk gene for late-onset Alzheimer's disease, the gene is neither necessary nor sufficient to cause AD and as much as 50 percent of the genetic risk effect remains unexplained," says senior study author Dr. Margaret A. Pericak-Vance from the Miami Institute for Human Genomics at the University of Miami in Florida.

To gain further insight into the genetics of late-onset Alzheimer's disease, Dr. Pericak-Vance and colleagues completed a sophisticated and comprehensive genetic analysis of 492 late-onset Alzheimer's disease patients and 498 control individuals.

The analysis was powerful enough to detect single nucleotide polymorphisms (SNPs) that are significantly more prevalent in individuals with Alzheimer's disease than they are in controls. A SNP is a variation of a single nucleotide of deoxyribonucleic acid (DNA).

The researchers confirmed the known apolipoprotein E association and identified a new association with a SNP on chromosome 12q13. The SNP is close to the gene for the vitamin D receptor, which has previously been linked with memory performance.

"There is no known connection between this SNP and the vitamin D receptor, but the region between the two is largely uncharacterized, and it is possible that our SNP is in a region that may play some sort of regulatory role," offers Dr. Jonathan Haines, co-director of the project at Vanderbilt University's Center for Human Genetics Research.

The team also identified four other regions of interest and validated several candidate genes that exhibited a promising genome-wide association with Alzheimer's disease.

"Detailed functional examination of these signals and genes may lead to a better understanding of the complex pathophysiology of Alzheimer's disease," concludes Dr. Pericak-Vance.

The study is published by Cell Press in the January 2009 issue of the *American Journal of Human Genetics.*

Chapter 48

Genetics and Asthma

What Is Asthma?

Asthma is a chronic inflammatory disease of the airways associated with a narrowing of the airway passages, bronchial hyperresponsiveness, and reversible airway obstruction, and characterized by recurrent episodes of wheezing, breathlessness, chest tightness, and cough. Many different features of the disease are used to identify asthma patients for studies or as phenotypes in genetic association studies. For example, genetic association studies have evaluated evidence for susceptibility to eosinophilia, elevated immunoglobulin E levels, bronchial hyperresponsiveness, wheeze, and atopy. The variability in disease definition among genetic studies can make interpretation and comparison of study findings difficult.

The Burden of Asthma

Asthma is a significant public health problem, causing considerable morbidity and, in some cases, death. It is also a disease of considerable economic burden.

Approximately 20.3 million (7.2 percent) of U.S. adults had current asthma in 2001 and an estimated 31.3 million people had been diagnosed with asthma during their lifetime.

Excerpted from "Asthma Genomics: Implications for Public Health—A Public Health Perspective," Centers for Disease Control and Prevention, CDC Office of Public Health Genomics, April 2004. Reviewed June 8, 2007.

In 2001, asthma caused approximately two million emergency department visits, 465,000 hospitalizations, and nearly 4,500 deaths.

Collectively, people who have asthma experience well over one hundred million days of restricted activity each year, and asthma is believed to be one of the most common reasons that students miss school.

The combined direct and indirect costs for asthma in United States rose from approximately $10.7 billion in 1994 to approximately $12.7 billion in 1998.

Risk Factors for Asthma

Both genetic and environmental factors are known to play a role in asthma development and expression, although the exact "causes" of asthma are still unknown. Many factors have been hypothesized to affect the development and exacerbation of asthma. Some environmental risk factors that have been shown to be associated with asthma development and/or exacerbation include the following:

- Exposure to air pollutants such as ozone, particulate matter, sulfur dioxide, nitrogen dioxide, diesel particulates, traffic-related pollution, building products, and combustion byproducts

- Exposure to all allergens produced by dust mites, cockroaches, fungi and dampness, and animal dander

- Exposure to environmental tobacco smoke

- Ingestion of nonsteroidal anti-inflammatory drugs (NSAIDs), including aspirin

- Viral infection

Evidence of a Genetic Component to Asthma

Evidence from numerous studies, including some dating back to the 1920s, indicate that asthma is passed down in families, suggesting at least a partial genetic component to the disease. More recent studies provide stronger evidence for genetic susceptibility to asthma. For example, several chromosomal regions and candidate genes have been linked or associated with asthma. The specific effects of these genes have yet to be determined and their impact on public health has yet to be defined. However, genomics research into mechanisms of disease pathogenesis and the recognition of asthma as a chronic inflammatory disease of the airways has allowed for opportunities to better understand the effects of standard therapies and is likely to lead to new therapeutic approaches to asthma.

Asthma is a complex disease in which multiple genes with variable involvement interact with environmental factors. The considerable increase in knowledge of asthma genomics has not yet resulted in changes in strategies to prevent, diagnose, or treat asthma, but it is likely that there will be applications available in the near future. Potential applications include pharmacogenomics, targeted lifestyle and environment modifications for affected individuals, improved disease classification, and identification of unaffected individuals at risk for asthma, concurrent with prevention efforts. The first practical use of asthma genomics is mostly likely to occur in the field of pharmacogenomics. Public health can play an important role in ensuring that discoveries from the "genomics revolution" are applied appropriately to populations.

Chapter 49

Cancer and Genetics

Chapter Contents

Section 49.1

Breast Cancer

Excerpted from "Learning about Breast Cancer," National Human
Genome Research Institute, National Institutes of Health, April 22, 2008.

What do we know about heredity and breast cancer?

Breast cancer is a common disease. Each year, approximately two
hundred thousand women in the United States are diagnosed with
breast cancer, and one in nine American women will develop breast
cancer in her lifetime. But hereditary breast cancer—caused by a
mutant gene passed from parents to their children—is rare. Estimates
of the incidence of hereditary breast cancer range from between 5 and
10 percent to as many as 27 percent of all breast cancers.

In 1994, the first gene associated with breast cancer—BRCA1 (for
BReast CAncer1) was identified on chromosome 17. A year later, a
second gene associated with breast cancer—BRCA2—was discovered
on chromosome 13. When individuals carry a mutated form of either
BRCA1 or BRCA2, they have an increased risk of developing breast
or ovarian cancer at some point in their lives. Children of parents with
a BRCA1 or BRCA2 mutation have a 50 percent chance of inheriting
the gene mutation.

What do we know about hereditary breast cancer in Ashkenazi Jews?

In 1995 and 1996, studies of deoxyribonucleic acid (DNA) samples
revealed that Ashkenazi (Eastern European) Jews are ten times more
likely to have mutations in BRCA1 and BRCA 2 genes than the general population. Approximately 2.65 percent of the Ashkenazi Jewish population has a mutation in these genes, while only 0.2 percent
of the general population carries these mutations.

Further research showed that three specific mutations in these
genes accounted for 90 percent of the BRCA1 and BRCA2 variants
within this ethnic group. This contrasts with hundreds of unique
mutations of these two genes within the general population. However,

despite the relatively high prevalence of these genetic mutations in Ashkenazi Jews, only 7 percent of breast cancers in Ashkenazi women are caused by alterations in BRCA1 and BRCA2.

What other genes may cause hereditary breast cancer?

Not all hereditary breast cancers are caused by BRCA1 and BRCA2. In fact, researchers now believe that at least half of hereditary breast cancers are not linked to these genes. Scientists also now think that these remaining cases of hereditary breast cancer are not caused by another single, unidentified gene, but rather by many genes, each accounting for a small fraction of breast cancers.

Is there a test for hereditary breast cancer?

Hereditary breast cancer is suspected when there is a strong family history of breast cancer: occurrences of the disease in at least three first- or second-degree relatives (sisters, mothers, aunts). Currently the only tests available are DNA tests to determine whether an individual in such a high-risk family has a genetic mutation in the BRCA1 or BRCA2 genes.

When someone with a family history of breast cancer has been tested and found to have an altered BRCA1 or BRCA2 gene, the family is said to have a "known mutation." Positive test results only provide information about the risk of developing breast cancer. The test cannot tell a person whether or when cancer might develop. Many, but not all, women and some men who inherit an altered gene will develop breast cancer. Both men and women who inherit an altered gene, whether or not they develop cancer themselves, can pass the alteration on to their sons and daughters.

But even if the test is negative, the individual may still have a predisposition to hereditary breast cancer. Currently available technique can't identify all cancer-predisposing mutations in the BRCA1 and BRCA2 genes. Or, an individual may have inherited a mutation caused by other genes. And, because most cases of breast cancer are not hereditary, individuals may develop breast cancer whether or not a genetic mutation is present.

How do I decide whether to be tested?

Given the limitations of testing for hereditary breast cancer, should an individual at high risk get tested? Genetic counselors can help individuals and families make decisions regarding testing.

For those who do test positive for the BRCA1 or BRCA2 gene, surveillance (mammography and clinical breast exams) can help detect the disease at an early stage. A woman who tests positive can also consider taking the drug tamoxifen, which has been found to reduce the risk of developing breast cancer by almost 50 percent in women at high risk. Clinical trials are now under way to determine whether another drug, raloxifene, is also effective in preventing breast cancer.

Section 49.2

Colon Cancer

Excerpted from "Learning about Colon Cancer," National Human Genome Research Institute, National Institutes of Health, May 13, 2008.

What do we know about heredity and colon cancer?

Colon cancer, a malignant tumor of the large intestine, affects both men and women. In the year 2000, there were an estimated 130,200 cases diagnosed.

The vast majority of colon cancer cases are not hereditary. However, approximately 5 percent of individuals with colon cancer have a hereditary form. In those families, the chances of developing colon cancer is significantly higher than in the average person.

Scientists have discovered several genes contributing to a susceptibility to two types of colon cancer:

- **Familial adenomatous polyposis (FAP):** So far, only one FAP gene has been discovered—the APC gene on chromosome 5. But over three hundred different mutations of that gene have been identified. Individuals with this syndrome develop many polyps in their colon. People who inherit mutations in this gene have a nearly 100 percent chance of developing colon cancer by age forty.

- **Hereditary nonpolyposis colorectal cancer (HNPCC):** Individuals with an HNPCC gene mutation have an estimated 80 percent lifetime risk of developing colon or rectal cancer.

However, these cancers account for only 3 to 5 percent of all colorectal cancers. So far, four HNPCC genes have been discovered:

- hMSH2 on chromosome 2, which accounts for 60 percent of HNPCC colon cancer cases

- hMLH1 on chromosome 3, which accounts for 30 percent of HNPCC colon cancer cases

- hPMSI on chromosome 2, which accounts for 5 percent of HNPCC colon cancer cases

- hPMS2 on chromosome 7, which accounts for 5 percent of HNPCC colon cancer cases

Together, FAP and HNPCC gene mutations account for approximately 5 percent of all colorectal cancers. These hereditary cancers typically occur at an earlier age than sporadic (noninherited) cases of colon cancer. The risk of inheriting these mutated genes from an affected parent is 50 percent for both males and females.

The genes that cause these two syndromes were relatively easy to discover because they exert strong effects. Other genes that cause susceptibility to colon cancer are harder to discover because the cancers are caused by an interplay among a number of genes, which individually exert a weak effect.

Is there a test for hereditary colon cancer?

Gene testing can identify some individuals who carry genes for FAP and some HPNCC cases of colon cancer. However, the tests are not perfect at this point in time. So, some families may have alterations in the FAP or HNPCC gene that cannot be detected.

The test for FAP syndrome involves examining deoxyribonucleic acid (DNA) in blood cells called lymphocytes (white blood cells), looking for mutations in the APC gene. No treatment to reduce cancer risk is currently available for people with FAP. But for those who test positive, frequent surveillance can detect the cancer at an early, more treatable stage. Because of the early age at which this syndrome appears, the test may be offered to people under eighteen who have a parent known to carry the mutated gene.

Researchers hope that an easier test, now experimental, will become available in three to five years. This new test examines a stool sample and looks for cancer cells sloughed off by the APC gene.

Genetic tests for HNPCC are of limited value since the current test can identify only a few mutations on two genes that cause HNPCC (hMSH2 and hMLH1). There are no clinical tests for the other two HNPCC genes.

Because of the limitations of available tests for hereditary colon cancer, testing is not recommended for the general population. However, individuals in families at high risk may consider testing. Genetic counselors can help individuals make decisions regarding testing.

Section 49.3

Lung Cancer

Reprinted from "Large-Scale Genetic Study Sheds New Light on Lung Cancer, Opens Door to Individualized Treatment Strategies," National Human Genome Research Institute, National Institutes of Health, October 22, 2008.

A multi-institution team, funded by the National Human Genome Research Institute (NHGRI) of the National Institutes of Health (NIH) recently reported results of the largest effort to date to chart the genetic changes involved in the most common form of lung cancer, lung adenocarcinoma. The findings should help pave the way for more individualized approaches for detecting and treating the nation's leading cause of cancer deaths.

In a paper published in the October 23, 2008, issue of the journal *Nature*, the Tumor Sequencing Project (TSP) consortium identified twenty-six genes that are frequently mutated in lung adenocarcinoma—an achievement that more than doubles the number of genes known to be associated with the deadly disease. But the pioneering effort involved far more than just tallying up genes. Using a systematic, multidisciplinary approach, the TSP team also detailed key pathways involved in the disease, and described patterns of genetic mutations among different subgroups of lung cancer patients, including smokers and never-smokers.

More than 1,000,000 people worldwide die of lung cancer each year, including more than 150,000 in the United States. Lung adenocarcinoma is the most frequently diagnosed form of lung cancer. The average five-year survival rate currently is about 15 percent, with survival being longest among people whose cancer has been detected early.

"By harnessing the power of genomic research, this pioneering work has painted the clearest and most complete portrait yet of lung cancer's molecular complexities. This big picture perspective will help to focus our research vision and speed our efforts to develop new strategies for disarming this common and devastating disease," said NHGRI acting director Alan E. Guttmacher, M.D.

Like most cancers, lung adenocarcinoma arises from changes that accumulate in people's deoxyribonucleic acid (DNA) over the course of their lives. However, little is known about the precise nature of these DNA changes, how they occur, and how they disrupt biological pathways to cause cancer's uncontrolled cell growth. To gain a more complete picture, researchers have joined together to form TSP and other large, collaborative projects that are using new tools and technologies to examine the complete set of DNA, or genome, found in various types of cancer.

"We found lung adenocarcinoma to be very diverse from a genetic standpoint. Our work uncovered many new targets for therapy of this deadly disease—oncogenes that drive particular forms of lung adenocarcinoma and tumor suppressor genes that would ordinarily prevent cancer cell growth," said Matthew Meyerson, M.D., Ph.D., a senior author of the paper. Dr. Meyerson is a senior associate member of the Broad Institute of the Massachusetts Institute of Technology (MIT) and Harvard and an associate professor at the Dana-Farber Cancer Institute and Harvard Medical School.

In the new study, the TSP team purified DNA from tumor samples and matching noncancerous tissue donated by 188 patients with lung adenocarcinoma. Next, they sequenced the DNA to look for mutations in 623 genes with known or potential relationships to cancer. Prior to the study, fewer than a dozen genes had been implicated in lung adenocarcinoma. The latest research identified 26 new genes that are mutated in a significant number of samples. Most of these genes had not previously been associated with lung adenocarcinoma.

Among the genes newly implicated in lung adenocarcinoma are the following:

- **Neurofibromatosis 1 (NF1):** Mutations in this gene have previously been shown to cause neurofibromatosis 1, a rare inherited disorder characterized by unchecked growth of tissue of the nervous system.

461

- **Ataxia telangiectasia mutated (ATM):** ATM mutations have previously been shown to play a role in ataxia telangiectasia, which is a rare inherited neurological disorder of childhood, and in various types of leukemia and lymphoma.

- **Retinoblastoma 1 (RB1):** Past research has tied RB1 mutations to retinoblastoma, a relatively uncommon type of childhood cancer that originates in the eye's retina.

- **Adenomatosis polyposis coli (APC):** Mutations of this gene are common in colon cancer.

- **Ephrin receptors A3 and A5 (EPHA3 and EPHA5), neurotrophin receptors (NTRK1 and NTRK3), and other receptor-coupled tyrosine kinases (ERBB4, KDR and FGFR4):** These genes code for cell receptors coupled to members of the tyrosine kinase family of enzymes, which are considered prime targets for new cancer therapies.

After identifying the genetic mutations, the team went on to examine their impacts on biological pathways and determine which of those pathways were most crucial in lung adenocarcinoma. Such research is essential to efforts to develop new and better treatments for cancer.

For example, TSP researchers found more than two-thirds of the 188 tumors studied had at least one gene mutation affecting the mitogen-activated protein kinase (MAPK) pathway, indicating it plays a pivotal role in lung cancer. Based on those findings, the researchers suggested new treatment strategies for some subtypes of lung adenocarcinoma might include compounds that affect the MAPK pathway. One such group of compounds, called mitogen-activated ERK kinase (MEK) inhibitors, has produced promising results in mouse models of colon cancer.

Likewise, the TSP's finding that more than 30 percent of tumors had mutations affecting the mammalian target of rapamycin (mTOR) pathway raises the possibility that the drug rapamycin might be tested in lung adenocarcinoma. Rapamycin is an mTOR-inhibiting compound approved for use in organ transplants and renal cancer.

In addition, the genetic findings suggest that certain lung cancer patients might benefit from chemotherapy drugs currently used to treat other types of cancer. For example, chemotherapy drugs known to inhibit the kinase insert domain receptor (KDR), such as sorafenib and sunitinib, might be tested in the relatively small percentage of lung adenocarcinoma patients whose tumors have mutations that activate the KDR gene.

In their *Nature* paper, TSP researchers also analyzed the patterns of genetic changes seen among different subgroups of lung adenocarcinoma patients, including smokers.

About 90 percent of lung cancer patients have significant histories of cigarette smoking, but 10 percent report no use of tobacco. In the TSP study, the number of genetic mutations detected in tumor samples from smokers was significantly higher than in tumors from never-smokers. Smokers' tumors contained as many as forty-nine mutations, while none of the never-smokers' tumors had more than five mutations. More work is needed to determine what these differences may mean for the management of lung cancer. However, doctors do know that in some other types of cancer, high mutation levels may cause a tumor to spread rapidly and/or be resistant to treatment.

"Our findings underscore the value of systematic, large-scale studies for exploring cancer. We now must move forward to apply this approach to even larger groups of samples and a wider range of cancers," said Richard K. Wilson, Ph.D., a senior author of the paper and director of the Genome Sequencing Center at Washington University School of Medicine, St. Louis.

The TSP team also included researchers from Baylor College of Medicine, Houston; Brigham and Women's Hospital, Boston; Memorial Sloan-Kettering Cancer Center, New York; the University of Cologne, Germany; the University of Michigan, Ann Arbor; and the University of Texas M.D. Anderson Cancer Center, Houston.

"Clearly, much still remains to be discovered. We have just begun to realize the tremendous potential of large-scale, genomic studies to unravel the many mysteries of cancer," said Richard Gibbs, Ph.D., a co-author of the lung adenocarcinoma paper and director of the Human Genome Sequencing Center at Baylor College of Medicine.

The TSP data are complementary to those from other large-scale cancer genome studies, such as The Cancer Genome Atlas (TCGA) project funded by NHGRI and the National Cancer Institute (NCI). In its pilot phase, TCGA is focusing on the most common form of brain tumor, called glioblastoma; a type of lung cancer called squamous cell lung cancer; and ovarian cancer. The first results from TCGA's glioblastoma study were published in the advance online edition of *Nature* on September 4, 2008, and published in *Nature*'s print edition on October 23, 2008.

The co-publication of these comprehensive cancer genome studies should provide hope to millions of people and families living with cancer. By applying advanced genomic tools to the complexities of cancer, these studies have helped to untangle the biological roots of these diseases, which will accelerate efforts by the worldwide scientific community to improve outcomes for cancer patients.

Section 49.4

Prostate Cancer

Excerpted from "Learning about Prostate Cancer," National Human Genome Research Institute, National Institutes of Health, April 15, 2008.

What is prostate cancer?

Prostate cancer is the most common cancer in American men aside from skin cancer. One in six American men will develop prostate cancer during their lifetime. However, there are many other men who have prostate cancer who do not develop symptoms and who are never diagnosed with prostate cancer.

Most often prostate cancers happen in men who are older than age sixty-five. At this time, more than two million men in the United States who have had prostate cancer at some point during their lives are still living.

What is the prostate?

The prostate is a small gland shaped like a walnut that is in the center of a man's body within the pelvis. The prostate makes a milky fluid that carries sperm during ejaculation. It is wrapped around the tube that carries urine out of the body (the urethra). It sits just below the bladder.

What are the risk factors for prostate cancer?

Age: A man's age is the strongest risk factor for prostate cancer. It is rare for a man to develop prostate cancer before the age of forty. After age fifty the chance of having prostate cancer increases rapidly.

African American background: Prostate cancer is more common in African American men than in men of other racial backgrounds. African American men are more often diagnosed with prostate cancer when it is in advanced stages. They are more than two times more likely to die from prostate cancer than white men. Hispanic/Latino and Asian American men are less likely to develop prostate cancer.

Family history of prostate cancer: Prostate cancer is known to run in families. Men who have a father or a brother who has had prostate cancer have twice the risk of developing prostate cancer than a man without a family history of the disease. One in ten men who get prostate cancer has hereditary prostate cancer—cancer that is caused by genes inherited from their parents. Hereditary prostate cancer is of concern when a man has one of the following:

- Three or more close relatives—father, brother, son—who have prostate cancer

- Family members with prostate cancer in three generations, one after the other, in the mother's or father's family

- At least two family members who have prostate cancer at age fifty-five or younger

Environmental factors: Environmental risk factors are associated with developing prostate cancer. These are as follows:

- *Geographic location:* Where a man lives. For example, there are more white men who develop prostate cancer living in the northwest region of the United States and in New England.

- A *high-fat diet.*

- *Eating foods with a lot of calories.*

- A *sedentary lifestyle:* Getting little exercise.

What is known about genetic factors and prostate cancer risk?

Research studies are helping scientists to understand the genetic factors that have a role in inherited risk for prostate cancer. Certain gene changes (mutations) have been found to increase the risk for prostate cancer, and research is ongoing regarding combinations of genetic changes that increase prostate cancer risk. More research is required to fully determine the genetic risk factors for prostate cancer.

Is genetic testing available now for prostate cancer?

Genetic testing is available for certain genes that can cause prostate cancer. Men from families with prostate cancer, breast cancer, or ovarian cancer can talk with their doctors about their risk and genetic counseling. Genetic counselors can take a detailed family history and talk about their risk for prostate cancer, and whether genetic testing is appropriate for them.

There are companies that will soon be marketing and selling genetic tests that will predict a man's risk of developing prostate cancer. It is important for you to talk with your doctor or a genetic counselor about this testing before you decide to have it to make sure that the testing will give you helpful information.

How is prostate cancer diagnosed and treated?

Symptoms: The symptoms of prostate cancer may include problems with urination and sexual function. As the prostate grows larger it can squeeze the urethra and cause frequent, small urination, difficulty beginning urination, or even an inability to urinate. The flow of urine can start and stop, be weak, or create pain or a burning feeling. Erection may hurt and there can be blood in the urine or semen. Pain may also occur in the back, hips, or upper thighs.

Diagnosis of prostate cancer: The blood level of prostate specific antigen (PSA), an enzyme made by the prostate gland, and a digital rectal examination (DRE) are two tests that are currently used for the detection of prostate cancer. If the level of PSA in the blood is higher than normal, or if the digital rectal exam finds any enlargement or unusual lumps in the prostate, it can mean that a man has prostate cancer.

The diagnosis of prostate cancer is then made by a biopsy (taking a small piece of tissue) of the prostate.

In the future, diagnosis of prostate cancer may be based in part on genetic changes that are found in the prostate gland.

Treatment of prostate cancer: Treatment of prostate cancer depends on when the diagnosis is made and how severe the disease is at that time. Small clusters of early-stage prostate cancer can be found in many men in a form that is harmless. In this situation, the doctor may take a "wait and watch approach" to these early cancers, and follow the man with regular PSA blood tests and physical exams. Often the disease can be managed this way for years, as long as the progression is slow.

Surgery may be another treatment used if the tumor has not spread to other parts of the body and the man is healthy enough to handle the operation.

If the prostate is enlarged and there is a mass that the doctor can feel, then surgery may be done to remove as much of the prostate, the tumor, and tissue around the prostate to check if the cancer cells have spread (called metastasis). Sometimes the surgery can cause nerve damage that impairs sexual function. Improvements in surgical techniques have lowered that risk and surgeons are now better able to preserve sexual function.

Radiation therapy is sometimes used after surgery or instead of surgery. This treatment is aimed directly at the tumor to kill the cancer cells. It is also used in later stages of prostate cancer to relieve pain.

When the prostate cancer is in advanced stages, hormonal therapy along with surgery or other medical treatment is used to lower the activity of male hormones (androgens) that cause tumor growth. Hormonal therapy can be effective for months to years, holding the disease at bay, but the effectiveness of this treatment may lessen over time. The side effects from hormonal therapy include impotence, decreased sexual desire, smaller muscle mass, and tenderness or enlargement of breast tissue.

Chemotherapy is usually reserved for prostate cancer recurrence or advanced disease. Chemotherapy can help to keep the disease stable and stop growth of the prostate. It is used in men who have had surgery, but whose prostate cancer may come back; in men who have had surgery and/or radiation; or in men whose prostate cancer has spread and hormone treatment is no longer working.

Section 49.5

Skin Cancer

Excerpted from "Learning about Skin Cancer," National
Human Genome Research Institute, National Institutes of Health,
May 30, 2008.

Skin cancer is the most common type of cancer in the United States. An estimated 40 to 50 percent of Americans who live to age sixty-five will have skin cancer at least once. The most common skin cancer is basal cell carcinoma, which accounts for more than 90 percent of all skin cancers in the United States.

The most virulent form of skin cancer is melanoma. In some parts of the world, especially in Western countries, the number of people who develop melanoma is increasing faster than any other cancer. In the United States, for example, the number of new cases of melanoma has more than doubled in the past twenty years.

What are the most common forms of skin cancer?

Three types of skin cancer are the most common:

- Basal cell carcinoma is a slow-growing cancer that seldom spreads to other parts of the body. Basal cells, which are round, form the layer just underneath the epidermis, or outer layer of the skin.

- Squamous cell carcinoma spreads more often than basal cell carcinoma, but still is considered rare. Squamous cells, which are flat, make up most of the epidermis.

- Melanoma is the most serious type of skin cancer. It occurs when melanocytes, the pigment cells in the lower part of the epidermis, become malignant, meaning that they start dividing uncontrollably. If melanoma spreads to the lymph nodes it may also reach other parts of the body, such as the liver, lungs, or brain. In such cases, the disease is called metastatic melanoma.

What are the symptoms of skin cancer?

The most commonly noticed symptom of skin cancer is a change on the skin, especially a new growth or a sore that doesn't heal. Both basal and squamous cell cancers are found mainly on areas of the skin that are exposed to the sun—the head, face, neck, hands, and arms. However, skin cancer can occur anywhere.

For melanoma, the first sign often is a change in the size, shape, color, or feel of an existing mole. Melanomas can vary greatly in the way they look, but generally show one or more of the "ABCD" features:

- Their shape may be asymmetrical.

- Their borders may be ragged or otherwise irregular.

- Their color may be uneven, with shades of black and brown.

- Their diameter may change in size.

What do we know about the causes and heredity of skin cancer?

Ultraviolet (UV) radiation from the sun is the main cause of skin cancer, although artificial sources of UV radiation, such as sunlamps and tanning booths, also play a role. UV radiation can damage the deoxyribonucleic acid (DNA), or genetic information, in skin cells, creating "misspellings" in their genetic code and, as a result, alter the function of those cells.

Cancers generally are caused by a combination of environmental and genetic factors. With skin cancer, the environment plays a greater role, but individuals can be born with a genetic disposition toward or vulnerability to getting cancer. The risk is greatest for people who have light-colored skin that freckles easily—often those who also have red or blond hair and blue or light-colored eyes—although anyone can get skin cancer.

Skin cancer is related to lifetime exposure to UV radiation, therefore most skin cancers appear after age fifty. However, the sun's damaging effects begin at an early age. People who live in areas that get high levels of UV radiation from the sun are more likely to get skin cancer. For example, the highest rates of skin cancer are found in South Africa and Australia, areas that receive high amounts of UV radiation.

About 10 percent of all patients with melanoma have family members who also have had the disease. Research suggests that a mutation in the CDKN2 gene on chromosome 9 plays a role in this form of melanoma. Studies have also implicated genes on chromosomes 1 and 12 in cases of familial melanoma.

Can I do anything to prevent or test for skin cancer?

When it comes to skin cancer, prevention is your best line of defense. Protection should start early in childhood and continue throughout life. Suggested protections include the following:

- Whenever possible, avoid exposure to the midday sun.

- Wear protective clothing—for example, long sleeves and broad-rimmed hats.

- Use sunscreen lotions with an sun protection factor (SPF) of at least 15.

- If a family member has had melanoma, have your doctor check for early warning signs regularly.

How is skin cancer treated?

Melanoma can be cured if it is diagnosed and treated when the tumor has not deeply invaded the skin. However, if a melanoma is not removed in its early stages, cancer cells may grow downward from the skin surface. When a melanoma becomes thick and deep, the disease often spreads to other parts of the body and is difficult to control.

Surgery is the standard treatment for melanoma, as well as other skin cancers. However, if the cancer has spread to other parts of the body, doctors may use other treatments, such as chemotherapy, immunotherapy, radiation therapy, or a combination of these methods.

Chapter 50

Heredity and Crohn Disease

What is Crohn disease?

Crohn disease, an idiopathic (of unknown cause), chronic inflammatory disorder of the bowel, involves any region of the gastrointestinal tract from the mouth to the anus. The swelling and inflammation can go deeply into the lining of the bowel. This can be very painful and can cause diarrhea, abdominal pain, nausea, and decreased appetite. The inflammatory process tends to be eccentric and segmental, often with skip areas (normal regions of bowel between inflamed areas).

Complications of Crohn disease include: blockage of the intestine; sores and ulcers in the affected area or surrounding tissues such as the bladder; tunnels around the anus and rectum called fistulas; nutritional deficiencies; anemia; arthritis; skin problems; kidney stones, gallstones, or other diseases of the liver and biliary system.

Both men and women can have Crohn disease. It can also run in families. About 20 percent (one in five) of people who have Crohn disease have a blood relative with some form of inflammatory bowel disease, usually a brother or a sister, and sometimes a parent and child.

Crohn disease is usually diagnosed in people between the ages of twenty and thirty. About 25 percent of new Crohn disease diagnoses are made in persons who are younger than twenty years of age.

Excerpted from "Learning about Crohn's Disease," National Human Genome Research Institute, National Institutes of Health, November 7, 2008.

When given proper medical care, most people who have Crohn disease are able to lead long and productive lives. New medications and research into the causes of Crohn disease are helping to increase the quality of life for people who have Crohn disease.

What are the symptoms of Crohn disease?

The symptoms of Crohn disease include the following:

- Abdominal pain, often in the lower right area
- Diarrhea
- Rectal bleeding
- Weight loss
- Arthritis
- Skin problems
- Fever

Rectal bleeding may be serious and continuous enough to cause anemia (low red blood count).

Children who have Crohn disease may have delayed development and stunted growth.

The range and severity of the symptoms of Crohn disease varies among individuals.

How is Crohn disease diagnosed?

Crohn disease is diagnosed by a thorough physical exam and a series of tests.

Blood tests may be done to do the following:

- Check for anemia
- Check for a high white blood cell count and sedimentation rate which are signs of swelling (inflammation) in the body

Other tests that may be done include the following:

- A stool sample to check to see if there is any bleeding or infection in the intestines.
- An x-ray called an upper gastrointestinal (GI) series with small bowel follow-through to look at the small intestine.

- A visual exam of the colon using sigmoidoscopy or colonoscopy that allows the doctor to see any inflammation or bleeding in the colon.

What is the treatment for Crohn disease?

There is currently no cure for Crohn disease. The treatment for Crohn disease usually involves medical care over a long period of time, with regular visits to the doctor to monitor the condition.

Treatment includes: drugs, nutrition supplements, and surgery, or a combination of these treatments. The goal of treatment is to control the swelling (inflammation), correct any nutritional deficiencies, and relieve symptoms such as abdominal pain, diarrhea, and rectal bleeding.

Drug therapy for Crohn disease includes the following:

- Anti-inflammation drugs such as sulfasalazine

- Cortisone or steroids (corticosteroids) such as prednisone

- Immune system suppressors, such as 6-mercaptopurine or a related drug, azathioprine

- Infliximab (Remicade®), a drug that is the first of a group of medications that blocks the body's inflammation process

- Antibiotics to treat bacterial overgrowth in the intestine or before surgery

- Anti-diarrhea medications and fluid replacements

Nutrition supplements may be recommended especially for children whose growth has been slowed. For some patients, this nutrition is given intravenously through a small tube in the arm.

While a patient may require colectomy for uncontrolled bleeding, this is increasingly rare in Crohn, especially with new immune therapies.

Is Crohn disease inherited?

There appears to be a risk for inheriting Crohn disease, especially in families of Jewish ancestry.

Children who have one parent with Crohn disease have a 7 to 9 percent lifetime risk of developing the condition. They also have a 10 percent chance to develop some form of inflammatory bowel disease. When both parents have inflammatory bowel disease, the risk for their children to develop Crohn disease is 35 percent.

Chapter 51

Genetics and Mental Illness

Chapter Contents

Section 51.1

Family History of Mental Illness

Reprinted from "Family History of Mental Illness," © 2008 Emory University School of Medicine Department of Human Genetics. Reprinted with permission. For additional information, visit the Department of Genetics website at http://www.genetics.emory.edu.

Mental illness is a category of diseases/disorders known to cause mild to severe disturbances in thought and/or behavior, which can result in an inability to cope with the ordinary demands and routines of life. There are more than two hundred classified forms of mental illness. Common disorders are depression, bipolar disorder, dementia, schizophrenia, and anxiety disorders. Symptoms may include changes in mood, personality, personal habits, and/or social withdrawal. With treatment, many individuals learn to cope or recover from a mental illness or emotional disorder.

Mental disorders are common in the United States and around the world. An estimated 57.5 million Americans eighteen years of age and older—approximately one in four adults—are diagnosed with a mental disorder in a given year. In addition, mental disorders are the leading cause of disability in the United States and Canada for ages fifteen to forty-four years. Many people suffer from more than one mental disorder. Approximately 45 percent of those with a mental disorder meet the criteria for two or more disorders.

Mental illnesses are multifactorial illnesses (caused by the interaction of various genetic and environmental factors). Causes may include a reaction to environmental stresses, genetic factors, biochemical imbalances, or a combination of these. Because genetic factors are involved, when one family member is affected, other close relatives may be at increased risk. At this time, no genetic tests are available for mental illness, and therefore prenatal diagnosis is not possible.

Mood Disorders

Mood disorders include major depressive disorder, dysthymia (a milder, but longer lasting form of depression), and bipolar disorder.

Approximately 20.9 million American adults (9.5 percent of the U.S. adult population) have a mood disorder. The median age of onset for mood disorders is thirty years.

Depression: Major depressive disorder is the leading cause of disability in the United States for ages fifteen to forty-four. While major depressive disorder can occur at any age, the median age of onset is thirty-two years. Major depressive disorder is more prevalent in women than in men. Recurrence risks for first-degree relatives (children, parents, siblings) are approximately 10 percent for individuals with depression (two to four times the general population risk); however, this risk could be higher depending on the family history, number of affected family members, and age of onset. Relatives of individuals diagnosed with depression earlier in life are at a greater risk to develop depression than relatives of individuals diagnosed later in life.

Bipolar disorder: More than two million American adults, or about 1 percent of the population age eighteen and older in any given year, have bipolar disorder. Bipolar disorder is also known as manic depression. The illness causes a person's mood to swing from excessively "high" (mania) to irritable, sad, and/or hopeless (depression), with periods of a normal mood in between. The median age of onset for bipolar disorder is twenty-five years.

Schizophrenia

Schizophrenia is a disorder in which a person may have difficulty distinguishing between what is real and what is imaginary; may be unresponsive or withdrawn; and may have difficulty expressing normal emotions in social situations. Schizophrenia is not split personality or multiple personality. Most people with schizophrenia are not violent and do not pose a danger to others. Schizophrenia is not caused by childhood experiences, poor parenting, or lack of willpower, nor are the symptoms identical for each person. Schizophrenia often appears in men in their late teens or early twenties, while women are generally affected in their twenties or early thirties. Schizophrenia affects men and women with equal frequency. There is a slight increase in the risk of schizophrenia in the siblings of patients with other types of psychosis.

Anxiety Disorders

Anxiety disorders include panic disorder, obsessive-compulsive disorder, post-traumatic stress disorder, generalized anxiety disorder, and phobias (social phobia, agoraphobia, and specific phobias). Approximately forty million Americans have an anxiety disorder. Most people with an anxiety disorder also have another mood disorder. Nearly three-quarters of those with an anxiety disorder will have their first episode by 21.5 years of age.

Section 51.2

New Research on Genetic Ties to Mental Illness

Genetic Risk Factors for Eating Disorders

Until recently, it was generally believed that eating disorders such as anorexia nervosa and bulimia nervosa resulted solely from environmental influences such as peer pressure and certain perceived expectations of society.

But research at Michigan State University has found that there are genetic risk factors at work as well.

The research of Kelly Klump, an MSU associate professor of psychology, published in the May 2007 issue of *Psychological Medicine*, indicates that the origin of eating disorders has biological roots, similar to how bipolar disorder and schizophrenia are thought to have biological causes.

Specifically, Klump's work found that when girls enter puberty their chances of developing such a disease grow rapidly.

"During puberty, there is an increased risk for developing an eating disorder," said Klump. "Up to 50 percent of this risk can be attributed to genetic factors that emerge during puberty."

Klump's research looked at more than five hundred female fourteen-year-old twins who were examined using sophisticated statistical modeling techniques. It was found that before puberty, environmental factors alone contribute to the development of various eating disorders.

As puberty progresses, the genetic risk is activated and increases in importance to accounting for more than half the risk for eating pathology.

These findings extend previous research by Klump in which she found that at age eleven there were no genetic influences on disordered eating. However, by age seventeen the heritability of disordered eating was more than 50 percent. The recent findings implicate puberty in the dramatic increase in genetic effects across time.

The female twins were part of the Minnesota Twin Family Study. An ongoing research project at the University of Minnesota, the project seeks to identify the genetic and environmental influences on the development of psychological disorders. More than eight thousand twins and their family members have participated in the project.

"This research underscores a need to fund future research in eating disorders," said Klump, who also is the president of the Academy for Eating Disorders. "There is a significant biological and psychological component to eating disorders that needs to be further examined."

The study was funded by grants from the National Institute of Mental Health, National Institute on Drug Abuse, and National Institute on Alcohol Abuse and Alcoholism.

Seasonal Affective Disorder May Be Linked to Genetic Mutation

With the days shortening toward winter, many people will begin to experience the winter blahs. For some, the effect can be devastating.

About 6 percent of the U.S. population suffers from seasonal affective disorder, or SAD, a sometimes-debilitating depression that begins in the fall and continues through winter. Sufferers may even find it difficult to get out of bed in the morning.

The disorder, which is not well understood, is often treated with "light therapy," where a SAD patient spends time each morning before a bank of bright lights in an effort to trick the brain into believing that the days are not so short or dim.

A new study indicates that SAD may be linked to a genetic mutation in the eye that makes a SAD patient less sensitive to light.

"These individuals may require brighter light levels to maintain normal functioning during the winter months," said Ignacio Provencio, a University of Virginia biology professor who studies the genetics of the body's biological clock, or circadian rhythms.

Provencio and his colleagues have discovered that melanopsin, a photopigment gene in the eye, may play a role in causing SAD in people with a recently discovered mutation.

"We believe that the mutation could contribute to increasing the amount of light needed for normal functioning during winter for people with SAD," Provencio said. "Lack of adequate light may be a trigger for SAD, but not the only explanation for the disorder."

The findings are published in the online edition of the *Journal of Affective Disorders*, and will appear later in the print version.

The study was conducted with several other institutions, including the National Institute of Mental Health. It involved 220 participants, 130 of whom had been diagnosed with SAD and 90 participants with no history of mental illness.

Using a genetics test, the study authors found that 7 of the 220 participants carried two copies of the mutation that may be a factor in causing SAD, and, strikingly, all seven belonged to the SAD group.

"While a person diagnosed with SAD does not necessarily carry the melanopsin mutation, what we found strongly indicates that people who carry the mutation could very well be diagnosed with SAD," Provencio said. "We think that if an individual has two copies of this gene, he or she has a reasonable chance of having the disorder."

The researchers found that a person with two copies of the gene is five times more likely to have symptoms of SAD than a person without the mutation.

"That is a very high effect for a mental illness, because most mental illnesses have many potential causes," Provencio noted. "A mental illness may arise from many mutations, and we have found one that has a clear link."

The melanopsin gene encodes a light-sensitive protein that is found in a class of photoreceptors in the retina that are not involved with vision, but are linked to many nonvisual responses, such as the control of circadian rhythms, the control of hormones, the mediation of alertness, and the regulation of sleep.

The mutation in this gene may result in aberrant regulation of these responses to light, leading to the depressive symptoms of SAD. About 29 percent of SAD patients come from families with a history of the disorder, suggesting a genetic or hereditary link.

"The finding suggests that melanopsin mutations may predispose some people to SAD, and that if you have two copies of this mutation, there is a very high probability that you will be afflicted," Provencio said. "An eventual understanding of the mechanisms underlying the pathological response to light in SAD may lead to improved treatments."

Provencio added that the finding, with further study, could also lead to improved testing for SAD.

Provencio's colleague and lead author in the study is Kathryn Roecklein, an assistant professor of psychology at the University of Pittsburgh.

Competing Genes Linked to Mental Illness

A genetic "tug of war" between a mother and father's genes may be behind such mental disorders as autism and schizophrenia.

Simon Fraser University evolutionary biologist Bernard Crespi and colleague Christopher Badcock, a sociologist at the London School of Economics, have published a sweeping new theory of brain development that could change how mental disorders are understood.

In a new article, *The New York Times* suggests their ideas, rooted in science, provide psychiatry with "perhaps its grandest working theory since Freud, and one that is grounded in work at the forefront of science."

The research, published recently in *Nature* and in *Behavioural and Brain Sciences*, proposes that genes passed on from either parent can steer brain development in certain directions. A strong bias toward the father leads to development along a more methodical leaning, and what researchers refer to as the autistic spectrum. A bias toward the mother leads to a hypersensitivity to mood changes, and what researchers call the psychotic spectrum, increasing the risk of developing schizophrenia and mood problems later in life.

Even if the theory is flawed observers say it is likely to provide new insights into the biology of mental illness.

Crespi says the empirical implications are "absolutely" huge. "If you get a gene linked to autism, for instance, you'd want to look at that same gene for schizophrenia. If it is a social brain gene, then it would be expected to have opposite effects on these disorders, whether gene expression was turned up or turned down."

481

Crespi, the recipient of a Killam teaching award in 2005, published findings in 2007 in the *Proceedings of the Royal Society B* that suggest schizophrenia may be a by-product of natural selection in human evolution.

Chapter 52

Diabetes: Research Reveals Genetic Link

Major Collaboration Uncovers Surprising New Genetic Clues to Diabetes

An international team that included scientists from the National Human Genome Research Institute (NHGRI), part of the National Institutes of Health (NIH), has reported it has identified six more genetic variants involved in type 2 diabetes, boosting to sixteen the total number of genetic risk factors associated with increased risk of the disease. None of the genetic variants uncovered by the new study had previously been suspected of playing a role in type 2 diabetes. Intriguingly, the new variant most strongly associated with type 2 diabetes also was recently implicated in a very different condition: prostate cancer.

The unprecedented analysis, published on March 30, 2008, in the advance online edition of *Nature Genetics*, combined genetic data from more than seventy thousand people. The work was carried out through the collaborative efforts of more than ninety researchers at more than forty centers in Europe and North America.

"None of the genes we have found was previously on the radar screen of diabetes researchers," said one of the paper's senior authors,

Reprinted from the following documents from the National Human Genome Research Institute: "Major Collaboration Uncovers Surprising New Genetic Clues to Diabetes," March 30, 2008, and "Researchers Identify New Genetic Risk Factors for Type 2 Diabetes," April 26, 2007.

Mark McCarthy, M.D., of the University of Oxford in England. "Each of these genes, therefore, provides new clues to the processes that go wrong when diabetes develops, and each provides an opportunity for the generation of new approaches for treating or preventing this condition."

When considered individually, the genetic variants discovered to date account for only small differences in the risk of developing type 2 diabetes. But researchers say when all of the variants are analyzed together, some significant differences in risk are likely to emerge. "By combining information from the large number of genes now implicated in diabetes risk, it may be possible to use genetic tools to identify people at unusually high or low risk of diabetes. However, until we know how to use this information to prompt beneficial changes in people's treatment or lifestyle, widespread genetic testing would be premature," said another senior author, David Altshuler, M.D., Ph.D., of Massachusetts General Hospital in Boston and the Broad Institute of Massachusetts Institute of Technology and Harvard in Cambridge, Massachusetts.

Type 2 diabetes affects more than two hundred million people worldwide, including nearly twenty-one million people in the United States. Previously known as adult-onset, or non-insulin-dependent diabetes mellitus (NIDDM), type 2 diabetes usually appears after age forty, often in overweight, sedentary people. However, a growing number of younger people—and even children—are developing the disease.

Diabetes is a major cause of heart disease and stroke in U.S. adults, as well as the most common cause of blindness, kidney failure, and amputations not related to trauma. Type 2 diabetes is characterized by the resistance of target tissues to respond to insulin, which controls glucose levels in the blood; and a gradual failure of insulin-secreting cells in the pancreas.

"These new variants, along with other recent genetic findings, provide a window into disease causation that may be our best hope for the next generation of therapeutics. By pinpointing particular pathways involved in diabetes risk, these discoveries can empower new approaches to understanding environmental influences and to the development of new, more precisely targeted drugs," said NHGRI director Francis S. Collins, M.D., Ph.D., who is a co-author of the study. Dr. Collins's laboratory is a participant in the FINRISK 2002 and Finland-United States Investigation of NIDDM Genetics (FUSION), which were among the studies that contributed data to the new analysis. FUSION is funded by NHGRI's Division of Intramural Research and the National Institute of Diabetes and Digestive and Kidney Diseases (NIDDK).

Researchers said more work is needed to understand the impact of their discovery that a genetic variant called JAZF1 appears to be involved in diabetes as well as prostate cancer. One of the study's lead authors, Eleftheria Zeggini, Ph.D., of the University of Oxford, said, "This is now the second example of a gene which affects both type 2 diabetes and prostate cancer. We don't yet know what the connections are, but this may have important implications for the future design of drugs for both of these conditions."

The research was conducted by the DIAbetes Genetics Replication And Meta-analysis (DIAGRAM) consortium, which brought together many groups active in the field of diabetes research. In the *Nature Genetics* paper, DIAGRAM researchers combined the data from three previously published genome-wide association studies in an effort to boost the statistical power of their searches—an approach that scientists refer to as meta-analysis. The strategy paid off, enabling researchers to identify six genetic variants associated with type 2 diabetes that had gone undetected in the smaller, individual studies.

Researchers Identify New Genetic Risk Factors for Type 2 Diabetes

In the most comprehensive look at genetic risk factors for type 2 diabetes to date, a U.S.-Finnish team, working in close collaboration with two other groups, has identified at least four new genetic variants associated with increased risk of diabetes and confirmed existence of another six. The findings of the three groups, published simultaneously on April 26, 2007, in the online edition of the journal *Science*, boost to at least ten the number of genetic variants confidently associated with increased susceptibility to type 2 diabetes—a disease that affects more than two hundred million people worldwide.

"This achievement represents a major milestone in our battle against diabetes. It will accelerate efforts to understand the genetic risk factors for this disease, as well as explore how these genetic factors interact with each other and with lifestyle factors," said National Institutes of Health (NIH) director Elias A. Zerhouni, M.D. "Such research is opening the door to the era of personalized medicine. Our current one-size-fits-all approach will soon give way to more individualized strategies based on each person's unique genetic make-up."

Led by Michael Boehnke, Ph.D., of the University of Michigan's School of Public Health, Ann Arbor; Francis Collins, M.D., Ph.D., of the National Human Genome Research Institute; Richard Bergman, Ph.D., of the University of Southern California, Los Angeles; Karen

Mohlke, Ph.D. of the University of North Carolina, Chapel Hill; and Jaakko Tuomilehto, M.D., Ph.D. of the University of Helsinki and National Public Health Institute in Finland; the U.S.-Finnish team received major support from the National Institute of Diabetes and Digestive and Kidney Diseases (NIDDK) and NHGRI's Division of Intramural Research, both part of the NIH. The laboratory analysis of genetic variants in the first stage of the study was conducted by the Center for Inherited Disease Research, using funding from NIH and The Johns Hopkins University in Baltimore.

The research was carried out in conjunction with the work of two other teams: the Diabetes Genetics Initiative, which is a collaboration of the Broad Institute of Harvard and the Massachusetts Institute of Technology (MIT), Cambridge, Massachusetts; Lund University, Malmo, Sweden; and Novartis, Basel, Switzerland; and the Wellcome Trust Case Control Consortium/U.K. Type 2 Diabetes Genetics Consortium. The Diabetes Genetics Initiative was led by David Altshuler, M.D., Ph.D., Broad Institute; Leif Groop, M.D., Ph.D., Lund University; and Thomas Hughes, Ph.D., Novartis. The British team was led by Mark McCarthy, M.D., FRCP, Oxford University, and Andrew Hattersley, D.M., FRCP, Peninsula Medical School, Plymouth.

"It's been a formidable challenge to identify the complex genetic factors involved in common diseases, such as type 2 diabetes. Now, thanks to the tools and technologies generated by the sequencing of the human genome and subsequent mapping of common human genetic variations, we finally are making significant progress," said NHGRI Director Collins, who led the NIH component of the Human Genome Project.

Type 2 diabetes affects nearly twenty-one million people in the United States and the incidence of the disease has skyrocketed in the United States and many other developed nations over the last thirty years. Diabetes is a major cause of heart disease and stroke, as well as the most common cause in U.S. adults of blindness, kidney failure, and amputations not related to trauma.

NIDDK director Griffin P. Rodgers, M.D., said, "These genetic findings are exciting news for diabetes research. While more work remains to be done, the newly identified genetic variants may point us in the direction of valuable new drug targets for the prevention or treatment of type 2 diabetes."

Previously known as adult-onset or non-insulin-dependent diabetes (NIDDM), type 2 diabetes usually appears after age forty, often in overweight, sedentary individuals. However, an increasing number of younger people and even children are developing the disease, which is characterized by the resistance of target tissues to respond to insulin and a gradual failure of insulin-secreting cells in the pancreas.

In addition to lifestyle factors like obesity, poor diet, and lack of exercise, doctors have long known that heredity plays a significant role in the risk of developing type 2 diabetes. People who have a parent or sibling with type 2 diabetes face a 3.5-times greater risk than people without a family history of the disease. However, researchers have only recently begun to zero in on particular genetic variants that increase or decrease susceptibility to the disease.

To make their discoveries, researchers used a relatively new, comprehensive strategy known as a genome-wide association study. "Genome-wide association studies offer a powerful way to uncover the genetic variations that contribute to diabetes, as well as other common conditions, such as asthma, arthritis, heart disease, cancer, and mental illnesses," Dr. Boehnke said. "Once susceptibility genes are identified, researchers then can use this information to develop better approaches to detecting, treating, and preventing disease."

To conduct a genome-wide association study, researchers use two groups of participants: a large group of people with the disease being studied and a large group of otherwise similar people without the disease. Utilizing deoxyribonucleic acid (DNA) purified from blood or cells, researchers quickly survey each participant's complete set of DNA, or genome, for strategically selected markers of genetic variation.

If certain genetic variations are found more frequently in people with the disease compared to healthy people, the variations are said to be associated with the disease. The associated genetic variations can serve as a strong pointer to the region of the genome where the genetic risk factor resides. However, the first variants detected may not themselves directly influence disease susceptibility, and the actual causative variant may lie nearby. This means researchers often need to take additional steps, such as sequencing every DNA base pair in that particular region of the genome, to identify the exact genetic variant that affects disease risk.

In the latest work, researchers began by scanning the genomes of more than 2,300 Finnish people who took part in the Finland-United States Investigation Of NIDDM Genetics (FUSION) and Finrisk 2002 studies. About half of the participants had type 2 diabetes and the other half had normal blood glucose levels.

"We thank all the Finnish citizens who participated in this study. Their generosity has created a lasting legacy that will help to reduce the terrible toll that diabetes is taking on the world's health," said

Dr. Tuomilehto of the Diabetes Unit in Finland's National Public Health Institute.

To validate their findings, the researchers compared their initial results with results from genome scans of three thousand Swedish and Finnish participants in the Diabetes Genetics Initiative and five thousand British participants in the Wellcome Trust Case Control Consortium, led by Peter Donnelly, D.Phil., Oxford University. After identifying promising leads through this approach, the three research teams jointly replicated their findings using smaller, more focused sets of genetic markers in additional groups totaling more than 22,000 people from Finland, Poland, Sweden, the United Kingdom and the United States. All told, the genomes of 32,554 people were tested for the study, making it one of the largest genome-wide association efforts conducted to date.

"This is a phenomenal accomplishment, in terms of both the breadth and depth of the research. By pulling together and sharing their data, these three groups were able to achieve far more than any one of them could have done alone," said Eric D. Green, M.D., Ph.D., director of NHGRI's Division of Intramural Research. "This is scientific collaboration at its best."

Ultimately, the researchers identified four new diabetes-associated variations, as well as confirmed previous findings that associated six other genetic variants with increased diabetes risk. The newly identified diabetes-associated variations lie in or near the following:

- **IGF2BP2:** This gene codes for a protein called insulin-like growth factor 2 mRNA binding protein 2. Insulin-like growth factor 2 is thought to play a role in regulating insulin action.

- **CDKAL1:** This gene codes for a protein called CDK5 regulatory subunit associated protein1-like1. The protein may affect the activity of the cyclin dependent kinase 5 (CDK5) protein, which stimulates insulin production and may influence other processes in the pancreas's insulin-producing cells, known as beta cells. In addition, excessive activity of CDK5 in the pancreas may lead to the degeneration of beta cells.

- **CDKN2A and CDKN2B:** The proteins produced by these two genes inhibit the activity of cyclin-dependent protein kinases, including one that has been shown to influence the growth of beta cells in mice. Interestingly, these genes have been heavily studied for their role in cancer, but their contribution to diabetes comes as a complete surprise.

- **Chromosome 11:** One intriguing association is located in a region of chromosome 11 not known to contain any genes. Researchers speculate that the variant sequences may regulate the activity of genes located elsewhere in the genome, but more work is needed to determine the exact relationships to pathways involved in type 2 diabetes.

The genetic variants associated with diabetes that were confidently confirmed by the new research are: TCF7L2, SLC30A8, HHEX, PPARG, KCNJ11, and FTO. A variant in FTO was recently associated with increased risk of obesity (T. Frayling et al. A Common Variant in the FTO Gene Is Associated with Body Mass Index and Predisposes to Childhood and Adult Obesity. *Science Express*, Published online April 12, 2007). The latest study found that variations in or near the FTO gene are also associated with greater risk of type 2 diabetes, which is likely related to an increased predisposition to obesity.

When the genomes of the Finnish participants were scanned for all ten diabetes-associated genetic variants, researchers could identify individuals whose genetic profiles placed them at increased risk for type 2 diabetes—including one subset of people who faced a risk four times higher than those at the lowest genetic risk. This "could potentially have value in a personalized preventive medicine program," the researchers wrote.

However, the researchers emphasized that their predictions of disease risk need to be interpreted with caution because the diabetes group in their sample was "enriched" with people who had affected siblings and because the healthy group excluded people who had impaired glucose tolerance or impaired fasting glucose.

Chapter 53

Genetics and Heart Disease

Chapter Contents

Section 53.1

Cardiovascular Disease and Genetics: What Is the Connection?

Heart disease is the leading cause of death for all people in the United States. While most people know some of the risk factors for heart disease—such as obesity, smoking, and high blood pressure—there is also a genetic component to your risk. It is important to know that a genetic predisposition does *not* doom you to cardiovascular disease! You still have many tools to control your health—along with an added incentive to do so.

First, some definitions: Cardiovascular disease includes disorders of the heart and blood vessel system. Cardiovascular diseases include heart disease, stroke, high blood pressure, and rheumatic heart disease. Heart disease means that the arteries that supply blood to the heart become narrowed and hardened due to a buildup of plaque resulting in decreased blood flow to the heart. This plaque is the accumulation of fat and cholesterol. If an artery becomes totally blocked with plaque, oxygen and nutrients are prevented from getting to the heart (heart attack) and the heart muscle may be permanently damaged. Although there are surgical procedures that can help restore blood flow to the heart, the arteries remain damaged.

Who is at risk?

It is important to acknowledge that many people are not aware of their risk for cardiovascular disease. Some common risk factors are high blood pressure, diabetes, smoking, obesity, physical inactivity, having a family history of early heart disease, and age (forty-five for men, fifty-five for women). Women who have gone through early menopause, either naturally or because they have had a hysterectomy, are twice as likely to develop heart disease as women of the same age who have not yet gone through menopause.

What does family history have to do with it?

Heart disease is multifactorial—meaning both genetics and environment affect your health. There are probably several hundred genes that influence cardiovascular health, and testing for every one of them is not practical—nor would it be helpful, since many of the genes interact with each other. Taking your family history, however, is both free and full of information about not only your risk for heart disease, but other multifactorial diseases as well. If your father or brother had a heart attack before age fifty-five, or if your mother or sister had one before age sixty-five, you are more likely to get heart disease yourself. Although you can't change your family history, you can be aware of it and use your knowledge to change your behavior. You can also use your family history to help educate other family members about their risks and how to improve their risk. Family members often share the same nongenetic risk factors such as a sedentary lifestyle, tobacco use, and poor diet. Working as a team to correct these factors can increase each individual's chance of success.

A small number of families have autosomal dominant genetic mutations that affect cholesterol transport and use in the body. These mutations predispose to a very high risk for heart disease. All of our genes come in pairs. Autosomal dominant means that a single change on one gene causes a change in the gene's function, leading to disease. About one in five hundred people have a gene change that predisposes them to familial hypercholesterolemia (FH). This is an autosomal dominant gene change that causes high cholesterol, which leads to heart attacks at a mean age of forty years for men and fifty years for women. About one in one hundred people have an autosomal dominant gene change that causes familial combined hyperlipidemia (FCH), in which individuals have elevated triglycerides, cholesterol, or both. About 15 percent of people who have a heart attack before age sixty have FCH.

What can you do?

First, talk to your doctor about the risk factors that you can control. Quitting smoking, starting an exercise program, and eating a healthy diet are the obvious first steps. Reviewing your family history and screening for high cholesterol and diabetes can help you and your physician fine-tune your health program. Your physician may recommend further screening or diagnostic tests, depending on your current and past health status. Last, acknowledge your family history without using it as an excuse for heart disease. Your genes do not equal your health destiny! Know that you have the privilege, ability, and responsibility to maximize your cardiovascular health, as well as the chance to talk with family and friends about their health.

Section 53.2

New Research in the Genetics of Heart Disease

"New Genetic Variants Associated with Risk for Coronary Artery Disease" is excerpted from "International Effort Finds New Genetic Variants Associated with Lipid Levels, Risk for Coronary Artery Disease," National Human Genome Research Institute, January 13, 2008. "Researchers Identify Gene Mutation Related to Atrial Fibrillation" is reprinted with permission from "UI Helps Identify Gene Mutation Related to Atrial Fibrillation," © 2008 University of Iowa.

New Genetic Variants Associated with Risk for Coronary Artery Disease

Environmental and genetic factors influence a person's blood fat, or lipid levels, important risk factors for coronary artery disease (CAD). While there is some understanding of the environmental contribution, the role of genetics has been less defined. Now, in an international collaboration supported primarily by the National Institutes of Health (NIH), scientists have discovered more than twenty-five genetic variants in eighteen genes connected to cholesterol and lipid levels. Seven of the eighteen genes previously had not been connected to these levels, while the eleven others confirm previous discoveries. In the investigation, published online January 13, 2008, and in the February 2008 print issue of *Nature Genetics*, the associated genes were found through studies of more than twenty thousand individuals and more than two million genetic variants, spanning the entire genome. These variants potentially open the door to strategies for the treatment and prevention of CAD.

"Heart disease is a leading cause of illness, disability, and death in industrialized countries, particularly for older people," says National Institute on Aging (NIA) director Richard J. Hodes, M.D. "We know that certain lifestyle factors like smoking, diet, and physical activity greatly affect a person's lipid profiles. This study is an important, basic step in finding the genes that influence lipid levels and heart disease so that we can better understand the genetic contribution to cardiovascular risk."

Cristen Willer, Ph.D., at the University of Michigan's School of Public Health, Ann Arbor, and Serena Sanna, Ph.D., at the C.N.R. Institute of Neurogenetics and Neuropharmacology, Monserrato, Italy, and other members of the SardiNIA Study of Aging, including investigators at NIA, conducted the study, along with members of the Finland-United States Investigation of Non-Insulin-Dependent Diabetes Mellitus Genetics (FUSION) study, which included investigators in North Carolina, Michigan, Finland, Los Angeles, and from the National Human Genome Research Institute (NHGRI). SardiNIA and FUSION investigators also coordinated the efforts of other groups in France, the United Kingdom, and across the United States.

The purpose of the study was to identify comprehensively genetic variants that influence lipid levels and to examine the relationships between these genetic variants and risk of CAD. High levels of low-density lipoprotein (LDL) ("bad" cholesterol) appear to increase the risk of CAD by narrowing or blocking arteries that carry blood to the heart. High levels of high-density lipoprotein (HDL) ("good" cholesterol) appear to lower the risk. High levels of triglycerides, which make up a large part of the body's fat and are also found in the bloodstream, are also associated with increased risk of CAD.

To identify genetic variants that play a role in lipid levels, researchers turned to a relatively new approach, known as a genome-wide association study (GWAS). The GWAS strategy enables researchers to survey the entire human genetic blueprint, or genome, not just the genetic variants in a few genes. The human genome contains approximately three billion base pairs, or letters, of deoxyribonucleic acid (DNA). Small, single-letter variations naturally occur about once in every one thousand letters of the DNA code. Most of these genetic variants have not yet been associated with particular traits or disease risks. However, in some instances, people with a certain trait, such as higher levels of LDL cholesterol, tend to have one version of the variant, while those with lower levels are more likely to have the other version. In such instances, researchers may infer that there is an association between the values of the trait and the variants in the gene.

Typically, GWAS studies have been carried out in samples where all individuals are examined with the same gene chip, an experimental device that allows investigators to measure more than one hundred thousand genetic variants in a single experiment. But in this study, investigators developed and employed new statistical methods that allowed them to combine data across different gene chips and thus examine much larger numbers of participants.

With the statistical power gained by new programs that facilitated pooling of the large SardiNIA, FUSION, and Diabetes Genetic Initiative (DGI) datasets, researchers were able to identify variations in eighteen genes that influence HDL, LDL, and/or triglyceride levels. This list of lipid-associated genes is substantially longer than what was generated by analyses of individual datasets, which had only pointed to one to three genes each. Of the seven newly implicated genes, two were associated with HDL levels, one with LDL levels, three with triglyceride levels, and one with both triglycerides and LDL levels.

"These results are yet another example of how genome-wide association studies are opening exciting new avenues for biomedical research," says NHGRI director Francis S. Collins, M.D., Ph.D., who is a coauthor of the study and an investigator in NHGRI's Genome Technology Branch. "While some of the genetic variants we identified are known to play a well-established role in lipid metabolism, others have no obvious connection. Further studies to identify the precise genes and biological pathways involved could shed new light on lipid metabolism."

Scientists estimate that the genetic contribution to lipid levels is about 30 to 40 percent; the genetic variants uncovered in the new study are responsible for about 5 to 8 percent of that contribution, the scientists note, which means there is more work to be done. "In this study we carried out a comprehensive search for common variants of large effect. The genetic factors still to be discovered might turn out to be common variants with smaller effects or rare variants with a large effect," says Karen L. Mohlke, Ph.D., of the University of North Carolina, Chapel Hill, who co-directed the study with Goncalo R. Abecasis, Ph.D., of the University of Michigan's School of Public Health.

To determine if the genetic variants associated with lipid levels also influence risk of heart disease, the researchers compared their results with results from the Wellcome Trust Case Control Consortium's recent genome-wide association study of CAD involving fifteen thousand British individuals. They found that all gene variants associated with increased LDL levels also were more prevalent among people with CAD. People with the gene variant for high triglyceride levels also had an increased risk for CAD, although the relationship was not as strong. No relationship was found between HDL and CAD.

"It was surprising that while it was clear that genetic variants that increase your 'bad' cholesterol are also associated with increased risk of heart disease, we did not find that variants influencing your 'good' cholesterol were associated with decreased risk of coronary artery disease. Perhaps that result will lead us to re-examine the roles of good and bad cholesterol in susceptibility to heart disease," remarks Abecasis.

Identifying a correlation among genes influencing lipid levels and risk for coronary heart disease is a first step in a long path to potentially important clinical implications. "What we're looking for, ultimately, are novel therapeutics and/or lifestyle modifications that can be recommended to individuals to help manage blood lipid levels and reduce risk of heart disease," says David Schlessinger, Ph.D., chief of the NIA's Laboratory of Genetics and NIA project officer for SardiNIA.

This study also demonstrates the power of international collaboration in genetic analyses. None of the studies that cooperated to make this work possible were large enough to find all of these important associations alone. By working together, previously unsuspected genetic influences on lipid levels and heart disease were revealed.

Researchers Identify Gene Mutation Related to Atrial Fibrillation

Mayo Clinic and University of Iowa (UI) researchers have identified a new mechanism of atrial fibrillation, the most common form of cardiac arrhythmia (irregular heartbeat).

The researchers discovered a mutation in a gene that encodes a hormone originating in the atria of the heart, and they established the mutation as causative of atrial fibrillation. This discovery opens a new avenue to pursue for possible treatments.

The study was based on the analysis of genetic information from one Caucasian family and other control subjects, and investigations in animal models. The study results appeared online July 10, 2008, at the *New England Journal of Medicine* website.

"While the family members with atrial fibrillation have a rare mutation, the study findings provide insight into pathways that may be applicable to people in the general population with atrial fibrillation," said the study's primary author, Denice Hodgson-Zingman, M.D., assistant professor of internal medicine at the UI Roy J. and Lucille A. Carver College of Medicine.

"Atrial fibrillation is a significant public health concern. Nearly one in four people age seventy-five and older has the condition, and it is a major cause of stroke," said Hodgson-Zingman, who also is an electrophysiologist with UI Heart and Vascular Care.

The study indicates that disturbances in a pathway involving atrial natriuretic peptide (ANP) promotes atrial fibrillation. ANP is a hormone that regulates body water, sodium, and certain vascular effects.

"Usually inherited arrhythmias are associated with mutations in heart structural proteins or ion channels," Hodgson-Zingman said. "It is intriguing that we identified a circulating hormone as a cause of atrial fibrillation because this gives us a potential new target for developing treatments."

The senior author of the study, Timothy Olson, M.D., associate professor of medicine and pediatrics at Mayo Clinic, led a team of investigators that gathered and analyzed genetic data from the affected and unaffected family members and control subjects. They found that the eleven family members with atrial fibrillation had a shared mutation in the gene that encodes for ANP. The mutation was not found in family members without atrial fibrillation or in unrelated patients without the condition.

The team also determined that in patients with the mutation, the blood concentration of the abnormal peptide is much higher than that of normal ANP, which is present at typical levels (because the mutation is in only one of the two copies of the gene, the persons with the mutation also make normal ANP).

UI researchers Hodgson-Zingman and co-author Leonid Zingman, M.D., assistant professor of internal medicine at the UI Carver College of Medicine, used animal models to establish that mutated ANP causes changes in heart electrical function expected to promote atrial fibrillation, thus providing crucial evidence that the mutated ANP is not neutral or an incidental finding.

The study also suggests the mutant peptide appears in the plasma in high levels, either because it is not broken down or more of it is generated than normal. "It is more likely that the peptide is not broken down as quickly, but additional research is needed. It also is possible that when concentrations are abnormally elevated for long periods of time, they could have toxic effects on the heart," Hodgson-Zingman said.

The UI results also suggest that mutant ANP may be more potent in its cellular effects than non-mutant ANP.

"The potency issue is important because it suggests changes to the peptide could be used for therapeutic purposes. However, more studies would be needed to determine how the peptide binds to receptors and affects downstream mechanisms," Hodgson-Zingman said.

Atrial fibrillation occurs when rapid, irregular electrical activity occurs in the top two chambers of the heart (the atria). As a result, the chambers do not beat as they normally should but instead quiver.

"The chaotic activity results in less efficient blood flow and can lead to clot formation with consequent stroke, and to rapid, irregular beating in the lower chambers of the heart, causing further problems," Hodgson-Zingman said.

Currently, there is no cure for atrial fibrillation. Treatment for people with the condition focuses on preventing stroke through the use of aspirin or other blood thinners, and symptom control through medications or invasive procedures.

The study was supported by a grant from the National Institutes of Health. In addition, Olson received a Mayo Foundation award.

Chapter 54

Genetics and Hypertension

Chapter Contents

Section 54.1

Researchers Identify Gene Variant Linked to High Blood Pressure

Researchers at the University of Maryland School of Medicine have identified a common gene variant that appears to influence people's risk of developing high blood pressure, according to the results of a study published online December 29, 2008, in the *Proceedings of the National Academy of Sciences* (*PNAS*).

The STK39 gene is the first hypertension susceptibility gene to be uncovered through a new technique called a genome-wide association study and confirmed by data from several independent studies. Located on chromosome 2, the gene produces a protein that helps to regulate how the kidneys process salt, which plays a key role in determining blood pressure.

"This discovery has great potential for enhancing our ability to tailor treatments to the individual—what we call personalized medicine—and to more effectively manage patients with hypertension. We hope that it will lead to new therapies to combat this serious public health problem worldwide," says the senior author, Yen-Pei Christy Chang, Ph.D., an assistant professor of medicine and of epidemiology and preventive medicine at the University of Maryland School of Medicine.

But, Dr. Chang says, more research is needed. "Hypertension is a very complex condition, with numerous other genetic, environmental, and lifestyle factors involved. The STK39 gene is only one important piece of the puzzle," she says. "We want to determine how people with different variations of this gene respond to diuretics and other medications, or to lifestyle changes, such as reducing the amount of salt in their diet. This information might help us discover the most effective way to control an individual patient's blood pressure."

One in four Americans has elevated blood pressure, or hypertension, which can lead to death or result in complications, such as cardiovascular disease, stroke, and end-stage kidney disease. Doctors consider the ideal systolic and diastolic blood pressure to be less than 120/80. (The numbers reflect the pressure of the blood against the arteries when the heart beats and is at rest.) When blood pressure is elevated, doctors recommend lifestyle changes or prescribe medications, such as diuretics, which force the kidneys to remove water from the body, in order to treat the condition. However, patients respond differently to treatments and finding the best treatment among all the possible ones for specific patients is still a "try and see" process, according to Dr. Chang.

Scientists believe multiple genes are involved in the most common form of high blood pressure called essential hypertension. But because so many factors affect blood pressure, including diet, exercise, and stress levels, it has been difficult to pinpoint a specific gene or group of genes, says the lead author, Ying Wang, Ph.D., a researcher at the University of Maryland School of Medicine.

The University of Maryland researchers identified the link between the STK39 gene and blood pressure by analyzing the deoxyribonucleic acid (DNA) of 542 members of the Old Order Amish community in Lancaster County, Pennsylvania, scanning approximately one hundred thousand genetic markers across the entire genome for variants known as single nucleotide polymorphisms, or SNPs, associated with systolic and diastolic blood pressure. The researchers found strong association "signals" with common variants of the serine/threonine kinase gene, or STK39, and confirmed their findings in another group of Amish people and in four other groups of Caucasians in the United States and Europe.

People with one particular variant showed slight increases in blood pressure compared to those with a more common form of the gene and were more likely to develop hypertension, researchers found. The researchers estimate that about 20 percent of Caucasians in the general population have this variant of the STK39 gene.

"With this new 'scanning' approach—the genome-wide association study—we are able to uncover genes that have previously eluded us. The field of complex disease genetics has undergone a revolution in terms of discovering new genes and understanding the genetic basis of common adult-onset diseases," says co-author Alan R. Shuldiner, M.D., professor of medicine; head of the Division of Endocrinology, Diabetes and Nutrition; and director of the Program in Genetics and Genomic Medicine at the University of Maryland School of Medicine.

The study being published online in PNAS is titled, "Whole-genome association study identifies STK39 as a novel hypertension suscepti- bility gene." It will appear in the print edition of PNAS in early Janu- ary 2009.

The Amish are ideal for such studies because they are a geneti- cally homogeneous people whose forefathers came to Pennsylvania from Europe in the mid-1700s and share a similar diet and rural lifestyle. Because many in the Amish community don't have regular medical checkups, they often don't know they have high blood pres- sure or take medications for it, according to Dr. Chang. The Amish appear to have as much hypertension as other Caucasians. As a re- sult of the study, some of the participants learned that they had hy- pertension and were able to start treatment.

The research, which was funded by the National Institutes of Health, is a spin-off project of another University of Maryland study— the Amish Family Diabetes study—looking for genes that may cause type 2 diabetes. Researchers at the School of Medicine already have identified a number of genes that may play a role in the development of this type of diabetes.

Since 1993, University of Maryland researchers, led by Dr. Shuldiner, have conducted more than a dozen studies of the Amish in Lancaster County, Pennsylvania, searching for genes that cause a variety of medical problems, including osteoporosis and obesity, as well as dia- betes and hypertension. More than four thousand members of the Amish community have participated in the studies.

Section 54.2

Rare Genetic Mutations Protect against Hypertension

Howard Hughes Medical Institute (HHMI) researchers have found that rare mutations in three genes contribute to blood pressure variation in the general population.

The scientists had previously shown that mutations in the three "salt handling" genes cause several rare diseases that are characterized by low blood pressure. By sequencing deoxyribonucleic acid (DNA) samples obtained from 3,125 people who are participating in the Framingham Heart Study, the researchers identified new functional mutations in these three genes that are likely to be carried by an estimated one hundred million people worldwide.

The Framingham Heart Study was begun in 1948 in an effort to identify common factors or characteristics that contribute to cardiovascular disease by following its development over a long period of time in a large group of participants who had not yet developed overt symptoms of cardiovascular disease or suffered a heart attack or stroke.

"We find that about 2 percent of the population has mutations in at least one of these three genes—although all of the identified mutations are individually very rare," said senior author Richard P. Lifton, a Howard Hughes Medical Institute researcher at Yale University School of Medicine. "Mutation carriers have reduced blood pressure, with a 60 percent reduction in the risk of hypertension at age sixty."

The findings, reported in the April 6, 2008, edition of the journal *Nature Genetics*, are important because they yield tantalizing new evidence about why some people seem to be less susceptible to developing high blood pressure, a condition that affects a billion people worldwide and contributes significantly to heart and kidney disease, and stroke.

505

"This study is an important milestone in the understanding of the genetic causes of hypertension," said Elizabeth G. Nabel, M.D., director of the National Heart, Lung, and Blood Institute (NHLBI) of the National Institutes of Health. "The discovery of a substantial blood pressure lowering effect of many rare mutations in genes involved in sodium handling—and the promise of future discoveries of other genetic mutations—has enormous potential public health impact."

What's more, by identifying the role played by rare genetic mutations in governing how the kidney regulates salt, the researchers have devised a general approach that may be broadly applicable to uncovering the genetic architecture of common conditions such as hypertension.

"This new study, for the first time, extends the findings from patients with rare Mendelian traits to the general population. The findings suggest that independently rare mutations that alter salt handling by the kidneys collectively account for a substantial fraction of the general population's variability in disease susceptibility," said Lifton.

Lifton noted that there are probably about one hundred million people worldwide who carry the mutations and are thus protected from hypertension. "The mutations we have identified have clinically meaningful effects to individual patients and suggest that independently rare mutations will collectively account for a substantial fraction of the population's variability in disease susceptibility," he said.

The researchers started by examining variations in three genes known to cause rare recessive diseases characterized by large reductions in blood pressure. The analysis was conducted on "salt handling" genes isolated from people involved in the Framingham Heart Study (FHS), which is directed by Daniel Levy of NHLBI. Levy is a co-author of the *Nature Genetics* report. Co-first authors Weizhen Ji and Jia Ni Foo are at Yale University School of Medicine.

Lifton's team zeroed in on the three salt-regulating genes—NCCT, NKCC2, and ROMK—which his group had previously linked to rare but serious human diseases, including Gitelman and Bartter syndromes. Both are conditions characterized by inherited low blood pressure caused by recessive mutations, where two defective copies of a gene are at play.

Salt handing is an essential function of the kidneys. Our kidneys process more than three pounds of salt per day, and genetic mutations that raise or lower the ability of the organ to absorb and process salt can manifest themselves in higher or lower blood pressure.

Lifton's group has searched worldwide for patients with very high or very low blood pressure due to mutations in single genes. Such patients are often identified through family histories of extreme blood pressure. To date, his group has found a score of gene mutations that lower or raise blood pressure, including those that cause the extreme low blood pressure found in patients with Gitelman and Bartter syndromes.

"We used knowledge of the spectrum of mutations that cause Gitelman and Bartter syndromes to sort among the hundreds of sequence changes we observed to identify those that are either known or highly likely to alter the function of the (gene) encoded proteins," Lifton explained.

By sequencing each of the three genes obtained from DNA samples from 3,125 participants in the Framingham Heart Study, and doing additional biochemical, genetic, and genomic analysis, the HHMI team found functional mutations in one of the genes in at least one of every sixty-four of the study's participants sampled.

"The results show that nearly 2 percent of the FHS cohort has a defective copy of one of these three genes," Lifton said. "Unlike patients with Gitelman and Bartter syndromes, these subjects have only one defective copy, not two."

Lifton's group then tracked the influence of the mutation on blood pressure in FHS subjects aged forty to sixty, a time of life when hypertension manifests itself and can pose serious health risks.

"We found that these mutation carriers have a 60 percent reduction in their risk of developing hypertension and have significantly lower blood pressure than those who do not have mutations," Lifton said. The influence of the mutation, he added, approximates effects achieved with drugs used to lower blood pressure.

The practical upshot of the new work, according to Lifton, could be potential new drugs to mimic the effects of the mutation by selectively inhibiting a single gene or several genes.

In addition, the study more broadly underscores the value of genetic analysis—resequencing of genes and genomes to ferret out functional mutations—for understanding individual risk of disease.

"A major question about the genetic underpinnings of hypertension and other common diseases has been whether these are accounted for by common or rare DNA variations," said Lifton. "Our study demonstrates the role of rare variation, showing that effects of rare mutations in these three genes cause relatively large effects, with clinically significant effects in individual patients. These findings suggest that much of the variation in common disease risk for hypertension and other diseases will be accounted for by rare (genetic) variants."

Section 54.3

Genetics Influence Reaction to Blood Pressure Medications

A person's genetic make-up seems to influence how he or she reacts to certain hypertension medications.

In the future, being able to match genes with medications may help save a patient's life, experts predict.

"This is potentially a very, very important observation. It's a large study with hard clinical endpoints," said Dr. Joshua M. Hare, chief of cardiology at the University of Miami Miller School of Medicine. "This is a beautiful example of what we anticipate personalized medicine to be," said Hare, who was not involved in the research.

Another expert agreed. Dr. Jeffery Vance, professor at the Miami Institute for Human Genomics, said that "This is where medicine is going. It's important that we've got big clinical trials [showing this]. They cost a lot of money but this shows that it's clearly worth it."

The gene variant identified in the new study is likely to be just one of several that play a role in hypertension, also known as high blood pressure.

"Hypertension is such a complex disease. There are many different mechanisms that help us regulate our blood pressure so we would not expect any one gene to have a really large effect for [such] a common condition like hypertension," noted study senior author Donna K. Arnett, professor and chair of the University of Alabama at Birmingham's Department of Epidemiology. "That we found this effect is important because we didn't think we would ever be able to do pharmacogenetics, given the complexity of hypertension."

According to background information with the study, published in the January 23, 2008, issue of the *Journal of the American Medical Association*, some sixty-five million people in the United States have hypertension. But only about two-thirds have their condition under control. Uncontrolled hypertension can lead to such problems as heart attack and stroke.

Previous studies have shown that the presence of certain gene characteristics can predict response to treatments such as angiotensin-converting enzyme (ACE) inhibitors, which are drugs used to control hypertension. But this information hasn't been adopted widely by doctors.

The new study focused on the NPPA (atrial natriuretic precursor A) gene, which is involved in forming atrial natriuretic polypeptide, which acts as a diuretic.

Specifically, the study authors wanted to see if people with hypertension and two different NPPA genotypes (known as NPPA G664A and NPPA T2238C) responded differently to different medications.

In all, 38,462 people with hypertension underwent genotyping (genetic testing) and were randomly assigned to receive a diuretic (chlorthalidone) or one of the following three drugs: a calcium channel blocker (amlodipine); an angiotensin-converting enzyme inhibitor (lisinopril); or an alpha-blocker (doxazosin).

People with the more common subtype of the NPPA gene responded better to the calcium channel blocker than the diuretic. There were no differences in response between the diuretic and the other two drugs studied, the researchers said.

People with the other genotype fared better on the diuretic.

"Eventually we should be able to utilize prescreening for treatment to determine which drug you may respond best to," Arnett said. "This is a small but important step toward personalized medicine."

Chapter 55

Heredity and Movement Disorders

Chapter Contents

Section 55.1

Essential Tremor

Essential tremor is a type of involuntary shaking movement in which no cause can be identified. Involuntary means you shake without trying to do so.

Causes

Essential tremor is the most common type of tremor. In general, tremors occur when there is a problem with the nerves supplying certain muscles. The specific cause for essential tremor is unknown. However, some research suggests that the cerebellum, the part of the brain that controls muscles movements, does not work correctly in patients with essential tremor.

Essential tremors can occur at any age but are most common in people older than sixty-five. There are several different types of essential tremor, including:

- essential tremor with head tremor;

- young-onset essential tremor (essential tremors that start at an earlier-than-usual age).

If an essential tremor occurs in more than one member of a family, it is called a familial tremor.

Symptoms

The tremors are usually most obvious in the hands, but may affect the arms, head, eyelids, or other muscles. The tremors rarely affect the legs or feet. People with essential tremors may have trouble holding or using small objects such as silverware or a pen.

The shaking usually involves small, rapid movements—more than five times a second.

The tremors may:

- occur when you move (action-related tremor), and may be less noticeable with rest;
- come and go, but generally get worse as you age;
- get worse with stress, caffeine, and certain medications;
- not affect both sides of the body the same way.

Exams and Tests

Your doctor can make the diagnosis by performing a physical exam and asking questions about your medical and personal history.

A physical exam will show shaking with movement. There are usually no problems with coordination or mental function.

Further tests may be needed to rule out other reasons for the tremors. Other causes of tremors may include:

- alcohol withdrawal;
- cigarette smoking;
- hyperthyroidism;
- pheochromocytoma;
- too much caffeine;
- use of certain medications;
- Wilson disease.

Blood tests and imaging studies (such as a computed tomography [CT] scan of the head, brain magnetic resonance imaging [MRI], and x-rays) are usually normal.

Treatment

Treatment may not be necessary unless the tremors interfere with your daily activities or cause embarrassment.

Medicines may help relieve symptoms. How well medicines work depend on the individual patient.

Two medications used to treat tremors include:

- propranolol, a drug that blocks the action of stimulating substances called neurotransmitters, particularly those related to adrenaline;

- primidone, an antiseizure drug that also control the function of some neurotransmitters.

The drugs can have significant side effects.
Side effects of propranolol include:

- fatigue;
- nose stuffiness;
- shortness of breath (people with asthma should not use this drug);
- slow heartbeat.

Side effects of primidone include:

- drowsiness;
- difficulty concentrating;
- nausea;
- problems with walking, balance, and coordination.

Other medications that may reduce tremors include:

- antiseizure drugs such as gabapentin and topiramate;
- mild tranquilizers such as alprazolam or clonazepam;
- blood pressure drugs called calcium-channel blockers such as flunarizine and nimodipine;
- Botox® injections, given in the hand, have been used to reduce tremors by weakening local muscles.

In severe cases, surgery to implant a stimulating device in the brain may be an option.

Outlook (Prognosis)

An essential tremor is not a dangerous condition, but some patients find the tremors annoying and embarrassing.

Possible Complications

Severe essential tremor can interfere with daily activities, especially fine motor skills such as writing. Sometimes the tremors affect the voice box, which occasionally leads to speech problems.

When to Contact a Medical Professional

Call for an appointment with your healthcare provider if essential tremor interferes with your ability to perform daily activities.

Call your healthcare provider if you are being treated for this condition and have side effects from the medication, such as fainting, very slow heart rate, confusion or changes in alertness, lack of coordination, problems walking, and prolonged nausea or vomiting.

Prevention

Stress and caffeine can make tremors worse. Avoid caffeinated drinks such as coffee, tea, and soda, and other stimulants. Exercise and counseling to reduce emotional stress may also help.

Alcoholic beverages in small quantities may decrease tremors but can lead to alcohol dependence and alcohol abuse, especially if you have a family history of such problems. How alcohol helps relieve tremors is unknown.

References

Jankovic J. Movement Disorders. In: Goetz CG. *Textbook of Clinical Neurology*. 3rd ed. St. Louis, Mo: WB Saunders; 2007: chap. 34.

Section 55.2

Heredity and Parkinson Disease

Reprinted from "Learning about Parkinson's Disease,"
National Human Genome Research Institute, National Institutes
of Health, May 27, 2008.

What Do We Know about Heredity and Parkinson Disease?

Parkinson disease (PD) is a neurological condition that typically causes tremor and/or stiffness in movement. The condition affects about 1 to 2 percent of people over the age of sixty years and the chance of developing PD increases as we age. Most people affected with PD are not aware of any relatives with the condition but in a number of families, there is a family history. When three or more people are affected in a family, especially if they are diagnosed at an early age (under fifty years) we suspect that there may be a gene making this family more likely to develop the condition.

Genetics: The Basics

Our genetic material is stored in the center of every cell in our bodies (skin cells, hair cells, blood cells). This genetic material comes in individual units called genes. We all have thousands of genes. Genes carry the information the body needs to make proteins, which are the substances in the body that actually carry out all the functions we need to live and grow. Our genes affect many things about us: our height, eye color, why we respond to some medications better than others, and our likelihood of developing certain conditions. We have two copies of every gene: we inherit one copy, one member of each pair, from our mother and the other from our father. We then pass only one copy of a gene from each pair of genes to the next generation. Whether we pass on the gene we got from our father or the one from our mother is purely by chance, like flipping a coin heads or tails.

We all have genes that don't work properly. In most cases the other copy of the gene makes up for the one that does not work properly and we are healthy. A problem only arises if we meet someone else who has a nonworking copy of the same gene and we have a child who inherits two nonworking copies of that gene. This is called recessive inheritance.

Sometimes if one of our genes is not working properly the other copy of the gene cannot make up for it and that causes a condition or an increased risk of developing a condition. Each time we have a child we randomly pass on one copy of each gene. If the child inherits the copy that doesn't work properly, they too may develop the condition. This is called dominant inheritance.

What Genes are Linked to Parkinson Disease?

In 1997, we studied a large family that came from a small town in Southern Italy in which PD was inherited from parent to child (dominant inheritance). We found the gene that caused their inherited Parkinson disease and it coded for a protein called alpha-synuclein. If one studies the brains of people with PD after they die, one can see tiny little accumulations of protein called Lewy bodies (named after the doctor who first found them). Research has shown that there is a large amount of alpha-synuclein protein in the Lewy bodies of people who have non-inherited PD as well as in the brains of people who have inherited PD. This immediately told us that alpha-synuclein played an important role in all forms of PD and we are still doing a lot of research to better understand this role.

Since 1997 four other genes have been found and they have been named parkin, DJ1, PINK1, and LRRK2. The first three genes were found in affected individuals who had siblings with the condition but whose parents did not have Parkinson disease (recessive inheritance). There is some research to suggest that these genes may also be involved in early-onset PD (diagnosed before the age of thirty) or in dominantly inherited PD but it is too early yet to be certain. The most recently discovered gene (LRRK2) has been reported in families with dominant inheritance. Changes in this gene may account for 5 to 10 percent of dominantly inherited Parkinson disease.

What Determines Who Gets Parkinson Disease?

In most cases inheriting a nonworking copy of a single gene will not cause someone to develop Parkinson disease. We believe that many other complicating factors such as additional genes and environmental factors determine who will get the condition, when they get it, and how it affects them. In the families we have studied, some people who inherit the gene develop the condition and others live their entire lives without showing any symptoms. There is a lot of research on genes and the environment that is attempting to understand how all these factors interact.

Genetic Testing in Parkinson Disease

Genetic testing has recently become available for the parkin and PINK1 genes. Parkin is a large gene and testing is difficult. At the current stage of understanding, testing is likely to give a meaningful result only for people who develop the condition before the age of thirty years. PINK1 appears to be a rare cause of inherited Parkinson disease. A small percentage (~2 percent) of those developing the condition at an early age appear to carry mutations in the PINK1 gene.

Chapter 56

Genetic Factors in Obesity

Chapter Contents

Section 56.1

Obesity and Genetics: What We Know and Do Not Know

Reprinted from "Obesity and Genetics: What We Know, What We Don't Know, and What It Means," Centers for Disease Control and Prevention, Office of Public Health Genomics, June 8, 2007.

Introduction

Rising rates of obesity seem to be a consequence of modern life, with access to large amounts of palatable, high-calorie food and limited need for physical activity. However, this environment of plenty affects different people in different ways. Some are able to maintain a reasonable balance between energy input and energy expenditure. Others have a chronic imbalance that favors energy input, which expresses itself as overweight and obesity. What accounts for these differences between individuals?

What We Know

Biological relatives tend to resemble each other in many ways, including body weight. Individuals with a family history of obesity may be predisposed to gain weight and interventions that prevent obesity are especially important.

In an environment made constant for food intake and physical activity, individuals respond differently. Some people store more energy as fat in an environment of excess; others lose less fat in an environment of scarcity. The different responses are largely due to genetic variation between individuals.

Fat stores are regulated over long periods of time by complex systems that involve input and feedback from fatty tissues, the brain, and endocrine glands like the pancreas and the thyroid. Overweight and obesity can result from only a very small positive energy input imbalance over a long period of time.

Rarely, people have mutations in single genes that result in severe obesity that starts in infancy. Studying these individuals is providing insight into the complex biological pathways that regulate the balance between energy input and energy expenditure.

Obese individuals have genetic similarities that may shed light on the biological differences that predispose to gain weight. This knowledge may be useful in preventing or treating obesity in predisposed people.

Pharmaceutical companies are using genetic approaches (pharmacogenomics) to develop new drug strategies to treat obesity.

The tendency to store energy in the form of fat is believed to result from thousands of years of evolution in an environment characterized by tenuous food supplies. In other words, those who could store energy in times of plenty were more likely to survive periods of famine and to pass this tendency to their offspring.

What We Don't Know

Why are biological relatives more similar in body weight? What genes are associated with this observation? Are the same genetic associations seen in every family? How do these genes affect energy metabolism and regulation?

Why are interventions based on diet and exercise more effective for some people than others? What are the biological differences between these high and low responders? How do we use these insights to tailor interventions to specific needs?

What elements of energy regulation feedback systems are different in individuals? How do these differences affect energy metabolism and regulation?

How can thousands of years of evolutionary pressure be countered? Can specific factors in the modern environment (other than the obvious) be identified and controlled to more effectively counter these tendencies?

Do additional obesity syndromes exist that are caused by mutations in single genes? If so, what are they? What are the natural history, management strategy, and outcome for affected individuals?

How do genetic variations that are shared by obese people affect gene expression and function? How do genetic variation and environmental factors interact to produce obesity? What are the biological features associated with the tendency to gain weight? What are environmental factors helpful in countering these tendencies?

Will pharmacologic approaches benefit most people affected with obesity? Will these drugs be accessible to most people?

How can thousands of years of evolutionary pressure be countered? Can specific factors in the modern environment (other than the obvious) be identified and controlled to more effectively counter these tendencies?

What It Means

For people who are genetically predisposed to gain weight, preventing obesity is the best course. Predisposed persons may require individualized interventions and greater support to be successful in maintaining a healthy weight.

Obesity is a chronic lifelong condition that is the result of an environment of caloric abundance and relative physical inactivity modulated by a susceptible genotype. For those who are predisposed, preventing weight gain is the best course of action.

Genes are not destiny. Obesity can be prevented or can be managed in many cases with a combination of diet, physical activity, and medication.

Section 56.2

Researchers Discover New Genetic Risk factors Involved in Adult and Childhood Obesity

Reprinted from "Researchers Discover New Genetic Risk Factors Involved in Adult and Childhood Obesity," National Human Genome Research Institute, National Institutes of Health, December 14, 2008.

An international consortium, in search of the genetic risk factors for obesity, has identified six new genetic variants associated with BMI, or body mass index, a measurement that compares height to weight. The results, funded in part by the National Institutes of Health (NIH), were published online in the journal *Nature Genetics* on December 14, 2008.

The effect of each individual genetic variant was modest and the authors state in the paper that their findings have uncovered only a small fraction of what are probably hundreds of regions in the human genome that are likely to have minor contributions to obesity. The paper estimates that the 1 percent of people harboring the most obesity-causing variants will be an average of ten pounds heavier than the 1 percent of individuals with the fewest variants, and four pounds heavier than a typical person.

"Obesity is a major public health concern, with myriad health consequences. Understanding obesity's biological basis is crucial to designing more effective treatment and prevention strategies to help control body weight," said Alan E. Guttmacher, M.D., acting director of the National Human Genome Research Institute (NHGRI). "Today's findings are a major step forward in understanding how the human body regulates weight."

The study, conducted by the Genetic Investigation of Anthropometric Traits (GIANT) consortium representing seventy-six international research organizations, was led by Joel Hirschhorn, M.D., Ph.D. of Children's Hospital Boston and the Broad Institute of Harvard and the Massachusetts Institute of Technology (MIT) and Goncalo R. Abecasis, Ph.D. of the University of Michigan's School of Public Health.

Coauthors included intramural researchers from the National Human Genome Research Institute, the National Institute of Aging, and the National Cancer Institute, all part of the NIH.

A large body of scientific evidence shows that obesity can predispose people to a variety of health problems, including diabetes, some cancers, stroke, high blood pressure, and coronary heart disease. It is estimated that nearly one-third of adults in the United States are considered obese, having a BMI of 30 or more. Genes regulate the fat-storing biological pathways in the body and these clearly vary among individuals. Obesity is also associated with more than one hundred thousand deaths each year in the U.S. population.

The research team tested and compared BMI data and genetic information from more than thirty-two thousand individuals of European ancestry pooled from fifteen genome-wide association studies identifying thirty-five genetic variants. These genetic variants were further tested for validation in more than fifty thousand additional individuals, also of European ancestry.

Genetic variants in six genes (TMEM18, KCTD15, GNPDA2, SH2B1, MTCH2, and NEGR1) were shown to be strongly associated with BMI. Four of the genetic variants were found to be associated with both adult and childhood obesity. In addition, the research team confirmed the association of variants in two genes (FTO and MC4R) that had previously been associated with BMI last year.

All six of the genetic variants were found to be activated in the central nervous system, specifically the brain and hypothalamus. Prior studies have demonstrated the role of the central nervous system in body weight regulation, including on appetite, energy expenditure, and other behavioral aspects.

In addition, the research team compared their results with a large genome-wide association study of BMI, led by deCODE Genetics in Iceland, which has an accompanying paper in the same issue of *Nature Genetics*. Where comparisons could be made, five of the genetic variants were confirmed in both data sets.

The GIANT researchers also compared their results to genome-wide association studies for known obesity complications, including type 2 diabetes, lipid levels, and coronary artery disease and found two of the genetic variants (in the GNPDA2 and TMEM18 genes) were associated with type 2 diabetes.

These results are intriguing and consistent with outcomes from family and twin studies which suggest that genetic factors may account for as much as 40 to 70 percent of BMI variation in the general population.

"We know that environmental factors, such as diet, play a role in obesity, but this research further provides evidence that genetic variation plays a significant role in an individual's predisposition to obesity, " said Eric D. Green, M.D., Ph.D., NHGRI scientific director. "It will be important to see what this team uncovers in follow-up studies and how this breakthrough contributes to our knowledge of the biology of human weight."

The GIANT consortium is currently pursuing large-scale studies to identify more genetic variants contributing to the risk of obesity in both adults and children. They hope to expand the study to examine the genetic information from more than one hundred thousand people, providing them with more statistical power for their findings. Additionally, they plan to study different ethnic populations as well as comparing people with extreme obesity to overweight and normal individuals.

In addition to NHGRI, the National Institute on Aging (NIA), and the National Cancer Institute (NCI), other NIH institutes who contributed funding to the study include the National Institute of Diabetes and Digestive and Kidney Diseases (NIDDK), the National Heart Lung and Blood Institute (NHLBI), and the National Institute of Mental Health (NIMH).

Chapter 57

Tourette Syndrome: Genetic Links

Tourette Syndrome: Frequently Asked Questions

What is Tourette syndrome?

Tourette syndrome (TS) is a neurological disorder characterized by repetitive, stereotyped, involuntary movements and vocalizations called tics. The disorder is named for Dr. Georges Gilles de la Tourette, the pioneering French neurologist who in 1885 first described the condition in an eighty-six-year-old French noblewoman.

The early symptoms of TS are almost always noticed first in childhood, with the average onset between the ages of seven and ten years. TS occurs in people from all ethnic groups; males are affected about three to four times more often than females. It is estimated that two hundred thousand Americans have the most severe form of TS, and as many as one in one hundred exhibit milder and less complex symptoms such as chronic motor or vocal tics or transient tics of childhood. Although TS can be a chronic condition with symptoms lasting a lifetime, most people with the condition experience their worst symptoms

"Tourette Syndrome: Frequently Asked Questions" is reprinted from "Tourette Syndrome Fact Sheet," National Institute of Neurological Disorders and Stroke, National Institutes of Health, NIH Publication No. 05-2163, July 15, 2008. "Scientists Discover First Gene for Tourette Syndrome" is reprinted from National Institute of Neurological Disorders and Stroke, National Institutes of Health, December 15, 2005.

527

in their early teens, with improvement occurring in the late teens and continuing into adulthood.

What are the symptoms?

Tics are classified as either simple or complex. Simple motor tics are sudden, brief, repetitive movements that involve a limited number of muscle groups. Some of the more common simple tics include eye blinking and other vision irregularities, facial grimacing, shoulder shrugging, and head or shoulder jerking. Simple vocalizations might include repetitive throat-clearing, sniffing, or grunting sounds. Complex tics are distinct, coordinated patterns of movements involving several muscle groups. Complex motor tics might include facial grimacing combined with a head twist and a shoulder shrug. Other complex motor tics may actually appear purposeful, including sniffing or touching objects, hopping, jumping, bending, or twisting. Simple vocal tics may include throat-clearing, sniffing/snorting, grunting, or barking. More complex vocal tics include words or phrases. Perhaps the most dramatic and disabling tics include motor movements that result in self-harm such as punching oneself in the face or vocal tics including coprolalia (uttering swear words) or echolalia (repeating the words or phrases of others). Some tics are preceded by an urge or sensation in the affected muscle group, commonly called a premonitory urge. Some with TS will describe a need to complete a tic in a certain way or a certain number of times in order to relieve the urge or decrease the sensation.

Tics are often worse with excitement or anxiety and better during calm, focused activities. Certain physical experiences can trigger or worsen tics, for example tight collars may trigger neck tics, or hearing another person sniff or throat-clear may trigger similar sounds. Tics do not go away during sleep but are often significantly diminished.

What is the course of TS?

Tics come and go over time, varying in type, frequency, location, and severity. The first symptoms usually occur in the head and neck area and may progress to include muscles of the trunk and extremities. Motor tics generally precede the development of vocal tics and simple tics often precede complex tics. Most patients experience peak tic severity before the mid-teen years with improvement for the majority of patients in the late teen years and early adulthood. Approximately

10 percent of those affected have a progressive or disabling course that lasts into adulthood.

Can people with TS control their tics?

Although the symptoms of TS are involuntary, some people can sometimes suppress, camouflage, or otherwise manage their tics in an effort to minimize their impact on functioning. However, people with TS often report a substantial buildup in tension when suppressing their tics to the point where they feel that the tic must be expressed. Tics in response to an environmental trigger can appear to be voluntary or purposeful but are not.

What causes TS?

Although the cause of TS is unknown, current research points to abnormalities in certain brain regions (including the basal ganglia, frontal lobes, and cortex), the circuits that interconnect these regions, and the neurotransmitters (dopamine, serotonin, and norepinephrine) responsible for communication among nerve cells. Given the often complex presentation of TS, the cause of the disorder is likely to be equally complex.

What disorders are associated with TS?

Many with TS experience additional neurobehavioral problems including inattention; hyperactivity and impulsivity (attention deficit hyperactivity disorder—ADHD) and related problems with reading, writing, and arithmetic; and obsessive-compulsive symptoms such as intrusive thoughts/worries and repetitive behaviors. For example, worries about dirt and germs may be associated with repetitive hand washing, and concerns about bad things happening may be associated with ritualistic behaviors such as counting, repeating, or ordering and arranging. People with TS have also reported problems with depression or anxiety disorders, as well as other difficulties with living, that may or may not be directly related to TS. Given the range of potential complications, people with TS are best served by receiving medical care that provides a comprehensive treatment plan.

How is TS diagnosed?

TS is a diagnosis that doctors make after verifying that the patient has had both motor and vocal tics for at least one year. The existence of other neurological or psychiatric conditions (including childhood-onset involuntary movement disorders such as dystonia, or psychiatric disorders characterized by repetitive behaviors/movements—for example, stereotypic behaviors in autism and compulsive behaviors in obsessive-compulsive disorder) can also help doctors arrive at a diagnosis. Common tics are not often misdiagnosed by knowledgeable clinicians. But atypical symptoms or atypical presentation (for example, onset of symptoms in adulthood) may require specific specialty expertise for diagnosis. There are no blood or laboratory tests needed for diagnosis, but neuroimaging studies, such as magnetic resonance imaging (MRI), computerized tomography (CT), and electroencephalogram (EEG) scans, or certain blood tests may be used to rule out other conditions that might be confused with TS.

It is not uncommon for patients to obtain a formal diagnosis of TS only after symptoms have been present for some time. The reasons for this are many. For families and physicians unfamiliar with TS, mild and even moderate tic symptoms may be considered inconsequential, part of a developmental phase, or the result of another condition. For example, parents may think that eye blinking is related to vision problems or that sniffing is related to seasonal allergies. Many patients are self-diagnosed after they, their parents, other relatives, or friends read or hear about TS from others.

How is TS treated?

Because tic symptoms do not often cause impairment, the majority of people with TS require no medication for tic suppression. However, effective medications are available for those whose symptoms interfere with functioning. Neuroleptics are the most consistently useful medications for tic suppression; a number are available but some are more effective than others (for example, haloperidol and pimozide). Unfortunately, there is no one medication that is helpful to all people with TS, nor does any medication completely eliminate symptoms. In addition, all medications have side effects. Most neuroleptic side effects can be managed by initiating treatment slowly and reducing the dose when side effects occur. The most common side effects of neuroleptics include sedation, weight gain, and cognitive dulling. Neurological side effects such as tremor, dystonic reactions (twisting movements or postures), parkinsonian-like symptoms, and other dyskinetic (involuntary) movements are less common and are readily managed with dose reduction. Discontinuing neuroleptics after long-term use must be done slowly to avoid rebound increases in tics and withdrawal dyskinesias. One form of withdrawal dyskinesia called tardive dyskinesia is a movement disorder distinct from TS that may result from the chronic use of neuroleptics. The risk of this side effect can be reduced by using lower doses of neuroleptics for shorter periods of time.

Other medications may also be useful for reducing tic severity, but most have not been as extensively studied or shown to be as consistently useful as neuroleptics. Additional medications with demonstrated efficacy include alpha-adrenergic agonists such as clonidine and guanfacine. These medications are used primarily for hypertension but are also used in the treatment of tics. The most common side effect from these medications that precludes their use is sedation.

Effective medications are also available to treat some of the associated neurobehavioral disorders that can occur in patients with TS. Recent research shows that stimulant medications such as methylphenidate and dextroamphetamine can lessen ADHD symptoms in people with TS without causing tics to become more severe. However, the product labeling for stimulants currently contraindicates the use of these drugs in children with tics/TS and those with a family history of tics. Scientists hope that future studies will include a thorough discussion of the risks and benefits of stimulants in those with TS or a family history of TS and will clarify this issue. For obsessive-compulsive symptoms that significantly disrupt daily functioning, the serotonin reuptake inhibitors (clomipramine, fluoxetine, fluvoxamine, paroxetine, and sertraline) have been proven effective in some patients.

Psychotherapy may also be helpful. Although psychological problems do not cause TS, such problems may result from TS. Psychotherapy can help the person with TS better cope with the disorder and deal with the secondary social and emotional problems that sometimes occur. More recently, specific behavioral treatments that include awareness training and competing response training, such as voluntarily moving in response to a premonitory urge, have shown effectiveness in small controlled trials. Larger and more definitive NIH-funded studies are underway.

Is TS inherited?

Evidence from twin and family studies suggests that TS is an inherited disorder. Although early family studies suggested an autosomal dominant mode of inheritance (an autosomal dominant disorder is one in which only one copy of the defective gene, inherited from one parent, is necessary to produce the disorder), more recent studies suggest that the pattern of inheritance is much more complex. Although there may be a few genes with substantial effects, it is also possible that many genes with smaller effects and environmental factors may play a role in the development of TS. Genetic studies also suggest that some forms of ADHD and OCD are genetically related to TS, but there is less evidence for a genetic relationship between TS and other neurobehavioral problems that commonly co-occur with TS. It is important for families to understand that genetic predisposition may not necessarily result in full-blown TS; instead, it may express itself as a milder tic disorder or as obsessive-compulsive behaviors. It is also possible that the gene-carrying offspring will not develop any TS symptoms.

The sex of the person also plays an important role in TS gene expression. At-risk males are more likely to have tics and at-risk females are more likely to have obsessive-compulsive symptoms.

People with TS may have genetic risks for other neurobehavioral disorders such as depression or substance abuse. Genetic counseling of individuals with TS should include a full review of all potentially hereditary conditions in the family.

What is the prognosis?

Although there is no cure for TS, the condition in many individuals improves in the late teens and early twenties. As a result, some may actually become symptom-free or no longer need medication for tic suppression. Although the disorder is generally lifelong and chronic, it is not a degenerative condition. Individuals with TS have a normal life expectancy. TS does not impair intelligence. Although tic symptoms tend to decrease with age, it is possible that neurobehavioral disorders such as depression, panic attacks, mood swings, and antisocial behaviors can persist and cause impairment in adult life.

What is the best educational setting for children with TS?

Although students with TS often function well in the regular classroom, ADHD, learning disabilities, obsessive-compulsive symptoms, and frequent tics can greatly interfere with academic performance or social adjustment. After a comprehensive assessment, students should be placed in an educational setting that meets their individual needs. Students may require tutoring, smaller or special classes, and in some cases special schools.

All students with TS need a tolerant and compassionate setting that both encourages them to work to their full potential and is flexible enough to accommodate their special needs. This setting may include a private study area, exams outside the regular classroom, or even oral exams when the child's symptoms interfere with his or her ability to write. Untimed testing reduces stress for students with TS.

What research is being done?

Within the federal government, the leading supporter of research on TS and other neurological disorders is the National Institute of Neurological Disorders and Stroke (NINDS). The NINDS, a part of the National Institutes of Health (NIH), is responsible for supporting and conducting research on the brain and central nervous system.

NINDS sponsors research on TS both in its laboratories at the NIH and through grants to major medical institutions across the country. The National Institute of Mental Health, the National Center for Research Resources, the National Institute of Child Health and Human Development, the National Institute on Drug Abuse, and the National Institute on Deafness and Other Communication Disorders also support research of relevance to TS. And another component of the Department of Health and Human Services, the Centers for Disease Control and Prevention, funds professional education programs as well as TS research.

Knowledge about TS comes from studies across a number of medical and scientific disciplines, including genetics, neuroimaging, neuropathology, clinical trials (medication and nonmedication), epidemiology, neurophysiology, neuroimmunology, and descriptive/diagnostic clinical science.

Genetic studies: Currently, NIH-funded investigators are conducting a variety of large-scale genetic studies. Rapid advances in the technology of gene finding will allow for genome-wide screening approaches in TS, and finding a gene or genes for TS would be a major step toward understanding genetic risk factors. In addition, understanding the genetics of TS genes will strengthen clinical diagnosis, improve genetic counseling, lead to the clarification of pathophysiology, and provide clues for more effective therapies.

Neuroimaging studies: Within the past five years, advances in imaging technology and an increase in trained investigators have led to an increasing use of novel and powerful techniques to identify brain regions, circuitry, and neurochemical factors important in TS and related conditions.

Neuropathology: Within the past five years, there has been an increase in the number and quality of donated postmortem brains from TS patients available for research purposes. This increase, coupled with advances in neuropathological techniques, has led to initial findings with implications for neuroimaging studies and animal models of TS.

Clinical trials: A number of clinical trials in TS have recently been completed or are currently underway. These include studies of stimulant treatment of ADHD in TS and behavioral treatments for reducing tic severity in children and adults. Smaller trials of novel approaches to treatment such as dopamine agonist and GABAergic medications also show promise.

Epidemiology and clinical science: Careful epidemiological studies now estimate the prevalence of TS to be substantially higher than previously thought with a wider range of clinical severity. Furthermore, clinical studies are providing new findings regarding TS and co-existing conditions. These include subtyping studies of TS and OCD, an examination of the link between ADHD and learning problems in children with TS, a new appreciation of sensory tics, and the role of co-existing disorders in rage attacks. One of the most important and controversial areas of TS science involves the relationship between TS and autoimmune brain injury associated with group A beta-hemolytic streptococcal infections or other infectious processes. There are a number of epidemiological and clinical investigations currently underway in this intriguing area.

Scientists Discover First Gene for Tourette Syndrome

A team of scientists has discovered the first gene mutation that may cause some cases of Tourette syndrome (TS), an inherited neuropsychiatric disorder known for involuntary muscle and vocal tics. The National Institute of Neurological Disorders and Stroke (NINDS), a part of the National Institutes of Health, provided funding for this research.

The team was led by NINDS grantee Matthew State, Ph.D., a geneticist at Yale School of Medicine. "We're delighted that our grant support to Dr. State contributed to the finding of the first gene for TS and hope for the speedy discovery of other genes that cause or contribute to this disorder," said Laura Mamounas, Ph.D., the NINDS program director for TS research. Findings appear in the October 14, 2005, issue of *Science*.

The gene, named SLITRK1, was found through genetic analysis of a boy with TS who was previously identified as having an "inversion" on chromosome 13—a portion of the chromosome had an orientation opposite that of the normal chromosome. He was the only family member with TS and the inversion, suggesting that these two events were related.

The team then screened SLITRK1 (found near where the boy's chromosome was abnormal) in 174 patients with TS and discovered an abnormality in the coding sequence of the gene in one family. The researchers also identified a separate mutated gene sequence in two unrelated individuals with the disorder. None of these mutations were identified among several thousand unaffected control individuals. Additional testing in cell cultures showed changes in protein expression or function, confirming the finding of the mutated gene.

"We now have an important clue to examine Tourette syndrome on a molecular and cellular level. Confirming this, in even a small number of TS patients, will pave the way for a deeper understanding of the disease process and offer a potential target for the development of drugs to treat the disorder," said Dr. State.

The normal SLITRK1 gene is involved with the growth of nerve cells and how they connect with other neurons. The mutated gene was found in regions of the brain (basal ganglia, cortex, and frontal lobes) previously identified as being associated with TS. Several chromosomal regions with breaks had previously been identified as possible sites of a TS-causing gene.

TS occurs in people from all ethnic groups; males are affected about three to four times more often than females. It is almost always noticed first in childhood, with the average onset between the ages of seven and ten years. An estimated two hundred thousand Americans have the most severe form of TS, and as many as one in one hundred have milder and less complex symptoms such as chronic motor or vocal tics or transient tics of childhood. Most people with TS experience their worst symptoms in their early teens, with improvement occurring in the late teens and continuing into adulthood.

The research team included scientists in the Tourette Syndrome Association's International Consortium for TS Genetics. In March 2000, the NINDS awarded the Consortium a five-year grant for $8.5 million to study the genetic causes of the disorder.

Part Five

Genetic Research

Chapter 58

The Human Genome Project

The Human Genome Project: An Overview

What is a genome?

A genome is an organism's complete set of deoxyribonucleic acid (DNA), including all of its genes. Each genome contains all of the information needed to build and maintain that organism. In humans, a copy of the entire genome—more than three billion DNA base pairs—is contained in all cells that have a nucleus.

What was the Human Genome Project and why has it been important?

The Human Genome Project was an international research effort to determine the sequence of the human genome and identify the genes that it contains. The project was coordinated by the National Institutes of Health and the U.S. Department of Energy. Additional contributors included universities across the United States and international partners in the United Kingdom, France, Germany, Japan, and China. The Human Genome Project formally began in 1990 and was completed in 2003, two years ahead of its original schedule.

"The Human Genome Project: An Overview" is excerpted from "The Human Genome Project," *Genetics Home Reference*, a service of the U.S. National Library of Medicine, January 2, 2009. "Potential Benefits of Human Genome Project Research" is reprinted from Human Genome Project Information, February 20, 2008.

The work of the Human Genome Project has allowed researchers to begin to understand the blueprint for building a person. As researchers learn more about the functions of genes and proteins, this knowledge will have a major impact in the fields of medicine, biotechnology, and the life sciences.

What were the goals of the Human Genome Project?

The main goals of the Human Genome Project were to provide a complete and accurate sequence of the three billion DNA base pairs that make up the human genome and to find all of the estimated twenty thousand to twenty-five thousand human genes. The project also aimed to sequence the genomes of several other organisms that are important to medical research, such as the mouse and the fruit fly.

In addition to sequencing DNA, the Human Genome Project sought to develop new tools to obtain and analyze the data and to make this information widely available. Also, because advances in genetics have consequences for individuals and society, the Human Genome Project committed to exploring the consequences of genomic research through its Ethical, Legal, and Social Implications (ELSI) program.

What did the Human Genome Project accomplish?

In April 2003, researchers announced that the Human Genome Project had completed a high-quality sequence of essentially the entire human genome. This sequence closed the gaps from a working draft of the genome, which was published in 2001. It also identified the locations of many human genes and provided information about their structure and organization. The project made the sequence of the human genome and tools to analyze the data freely available via the internet.

In addition to the human genome, the Human Genome Project sequenced the genomes of several other organisms, including brewers' yeast, the roundworm, and the fruit fly. In 2002, researchers announced that they had also completed a working draft of the mouse genome. By studying the similarities and differences between human genes and those of other organisms, researchers can discover the functions of particular genes and identify which genes are critical for life.

The project's Ethical, Legal, and Social Implications (ELSI) program became the world's largest bioethics program and a model for other ELSI programs worldwide.

What were some of the ethical, legal, and social implications addressed by the Human Genome Project?

The Ethical, Legal, and Social Implications (ELSI) program was founded in 1990 as an integral part of the Human Genome Project. The mission of the ELSI program was to identify and address issues raised by genomic research that would affect individuals, families, and society. A percentage of the Human Genome Project budget at the National Institutes of Health and the U.S. Department of Energy was devoted to ELSI research.

The ELSI program focused on the possible consequences of genomic research in four main areas:

- Privacy and fairness in the use of genetic information, including the potential for genetic discrimination in employment and insurance

- The integration of new genetic technologies, such as genetic testing, into the practice of clinical medicine

- Ethical issues surrounding the design and conduct of genetic research with people, including the process of informed consent

- The education of healthcare professionals, policymakers, students, and the public about genetics and the complex issues that result from genomic research

Potential Benefits of Human Genome Project Research

Rapid progress in genome science and a glimpse into its potential applications have spurred observers to predict that biology will be the foremost science of the twenty-first century. Technology and resources generated by the Human Genome Project and other genomics research are already having a major impact on research across the life sciences. The potential for commercial development of genomics research presents U.S. industry with a wealth of opportunities, and sales of deoxyribonucleic acid (DNA)–based products and technologies in the biotechnology industry are projected to exceed $45 billion by 2009 (Consulting Resources Corporation Newsletter, Spring 1999).

Some current and potential applications of genome research include the following:

- Molecular medicine

- Energy sources and environmental applications
- Risk assessment
- Bioarchaeology, anthropology, evolution, and human migration
- DNA forensics (identification)
- Agriculture, livestock breeding, and bioprocessing

Molecular Medicine

- Improved diagnosis of disease
- Earlier detection of genetic predispositions to disease
- Rational drug design
- Gene therapy and control systems for drugs
- Pharmacogenomics "custom drugs"

Technology and resources promoted by the Human Genome Project are starting to have profound impacts on biomedical research and promise to revolutionize the wider spectrum of biological research and clinical medicine. Increasingly detailed genome maps have aided researchers seeking genes associated with dozens of genetic conditions, including myotonic dystrophy, fragile X syndrome, neurofibromatosis types 1 and 2, inherited colon cancer, Alzheimer disease, and familial breast cancer.

On the horizon is a new era of molecular medicine characterized less by treating symptoms and more by looking to the most fundamental causes of disease. Rapid and more specific diagnostic tests will make possible earlier treatment of countless maladies. Medical researchers also will be able to devise novel therapeutic regimens based on new classes of drugs, immunotherapy techniques, avoidance of environmental conditions that may trigger disease, and possible augmentation or even replacement of defective genes through gene therapy.

Energy and Environmental Applications

- Use microbial genomics research to create new energy sources (biofuels)
- Use microbial genomics research to develop environmental monitoring techniques to detect pollutants

- Use microbial genomics research for safe, efficient environmental remediation

- Use microbial genomics research for carbon sequestration

In 1994, taking advantage of new capabilities developed by the genome project, the Department of Energy (DOE) initiated the Microbial Genome Program to sequence the genomes of bacteria useful in energy production, environmental remediation, toxic waste reduction, and industrial processing. A follow-on program, Genomics: GTL builds on data and resources from the Human Genome Project, the Microbial Genome Program, and systems biology. GTL will accelerate understanding of dynamic living systems for solutions to DOE mission challenges in energy and the environment.

Despite our reliance on the inhabitants of the microbial world, we know little of their number or their nature: estimates are that less than 0.01 percent of all microbes have been cultivated and characterized. Microbial genome sequencing will help lay a foundation for knowledge that will ultimately benefit human health and the environment. The economy will benefit from further industrial applications of microbial capabilities.

Information gleaned from the characterization of complete microbial genomes will lead to insights into the development of such new energy-related biotechnologies as photosynthetic systems, microbial systems that function in extreme environments, and organisms that can metabolize readily available renewable resources and waste material with equal facility. Expected benefits also include development of diverse new products, processes, and test methods that will open the door to a cleaner environment. Biomanufacturing will use non-toxic chemicals and enzymes to reduce the cost and improve the efficiency of industrial processes. Microbial enzymes have been used to bleach paper pulp, stone wash denim, remove lipstick from glassware, break down starch in brewing, and coagulate milk protein for cheese production. In the health arena, microbial sequences may help researchers find new human genes and shed light on the disease-producing properties of pathogens.

Microbial genomics will also help pharmaceutical researchers gain a better understanding of how pathogenic microbes cause disease. Sequencing these microbes will help reveal vulnerabilities and identify new drug targets.

Gaining a deeper understanding of the microbial world also will provide insights into the strategies and limits of life on this planet.

Data generated in this young program have helped scientists identify the minimum number of genes necessary for life and confirm the existence of a third major kingdom of life. Additionally, the new genetic techniques now allow us to establish more precisely the diversity of microorganisms and identify those critical to maintaining or restoring the function and integrity of large and small ecosystems; this knowledge also can be useful in monitoring and predicting environmental change. Finally, studies on microbial communities provide models for understanding biological interactions and evolutionary history.

Risk Assessment

- Assess health damage and risks caused by radiation exposure, including low-dose exposures

- Assess health damage and risks caused by exposure to mutagenic chemicals and cancer-causing toxins

- Reduce the likelihood of heritable mutations

Understanding the human genome will have an enormous impact on the ability to assess risks posed to individuals by exposure to toxic agents. Scientists know that genetic differences make some people more susceptible and others more resistant to such agents. Far more work must be done to determine the genetic basis of such variability. This knowledge will directly address DOE's long-term mission to understand the effects of low-level exposures to radiation and other energy-related agents, especially in terms of cancer risk.

Bioarchaeology, Anthropology, Evolution, and Human Migration

- Study evolution through germline mutations in lineages

- Study migration of different population groups based on female genetic inheritance

- Study mutations on the Y chromosome to trace lineage and migration of males

- Compare breakpoints in the evolution of mutations with ages of populations and historical events

Understanding genomics will help us understand human evolution and the common biology we share with all of life. Comparative genomics between humans and other organisms such as mice already has led to similar genes associated with diseases and traits. Further comparative studies will help determine the yet-unknown function of thousands of other genes.

Comparing the DNA sequences of entire genomes of different microbes will provide new insights about relationships among the three kingdoms of life: Archaebacteria, eukaryotes, and prokaryotes.

DNA Forensics (Identification)

- Identify potential suspects whose DNA may match evidence left at crime scenes

- Exonerate persons wrongly accused of crimes

- Identify crime and catastrophe victims

- Establish paternity and other family relationships

- Identify endangered and protected species as an aid to wildlife officials (could be used for prosecuting poachers)

- Detect bacteria and other organisms that may pollute air, water, soil, and food

- Match organ donors with recipients in transplant programs

- Determine pedigree for seed or livestock breeds

- Authenticate consumables such as caviar and wine

Any type of organism can be identified by examination of DNA sequences unique to that species. Identifying individuals is less precise, although when DNA sequencing technologies progress further, direct characterization of very large DNA segments, and possibly even whole genomes, will become feasible and practical and will allow precise individual identification.

To identify individuals, forensic scientists scan about ten DNA regions that vary from person to person and use the data to create a DNA profile of that individual (sometimes called a DNA fingerprint). There is an extremely small chance that another person has the same DNA profile for a particular set of regions.

Agriculture, Livestock Breeding, and Bioprocessing

- Disease-, insect-, and drought-resistant crops

- Healthier, more productive, disease-resistant farm animals

- More nutritious produce

- Biopesticides

- Edible vaccines incorporated into food products

- New environmental cleanup uses for plants like tobacco

Understanding plant and animal genomes will allow us to create stronger, more disease-resistant plants and animals—reducing the costs of agriculture and providing consumers with more nutritious, pesticide-free foods. Already growers are using bioengineered seeds to grow insect- and drought-resistant crops that require little or no pesticide. Farmers have been able to increase outputs and reduce waste because their crops and herds are healthier.

Alternate uses for crops such as tobacco have been found. One researcher has genetically engineered tobacco plants in his laboratory to produce a bacterial enzyme that breaks down explosives such as TNT (trinitrotoluene) and dinitroglycerin. Waste that would take centuries to break down in the soil can be cleaned up by simply growing these special plants in the polluted area.

Chapter 59

After the Human Genome Project: What Are the Next Steps?

What are the next steps in genomic research?

Discovering the sequence of the human genome was only the first step in understanding how the instructions coded in deoxyribonucleic acid (DNA) lead to a functioning human being. The next stage of genomic research will begin to derive meaningful knowledge from the DNA sequence. Research studies that build on the work of the Human Genome Project are under way worldwide.

The objectives of continued genomic research include the following:

- Determine the function of genes and the elements that regulate genes throughout the genome.

- Find variations in the DNA sequence among people and determine their significance. The most common type of genetic variation is known as a single nucleotide polymorphism or SNP (pronounced "snip"). These small differences may help predict a person's risk of particular diseases and response to certain medications.

- Discover the three-dimensional structures of proteins and identify their functions.

Excerpted from "Genomic Research," *Genetics Home Reference*, a service of the U.S. National Library of Medicine, January 2, 2009.

- Explore how DNA and proteins interact with one another and with the environment to create complex living systems.

- Develop and apply genome-based strategies for the early detection, diagnosis, and treatment of disease.

- Sequence the genomes of other organisms, such as the rat, cow, and chimpanzee, in order to compare similar genes between species.

- Develop new technologies to study genes and DNA on a large scale and store genomic data efficiently.

- Continue to explore the ethical, legal, and social issues raised by genomic research.

What are single nucleotide polymorphisms (SNPs)?

Single nucleotide polymorphisms, frequently called SNPs (pronounced "snips"), are the most common type of genetic variation among people. Each SNP represents a difference in a single DNA building block, called a nucleotide. For example, a SNP may replace the nucleotide cytosine (C) with the nucleotide thymine (T) in a certain stretch of DNA.

SNPs occur normally throughout a person's DNA. They occur once in every three hundred nucleotides on average, which means there are roughly ten million SNPs in the human genome. Most commonly, these variations are found in the DNA between genes. They can act as biological markers, helping scientists locate genes that are associated with disease. When SNPs occur within a gene or in a regulatory region near a gene, they may play a more direct role in disease by affecting the gene's function.

Most SNPs have no effect on health or development. Some of these genetic differences, however, have proven to be very important in the study of human health. Researchers have found SNPs that may help predict an individual's response to certain drugs, susceptibility to environmental factors such as toxins, and risk of developing particular diseases. SNPs can also be used to track the inheritance of disease genes within families. Future studies will work to identify SNPs associated with complex diseases such as heart disease, diabetes, and cancer.

What are genome-wide association studies?

Genome-wide association studies are a relatively new way for scientists to identify genes involved in human disease. This method searches the genome for small variations, called single nucleotide polymorphisms or SNPs (pronounced "snips"), that occur more frequently in people with a particular disease than in people without the disease. Each study can look at hundreds or thousands of SNPs at the same time. Researchers use data from this type of study to pinpoint genes that may contribute to a person's risk of developing a certain disease.

Because genome-wide association studies examine SNPs across the genome, they represent a promising way to study complex, common diseases in which many genetic variations contribute to a person's risk. This approach has already identified SNPs related to several complex conditions including diabetes, heart abnormalities, Parkinson disease, and Crohn disease. Researchers hope that future genome-wide association studies will identify more SNPs associated with chronic diseases, as well as variations that affect a person's response to certain drugs and influence interactions between a person's genes and the environment.

What is the International HapMap Project?

The International HapMap Project is an international scientific effort to identify common genetic variations among people. This project represents a collaboration of scientists from public and private organizations in six countries. Data from the project is freely available to researchers worldwide. Researchers can use the data to learn more about the relationship between genetic differences and human disease.

The HapMap (short for "haplotype map") is a catalog of common genetic variants called single nucleotide polymorphisms or SNPs. Each SNP represents a difference in a single DNA building block, called a nucleotide. These variations occur normally throughout a person's DNA. When several SNPs cluster together on a chromosome, they are inherited as a block known as a haplotype. The HapMap describes haplotypes, including their locations in the genome and how common they are in different populations throughout the world.

The human genome contains roughly ten million SNPs. It would be difficult, time-consuming, and expensive to look at each of these changes and determine whether it plays a role in human disease. Using haplotypes, researchers can sample a selection of these variants instead of studying each one. The HapMap will make carrying out large-scale studies of SNPs and human disease (called genome-wide association studies) cheaper, faster, and less complicated.

The main goal of the International HapMap Project is to describe common patterns of human genetic variation that are involved in human health and disease. Additionally, data from the project will help researchers find genetic differences that can help predict an individual's response to particular medicines or environmental factors (such as toxins.)

What is pharmacogenomics?

Pharmacogenomics is the study of how genes affect a person's response to drugs. This relatively new field combines pharmacology (the science of drugs) and genomics (the study of genes and their functions) to develop effective, safe medications and doses that will be tailored to a person's genetic makeup.

Many drugs that are currently available are "one size fits all," but they don't work the same way for everyone. It can be difficult to predict who will benefit from a medication, who will not respond at all, and who will experience negative side effects (called adverse drug reactions). Adverse drug reactions are a significant cause of hospitalizations and deaths in the United States. With the knowledge gained from the Human Genome Project, researchers are learning how inherited differences in genes affect the body's response to medications. These genetic differences will be used to predict whether a medication will be effective for a particular person and to help prevent adverse drug reactions.

The field of pharmacogenomics is still in its infancy. Its use is currently quite limited, but new approaches are under study in clinical trials. In the future, pharmacogenomics will allow the development of tailored drugs to treat a wide range of health problems, including cardiovascular disease, Alzheimer disease, cancer, human immunodeficiency virus/acquired immunodeficiency syndrome (HIV/AIDS), and asthma.

Chapter 60

Over-the-Counter Genetic Tests: What You Need to Know

Could a simple medical test tell you if you are likely to get a particular disease? Could it evaluate your health risks and even suggest a specific treatment? Could you take this test in the privacy of your home, without a doctor's prescription or guidance? Some companies say genetic testing can do all this and more. They claim that at-home genetic testing can screen for diseases and provide a basis for choosing a particular diet, dietary supplement, lifestyle change, or medication. They sell their tests in supermarkets and drugstores, and they advertise their services in print, on television, and online.

The Federal Trade Commission (FTC) wants you to know the facts about the direct-to-consumers marketing of genetic tests. According to the Food and Drug Administration (FDA), which regulates the manufacturers of genetic tests; and the Centers for Disease Control and Prevention (CDC), which promotes health and quality of life, some of these tests lack scientific validity, and others provide medical results that are meaningful only in the context of a full medical evaluation. The FDA and CDC say that because of the complexities involved in both the testing and the interpretation of the results, genetic tests should be performed in a specialized laboratory, and the results should be interpreted by a doctor or trained counselor who understands the value of genetic testing for a particular situation.

Excerpted from "At Home Genetic Tests: A Healthy Dose of Skepticism May Be the Best Prescription," Federal Trade Commission, July 2006.

Genes and Genetic Tests

Inside the cells of your body, chromosomes carry your genetic blueprint. Your chromosomes, which are passed to you by your parents, contain genes made of DNA (deoxyribonucleic acid). Your genes determine characteristics like eye color or height, and contribute to your chances of getting certain diseases.

Genetic tests examine genes and DNA to see if they indicate particular diseases or disorders. Several different types of tests are available. Some look at the number and shape of chromosomes to see if there are obvious abnormalities. Others look for small unusual portions of individual proteins or sections of DNA. Typically, these tests require a blood sample or a swab from inside the cheek. In "at-home" tests, the sample is collected at your home and then sent to a laboratory for analysis. Prices of at-home genetic tests range from $295 to $1,200.

Interpreting Test Results

The results of genetic tests are not always "black and white." That makes interpretations and explanations difficult. In most cases, diseases occur as a result of interaction between our genes and the environment—for example, our lifestyle, foods we eat, elements we are exposed to such as sunlight, and tobacco. The interaction between these factors in contributing to health and disease can be very complicated. Even health care experts are just beginning to understand these issues. That's why it is important to gather and analyze this information with a qualified healthcare provider so you can be sure genetic data is accurate and correctly used.

Most genetic tests look at only a small number of the more than twenty thousand genes in the human body. A positive result means that the testing laboratory found unusual characteristics or changes in the genes it tested. Depending on the purpose of the test, a positive result may confirm a diagnosis, identify an increased risk of developing a disease, or indicate that a person is a carrier for a particular disease. It does not necessarily mean that a disease will develop, or if it does, that the disease will be progressive or severe.

A negative result means that the laboratory found no unusual characteristics or changes in the genes it tested. This could mean that a person doesn't have a particular disease, doesn't have an increased risk of developing the disease, or isn't a carrier of the disease. Or it could mean that the test missed the specific genetic changes associated with a particular disease.

In short, the FDA and CDC say that genetic testing provides only one piece of information about a person's susceptibility to disease. Other factors, like family background, medical history, and environment also contribute to the likelihood of getting a particular disease. In most cases, genetic testing makes the most sense when it is part of a physical exam that includes a patient's family background and medical history.

Company Claims

Be wary of claims about the benefits these products supposedly offer. Some companies claim that at-home genetic tests can measure the risk of developing a particular disease, like heart disease, diabetes, cancer, or Alzheimer disease. But the FDA and CDC say they aren't aware of any valid studies that prove these tests give accurate results. Having a particular gene doesn't necessarily mean that a disease will develop; not having a particular gene doesn't necessarily mean that the disease will not.

Some companies also may claim that a person can protect against serious disease by choosing special foods and nutritional supplements. Consequently, the results of their at-home tests often include dietary advice and sales offers for "customized" dietary supplements. But the advice rarely goes beyond standard sensible dietary recommendations. The FDA and CDC say they know of no valid scientific studies showing that genetic tests can be used safely or effectively to recommend nutritional choices.

Be skeptical of claims that the tests can assess a person's ability to withstand certain environmental exposures, like particular toxins or cigarette smoke. The FDA and CDC aren't aware of any valid scientific studies that show that genetic tests can be used to predict whether a person can withstand environmental exposures.

Recently, some companies have claimed their at-home tests can give information about how a person's body will respond to a certain treatment, and how well people will respond to a particular drug. This claim is based on current medical research that shows differences in drug effectiveness based on genetic makeup. But, say federal experts, while these tests may provide some information your doctor needs or uses to make treatment decisions for a specific condition, they are not a substitute for a physician's judgment and clinical experience.

If You're Considering an At-Home Genetic Test

According to the FDA and CDC, at-home genetic tests aren't a suitable substitute for a traditional healthcare evaluation. Medical exams that include conventional laboratory tests like blood chemistry and lipid profiles are a more appropriate starting point for diagnosing diseases and assessing preventive measures. Nevertheless, if you are considering using an at-home genetic test, here are some suggestions:

- Talk to your doctor or healthcare practitioner about whether it might provide useful information about your health, and if so, which test would be best. Make sure you understand the benefits and limits of any test before you buy it—or take it.

- Ask your doctor or a genetic counselor to help you understand your test results. Most companies that sell at-home genetic tests do not interpret the results.

- Discuss the results of your test with your doctor or healthcare practitioner before making dietary or other health-related decisions. Genetic test results can be complex and serious. You don't want to make any decisions based on incomplete, inaccurate, or misunderstood information.

- Protect your privacy. At-home test companies may post patient test results online. If the website is not secure, your information may be seen by others. Before you do business with any company online, check the privacy policy to see how they may use your personal information, and whether they share customer information with marketers.

- While most other home-use medical tests undergo FDA review to provide a reasonable assurance of their safety and effectiveness, no at-home genetic tests have been reviewed by the FDA, and the FDA has not evaluated the accuracy of their claims.

Chapter 61

Pharmacogenomics: Tailoring Medicine to the Individual

Chapter Contents

Section 61.1

What Is Pharmacogenomics?

Excerpted from "Pharmacogenomics,"
Human Genome Project Information, September 19, 2008.

What is pharmacogenomics?

Pharmacogenomics is the study of how an individual's genetic inheritance affects the body's response to drugs. The term comes from the words *pharmacology* and *genomics* and is thus the intersection of pharmaceuticals and genetics.

Pharmacogenomics holds the promise that drugs might one day be tailor-made for individuals and adapted to each person's own genetic makeup. Environment, diet, age, lifestyle, and state of health all can influence a person's response to medicines, but understanding an individual's genetic makeup is thought to be the key to creating personalized drugs with greater efficacy and safety.

Pharmacogenomics combines traditional pharmaceutical sciences such as biochemistry with annotated knowledge of genes, proteins, and single nucleotide polymorphisms.

What are the anticipated benefits of pharmacogenomics?

More powerful medicines: Pharmaceutical companies will be able to create drugs based on the proteins, enzymes, and ribonucleic acid (RNA) molecules associated with genes and diseases. This will facilitate drug discovery and allow drug makers to produce a therapy more targeted to specific diseases. This accuracy not only will maximize therapeutic effects but also decrease damage to nearby healthy cells.

Better, safer drugs the first time: Instead of the standard trial-and-error method of matching patients with the right drugs, doctors will be able to analyze a patient's genetic profile and prescribe the best available drug therapy from the beginning. Not only will this take the guesswork out of finding the right drug, it will speed recovery time and increase safety as the likelihood of adverse reactions is eliminated.

Pharmacogenomics has the potential to dramatically reduce the estimated one hundred thousand deaths and two million hospitalizations that occur each year in the United States as the result of adverse drug response.[1]

More accurate methods of determining appropriate drug dosages: Current methods of basing dosages on weight and age will be replaced with dosages based on a person's genetics—how well the body processes the medicine and the time it takes to metabolize it. This will maximize the therapy's value and decrease the likelihood of overdose.

Advanced screening for disease: Knowing one's genetic code will allow a person to make adequate lifestyle and environmental changes at an early age so as to avoid or lessen the severity of a genetic disease. Likewise, advance knowledge of a particular disease susceptibility will allow careful monitoring, and treatments can be introduced at the most appropriate stage to maximize their therapy.

Better vaccines: Vaccines made of genetic material, either deoxyribonucleic acid (DNA) or RNA, promise all the benefits of existing vaccines without all the risks. They will activate the immune system but will be unable to cause infections. They will be inexpensive, stable, easy to store, and capable of being engineered to carry several strains of a pathogen at once.

Improvements in the drug discovery and approval process: Pharmaceutical companies will be able to discover potential therapies more easily using genome targets. Previously failed drug candidates may be revived as they are matched with the niche population they serve. The drug approval process should be facilitated as trials are targeted for specific genetic population groups—providing greater degrees of success. The cost and risk of clinical trials will be reduced by targeting only those persons capable of responding to a drug.

Decrease in the overall cost of health care: Decreases in the number of adverse drug reactions, the number of failed drug trials, the time it takes to get a drug approved, the length of time patients are on medication, the number of medications patients must take to find an effective therapy, the effects of a disease on the body (through early detection), and an increase in the range of possible drug targets will promote a net decrease in the cost of health care.

Is pharmacogenomics in use today?

To a limited degree. The cytochrome P450 (CYP) family of liver enzymes is responsible for breaking down more than thirty different classes of drugs. DNA variations in genes that code for these enzymes can influence their ability to metabolize certain drugs. Less active or inactive forms of CYP enzymes that are unable to break down and efficiently eliminate drugs from the body can cause drug overdose in patients. Today, clinical trials researchers use genetic tests for variations in cytochrome P450 genes to screen and monitor patients. In addition, many pharmaceutical companies screen their chemical compounds to see how well they are broken down by variant forms of CYP enzymes.[2]

Another enzyme called TPMT (thiopurine methyltransferase) plays an important role in the chemotherapy treatment of a common childhood leukemia by breaking down a class of therapeutic compounds called thiopurines. A small percentage of Caucasians have genetic variants that prevent them from producing an active form of this protein. As a result, thiopurines elevate to toxic levels in the patient because the inactive form of TMPT is unable to break down the drug. Today, doctors can use a genetic test to screen patients for this deficiency, and the TMPT activity is monitored to determine appropriate thiopurine dosage levels.[3]

What are some of the barriers to pharmacogenomics progress?

Pharmacogenomics is a developing research field that is still in its infancy. Several of the following barriers will have to be overcome before many pharmacogenomics benefits can be realized:

- **Complexity of finding gene variations that affect drug response:** Single nucleotide polymorphisms (SNPs) are DNA sequence variations that occur when a single nucleotide (A, T, C, or G) in the genome sequence is altered. SNPs occur every one hundred to three hundred bases along the three-billion-base human genome, therefore millions of SNPs must be identified and analyzed to determine their involvement (if any) in drug response. Further complicating the process is our limited knowledge of which genes are involved with each drug response. Since many genes are likely to influence responses, obtaining the big picture on the impact of gene variations is highly time-consuming and complicated.

- **Limited drug alternatives:** Only one or two approved drugs may be available for treatment of a particular condition. If patients have gene variations that prevent them using these drugs, they may be left without any alternatives for treatment.

- **Disincentives for drug companies to make multiple pharmacogenomic products:** Most pharmaceutical companies have been successful with their "one size fits all" approach to drug development. Since it costs hundreds of millions of dollars to bring a drug to market, will these companies be willing to develop alternative drugs that serve only a small portion of the population?

- **Educating healthcare providers:** Introducing multiple pharmacogenomic products to treat the same condition for different population subsets undoubtedly will complicate the process of prescribing and dispensing drugs. Physicians must execute an extra diagnostic step to determine which drug is best suited to each patient. To interpret the diagnostic accurately and recommend the best course of treatment for each patient, all prescribing physicians, regardless of specialty, will need a better understanding of genetics.

References

1. J. Lazarou, B. H. Pomeranz, and P. N. Corey. Incidence of adverse drug reactions in hospitalized patients: a meta-analysis of prospective studies. *JAMA*. Apr 15, 1998. 279(15):1200–5.

2. J. Hodgson, and A. Marshall. Pharmacogenomics: will the regulators approve? *Nature Biotechnology*. 16: 243–46. 1998.

3. S. Pistoi. Facing your genetic destiny, part II. *Scientific American*. February 25, 2002.

Section 61.2

Pharmacogenetics: Frequently Asked Questions

Reprinted from "Frequently Asked Questions about
Pharmacogenetics," National Institute of General Medical Sciences,
National Institutes of Health, November 19, 2008.

What are pharmacogenomics and pharmacogenetics?

The terms *pharmacogenomics* and *pharmacogenetics* are often used
interchangeably to describe a field of research focused on how genes
affect individual responses to medicines. Whether a medicine works
well for you—or whether it causes serious side effects—depends, to a
certain extent, on your genes.

Just as genes contribute to whether you will be tall or short, black-
haired or blond, your genes also determine how you will respond to
medicines. Genes are like recipes—they carry instructions for making protein molecules. As medicines travel through your body, they
interact with thousands of proteins. Small differences in the composition or quantities of these molecules can affect how medicines do
their jobs.

These differences can be due to diet, level of activity, or the medicines a person takes, but they can also be due to differences in genes.
By understanding the genetic basis of drug responses, scientists hope
to enable doctors to prescribe the drugs and doses best suited for each
individual.

Aren't prescribed medicines already safe and effective?

While standard doses of most medicines work well for most people,
some medicines don't work at all in certain people or cause annoying
and sometimes dangerous side effects. For example, codeine is use-
less as a painkiller in nearly 10 percent of people, and an anticancer
drug, 6-mercaptopurine, is extremely toxic in a small fraction of the
population.

560

How do scientists gather pharmacogenetic information?

Many pharmacogenetic findings are based on knowledge of biochemical pathways within cells. For example, scientists already knew a lot about the enzymes that break down the anticancer drug irinotecan when its toxic effects in certain patients came to light. This knowledge allowed researchers to rapidly pinpoint a genetic variant of one of these enzymes as the cause of the dangerous reaction. Scientists have developed a genetic test for this variant so that doctors can adjust the dosage for those at risk for serious side effects.

Pharmacogenetic advances can also come from studies that accompany clinical drug trials. After obtaining permission from participants, some pharmaceutical companies collect deoxyribonucleic acid (DNA) samples from people in clinical trials. Scientists then analyze the samples together with results of the clinical trial to identify genetic variations that correlate with a drug's effectiveness or toxicity.

Pharmacogenetic researchers have already identified many genes whose variations affect drug responses. They also know where to look for the numerous others they are bound to discover in the future. The availability of the human genome sequence, which was completed in 2003, led to the HapMap project, an international effort to catalog common genetic differences among human beings. These resources are providing a treasure trove of genetic information that is expected to speed advances in pharmacogenetics.

In what ways can doctors use pharmacogenetics to help them treat their patients?

The right dose: Dosage is usually based on factors such as age, weight, and liver and kidney function. But for someone who breaks down a drug quickly, a typical dose may be ineffective. In contrast, someone who breaks down a drug more slowly may need a lower dose to avoid accumulating toxic levels of the drug in the bloodstream. A pharmacogenetic test can help reveal the right dose for individual patients.

The right drug—for cancer: Pharmacogenetics is used in targeted therapy for cancer to identify the best drug regimen for a particular tumor. Even tumors of the same type (such as lung, breast, or liver) vary at the genetic level. Cancer is fundamentally a genetic disease, but most of the genetic differences between cancer cells and normal cells are not inherited—they accumulate as the cancer develops.

Analyzing specific genes in a patient's tumor helps doctors identify the drug combination to which the tumor will most likely respond. For example, the breast cancer drug Herceptin® is only effective when the tumor cells have accumulated extra copies of the HER2 gene and have high levels of the protein this gene encodes on their surfaces.

The right drug—for human immunodeficiency virus (HIV): For patients with a bacterial or viral infection, analyzing the genes of the infectious agent can reveal the most suitable drug treatment. For example, the Food and Drug Administration (FDA) has approved a genotyping kit that detects genetic variations in HIV that make the virus resistant to some antiretroviral drugs. If drug resistance is discovered, doctors can prescribe other medications.

The right drug—for depression: Depression can be treated with a variety of different medicines, and it is often time-consuming and difficult to find the drug(s) that works best for each person. In the future, genetic testing may take some of the guesswork out of choosing a drug regimen. These tests are likely to involve analyzing a person's liver enzymes, especially those in the cytochrome P450 family, which are largely responsible for processing antidepressants.

Other tests that may prove useful to psychiatrists will detect differences in the molecules targeted by antidepressants, such as the serotonin transporters targeted by a large class of antidepressants called selective serotonin reuptake inhibitors (SSRIs). Scientists have uncovered evidence for a link between a person's response to SSRIs and variations in serotonin transporters and other biological molecules that act on serotonin.

The right drug—for cardiovascular disease: Statins, the most widely prescribed drugs worldwide, help prevent cardiovascular disease by reducing the level of "bad" cholesterol in the bloodstream. While statins work well for many patients, responses are highly variable and doctors must adjust the dosage for each person.

Researchers have discovered that variants in a number of molecules—including those that break down or transport statins, as well as the statins' molecular target in the cholesterol production pathway—contribute to the variable response among individuals. Using results of genetic tests, doctors may one day be able to prescribe the right dose from the start and more quickly reduce their patients' risk of dangerous cardiovascular events such as heart attack and stroke.

Does the U.S. Food and Drug Administration (FDA) require that doctors test patients for genetic differences before prescribing any drugs currently on the market?

The labels of more than twenty medications now mention the availability of tests for genetic variations that impact the drug's action. However, in many cases, such as the anticancer drugs azathioprine and irinotecan, which can build up to toxic levels in a small fraction of people, testing is optional.

How do I get a pharmacogenetic test?

Ask your doctor, who can order a test from a medical laboratory. Some major institutions, such as the Mayo Clinic, the Indiana University School of Medicine, and St. Jude Children's Hospital, also offer pharmacogenetic testing. If you take a test, a technician will draw a sample of your blood or rub a cotton swab along the inside of your cheek to collect cells. The lab will extract genetic material from the sample and carry out the test. These tests typically cost a few hundred dollars and may be covered by your health insurance company.

Cancer biopsy samples are also often subjected to genetic tests. The results can help guide therapy and predict the likelihood of recurrence. Several such tests have been approved by the FDA.

Are the results of pharmacogenetic tests confidential?

While pharmacogenetic tests are designed to help people, some fear that the results could be used against them, such as to discriminate against them in a job setting or to deny them health insurance coverage. A person's genetic information is protected through the Health Insurance Portability and Accountability Act (HIPAA), which was passed by Congress in 1996. Many states also have laws in place that protect the privacy of health information, including genetic data.

How will pharmacogenetics affect the design, development, and availability of new medicines?

Pharmacogenetic knowledge will enable pharmaceutical companies to design, develop, and market drugs for people with specific genetic profiles. Testing a drug only in those likely to benefit from it could streamline its development and maximize its therapeutic benefit.

The FDA, which monitors the safety of all drugs in the United States, considers pharmacogenetics to be a valuable tool in the development of new medical products. To date, the FDA has approved a number of genotyping kits relevant to pharmacogenetics, including one that screens for variants in the cytochrome P450 enzymes, which process many kinds of drugs. In most cases the FDA encourages, but does not require, companies to submit pharmacogenetic data with new drug applications. This data is only required for medicines that were developed based on pharmacogenetics.

How will pharmacogenetics affect the quality of health care?

In the future, pharmacogenetics will increasingly enable doctors to prescribe the right dose of the right medicine the first time for everyone. This would mean that patients will receive medicines that are safer and more effective, leading to better health care overall.

Also, if scientists could identify the genetic basis for certain toxic side effects, drugs could be prescribed only to those who are not genetically at risk for these effects. This could maintain the availability of potentially lifesaving medications that might otherwise be taken off the market.

What are some of the challenges that face pharmacogenetics?

While pharmacogenetics is expected to be a useful tool to find the best dose of the right medicine for each patient, doctors are unlikely to be able to rely on it alone. Other factors will remain important, and may sometimes overshadow pharmacogenetics. These other factors include characteristics of the disease itself as well as the patient's diet, weight, lifestyle, and other medicines he or she is taking.

As with many new medical advances, it will take time before pharmacogenetics enters the mainstream and becomes a standard tool for making treatment decisions. Overcoming this barrier may be particularly tricky for pharmacogenetics because most medicines work well for most people and adverse reactions are rare.

Another challenge facing pharmacogenetics is the number and complexity of interactions a drug has with biological molecules in the body. Variations in many different molecules may influence how someone responds to a medicine. Teasing out the genetic patterns associated with particular drug responses could involve some intricate and time-consuming scientific detective work.

While routine pharmacogenetic testing could ultimately save our health care system billions of dollars by improving drug effectiveness and safety, the savings could be offset by the additional cost of genetic tests.

What is the role of the National Institutes of Health (NIH)?

In April 2000, NIH launched the Pharmacogenetics Research Network (PGRN), a nationwide collaboration of hundreds of scientists focused on understanding how genes affect the way a person responds to medicines. Since its inception, PGRN scientists have studied genes and medications relevant to a wide range of diseases, including asthma, depression, cancer, and heart disease. A key component of the PGRN is the Pharmacogenetics Knowledge Base, an online resource that contains pharmacogenetic data from the PGRN and others, and is freely available to the research community.

The PGRN was launched with grants totaling $140 million over five years. An additional $150 million is allocated for the period of 2005–2009. The PGRN is funded largely through the National Institute of General Medical Sciences and the National Heart, Lung, and Blood Institute, with additional support from the National Cancer Institute, the National Library of Medicine, the National Institute of Environmental Health Sciences, the National Institute on Drug Abuse, the National Institute of Mental Health, the National Human Genome Research Institute, and the Office of Research on Women's Health.

NIH takes seriously the ethical and legal implications of pharmacogenetics research and is working closely with several task forces and associations to maximize the benefits of this research and to prevent any potential harm to individuals or society.

Chapter 62

Nutrigenomics: Developing Personalized Diets for Disease Prevention

Introduction

The marked difference among individuals in terms of their response to dietary factors has puzzled nutritional scientists over the last century. Nowhere are the differences most obvious than in the studies related to the effect of dietary fat. As summarized in an excellent review (Taubes, 2001), the effects of dietary fat content and fatty acid composition on health, obesity, and metabolic parameters (e.g., plasma cholesterol) in humans have been widely variable, and remain controversial despite a vast number of investigations. Although a genetic basis for some of these differences were suggested earlier, establishment of a definite genetic link was only possible after the completion of the Human Genome Project (Venter et al., 2001) and subsequent documentation of single nucleotide polymorphisms (SNPs) in candidate genes related to fatty acid, cholesterol, and lipoprotein metabolism (Ordovas, 2006; Ordovas et al., 2007). Today, there is wide support to the theory that genetic variation in selected SNPs, haplotypes, and copy number variants can have remarkable effect not only in our response to dietary components, but also on our

Excerpted from "Understanding the Nutrigenomic Definitions and Concepts at the Food-Genome Junction," by M. T. Ravi Subbiah, *OMICS: A Journal of Integrative Biology*, December 2008. Reprinted with permission. The publisher for this copyrighted material is Mary Ann Liebert, Inc. The complete text of this article is available at http://www.liebertonline.com/toc/omi/12/4.

food preferences and their optimal utilization (Ferguson, 2006). Furthermore, there are numerous scientific reports that illustrate that micronutrients and botanicals can interact with the genome, modify gene expression, alter protein and metabolite composition within cells, and even participate in the deoxyribonucleic acid (DNA) repair and replication process (French, 2008; Marambaud et al., 2005; Shay and Banz, 2005; Zheng and Chen, 2005). This has further increased expectations that one can tailor diet by incorporating dietary supplements or nutraceuticals targeted to an individual or to groups based on sex, ethnicity, or specific metabolic imbalance (Subbiah, 2007). This concept puts the nutritional genomic area at the food/gene interphase creating opportunities for industry to develop commercially viable supplements or nutraceuticals that can modify the expression of genes of interest. These developments have helped us to formulate the concept of nutritional genomics, providing a forum to further explore genome differences and their potential relationship to metabolic abnormalities and response to nutrients (Debusk et al., 2005; Kaput, 2007; Stover, 2006). In this regard, nutrigenomics parallels pharmacogenomics (personalizing drug therapy based on individual SNPs), which has made tremendous headway in recent years as a tool to reduce individual drug toxicity and design personalized medicine (Giacomino et al., 2007; Reiling and Hoffman, 2007).

Controversies and Concerns in Nutrigenomics

Although nutrigenomics promises us the ability to tailor diet based on our genes and genetic polymorphisms, there is a lot of controversy whether it can truly bring about meaningful change in reducing risk factors connected to a metabolic disease. Unlike pharmacogenomics, wherein a clinical improvement can be documented, nutritional changes are more complex, slower, and depend upon a number of other factors. Although there has been a number of genome-wide association studies related to nutrigenetics using a smaller number of subjects, large-scale dietary intervention studies that actually demonstrate positive modification of biomarkers in groups with genetic polymorphisms have been limited. This is understandable considering the cost, management, and significant occurrence of noncompliance problems due to differences in personal dietary habits and cultural factors. In this connection, there are three clinical trials underway overseas that could serve as important resources for validation of nutrigenetic concepts:

- The PREDIMED study in Spain (a multicenter project with more than nine thousand subjects with high cardiovascular risk) that compares the effect of Mediterranean diet with a low-fat diet exploring differences in cardiovascular outcomes (Estruck et al., 2006)

- The medi-RIVAGE study, with more than two hundred subjects, which compares the effect of Mediterranean diet and a low-fat diet on some nutrigenetic candidate genes and other phenotypical parameters (Vincent et al., 2004)

- The DIRECT study in Israel and its nutrigenetic component, which compares the efficacy of low-fat, Mediterranean, and low-carbohydrate regimens.

Although these studies primarily focused on cardiovascular biomarkers and body weight changes, the samples collected will serve as a valuable resource for collaborative studies on nutrigenetic SNP's, haplotypes, and other genetic markers. These international studies will also yield valuable information on how genetic makeup in culturally and ethnically diverse groups can influence response to nutrients and contribute to the initiation and/or progression of metabolic diseases.

Public interest in the use of nutraceuticals, functional foods, and dietary supplements as lifetime preventive measures for optimal health is at an all-time high. This is indicated by the magnitude of the market (50–75 billion dollars) projected for dietary supplements, nutraceuticals, and functional foods (Sloan, 2002). In order for the medical community to accept these products, it is essential that the products be clinically tested and a clear understanding of their composition, toxicity, and potential interaction with other drugs (Chan, 2003; Cronin, 2002) be clarified. For example, a study underway testing the efficacy of soy isoflavones for potential cardiovascular benefit (Rimbach et al., 2007) is an example of a well-controlled study that could be well accepted by the medical community. There is an urgent need to ensure that regulatory guidelines are in place to monitor clinical laboratories that offer nutrigenomic testing. This is of particular concern with laboratories offering online testing directly to the public (without a physician's request). Some important questions are: What specific type of genetic counseling will be offered? When offered, would genetic councilors be affiliated with the nutrigenomics companies (e.g., as their employees) or serve as independent councilors at arm's length from the industry to best inform the patients on predictive utility of nutrigenomics tests? Is it ethical for a diagnostic laboratory to recommend a particular nutraceutical product? Who will monitor these labs? These socioethical and legal aspects (Reilly and Debusk, 2008) related to genetic testing need clear state/federal guidelines and regulatory oversight.

Another important topic with regard to nutrigenomic testing as a preventive tool in early diagnosis of metabolic diseases is the cost, which can currently go more than $1,000 depending upon the number of tests. Will the insurance companies cover these costs? The rapid increase in the number of nutrigenomic tests discovered poses another problem in terms of cost and time. The availability of high throughput analytical techniques (that can run hundreds of SNPs in a day) might eventually lower cost and turnaround times. In the future, it is possible that metabolite profiling (metabolomics), which can identify key products of genotypic variation at the cellular level, might also find use in clinical laboratories.

Conclusion and Future Outlook

Nutrigenomics may lead to substantial advances in public health due to its strong focus on preventive medicine and study of both healthy individuals and patients. It is essential that validation of nutrigenomic concepts by large prospective population studies lay the groundwork for scientifically acceptable "nutrigenomic panels of tests" before they can be utilized in routine molecular diagnostic testing in the clinic. Sensitivity and specificity of nutrigenomics tests need to be discerned in different human populations. This information should be made available to the public and consumers in a form that is open, transparent, and accessible. It is interesting to note that France has recently introduced a National Nutrition and Health Program (Estaquio et al., 2008) to assess nutritional status and risk of major metabolic diseases, although the extent of genetic testing used is not very clear. Routine use of nutrigenomics in clinical labs, in turn, will demand a new brand of dietitians, genetic counselors, and nutritional scientists. These individuals will need to be equipped with substantial interdisciplinary expertise in genomics, proteomics, metabolomics, and omics technologies more generally. To this end, many of the high throughput omics biomarker technologies still remain in a very specialized research domain. Universities will play a significant leadership role in developing appropriately diversified curriculum and training programs to meet these growing educational demands in both health professional and graduate research programs. Industries will find opportunities in developing novel nutraceuticals, functional foods, and dietary supplements that can modify a given metabolic problem. The nutrigenomic approach to preventing disease will likely lead to a decrease in pharmaceutical use, and ultimately reduce national and international health care costs associated with chronic diseases. Public and patients, too, will be better informed on future disease liabilities and how best to reduce or prevent such health risks through personalized nutrition using nutrigenomic tests.

References

Chan, M. (2003). Herbal medicines: what work and how to use them safely. *Ohio Fam Phys* Fall, 20–23.

Cronin, J.R. (2002). Dietary supplements: safety, certification, labeling and efficacy. *Alternat Compliment Ther* 8, 141–148.

Debusk, R.M., Fogarty, C.P., Ordovas, J.M., and Kornman, K.S. (2005). Nutritional genomics in practice: where do we begin? *J Am Diet Assoc* 105, 589–598.

Estaquio, C., Castetbon, K., Kesse-Guyott, E., Bertrais, S., Deschamps, V., Dauchet, L., et al. (2008). The French "National Nutrition and Health Program" score is associated with nutritional status and risk of major chronic diseases. *J Nutr* 138, 946–953.

Estruck, R., Martinez Gonzalez, M.A., Corella, D., Salas-Salvado, J., Ruiz-Guitierez, V., Covas, M.I., et al. (2006). Effects of a Mediterranean-style diet on cardiovascular risk factors: a randomized trial. *Ann Intern Med* 145, 1–11.

Fenech, M. (2008). Genome health nutrigenomics and nutrigenetics: diagnosis and nutritional treatment of genome damage on an individual basis. *Food Chem. Toxicol* 46, 1365–1370.

Ferguson, L.R. (2006). Nutrigenomics: integrating genomic approaches into nutrition research. *Mol Diagn Ther* 10, 101–108.

Giacomino, K.M, Brett, C.M, Altman, R.B, Benowitz, N.L, Dolan, M.E, Flockhart, D.A, et. al. (2007). Pharmacogenetic research network: from SNP discovery to clinical drug response. *Clin Pharmacol Ther* 81, 328–345.

Kaput, J. (2007). Developing the promise of nutrigenomics through complete science and international collaborations. *Forum Nutr* 60, 209–223.

Marambaud, P., Zhao, H., and Davies, P. (2005). Resveratrol promotes clearance of Alzheimer's disease amyloid–beta peptides. *J Biol Chem* 280, 37377–37382.

Ordovas, J.M. (2006). Genetic interactions with diet influence the risk of cardiovascular disease. *Am J Clin Nutr* 83(Suppl), 443S–446S.

Ordovas, J.M., Kaput, J., and Corella, D. (2007). Nutrition in the genomics era: cardiovascular disease risk and the Mediterranean diet. *Mol Nutr Food Res* 51, 1293 1299.

Reilly, P.R., and Debusk, R.M. (2008). Ethical and legal issues in nutritional genomics. *J Amer Diet Assoc* 108, 36–40.

Relling, M.V., and Hoffman, J.M. (2007). Should pharmacogenetic studies be required for new drug approvals? *Clin Pharmacol Ther* 81, 425–428.

Rimbach, G., Boesch-Saadatmandi, C., Fuchs, D., Wenzel, U., Daniel, H., Hall, W.L., et al. (2007). Dietary isoflavones in the prevention of cardiovascular disease: a molecular perspective. *Food Chem Toxicol* 46, 1308–1319.

Shay, N.F., and Banz, W.J. (2005). Regulation of gene transcription by botanicals: novel regulatory mechanisms. *Annu Rev Nutr* 25, 297–315.

Sloan, A.E. (2002). The top 10 functional food trends: the next generation. Food Tech 56, 32–57. Stover, P.J. (2006). Influence of human genetic variation on nutritional requirements. *Amer J Clin Nutr* 83(Suppl), 436S–442S.

Subbiah, M.T.R. (2007). Nutrigenetics and nutraceuticals: the next wave riding on personalized medicine. *Transl Res* 149, 55–61.

Taubes, G. (2001). The soft science of dietary fat. *Science* 291, 2536–2545.

Venter, J.C., Adams, M.D., Myers, E.W., Peter, W., Mural, R.J., Sutton, G.G., et.al. (2001).The sequence of human genome. *Science* 291, 1304–1351.

Vincent, S., Geber, M., Bernard, M.C., De Foort, C., Loundou, A., Portugal, H., et.al. (2004). The Medi-RIVAGE study. Mediterranean diet, cardiovascular risks and gene polymorphisms: rationale, recruitment, design, dietary intervention and baseline characteristics of participants. *Public Health Nutr* 7, 531–542.

Zheng, S., and Chen, A. (2005). Curcumin suppresses the expression of extracellular matrix genes in activated hepatic stellate cells by inhibiting gene expression of connective tissue growth factor. *Am J Physiol (Gastrointest Liver Physiol)* 290, G883–G893.

Chapter 63

Gene Therapy:
Correcting Defective Genes

What is gene therapy?

Genes, which are carried on chromosomes, are the basic physical and functional units of heredity. Genes are specific sequences of bases that encode instructions on how to make proteins. Although genes get a lot of attention, it's the proteins that perform most life functions and even make up the majority of cellular structures. When genes are altered so that the encoded proteins are unable to carry out their normal functions, genetic disorders can result.

Gene therapy is a technique for correcting defective genes responsible for disease development. Researchers may use one of several approaches for correcting faulty genes:

- A normal gene may be inserted into a nonspecific location within the genome to replace a nonfunctional gene. This approach is most common.

- An abnormal gene could be swapped for a normal gene through homologous recombination.

- The abnormal gene could be repaired through selective reverse mutation, which returns the gene to its normal function.

- The regulation (the degree to which a gene is turned on or off) of a particular gene could be altered.

Excerpted from "Gene Therapy," Human Genome Project Information, September 19, 2008

How does gene therapy work?

In most gene therapy studies, a "normal" gene is inserted into the genome to replace an "abnormal," disease-causing gene. A carrier molecule called a vector must be used to deliver the therapeutic gene to the patient's target cells. Currently, the most common vector is a virus that has been genetically altered to carry normal human deoxyribonucleic acid (DNA). Viruses have evolved a way of encapsulating and delivering their genes to human cells in a pathogenic manner. Scientists have tried to take advantage of this capability and manipulate the virus genome to remove disease-causing genes and insert therapeutic genes.

Target cells such as the patient's liver or lung cells are infected with the viral vector. The vector then unloads its genetic material containing the therapeutic human gene into the target cell. The generation of a functional protein product from the therapeutic gene restores the target cell to a normal state.

Some of the different types of viruses used as gene therapy vectors are as follows:

- **Retroviruses:** A class of viruses that can create double-stranded DNA copies of their (ribonucleic acid) RNA genomes. These copies of its genome can be integrated into the chromosomes of host cells. Human immunodeficiency virus (HIV) is a retrovirus.

- **Adenoviruses:** A class of viruses with double-stranded DNA genomes that cause respiratory, intestinal, and eye infections in humans. The virus that causes the common cold is an adenovirus.

- **Adeno-associated viruses:** A class of small, single-stranded DNA viruses that can insert their genetic material at a specific site on chromosome 19.

- **Herpes simplex viruses:** A class of double-stranded DNA viruses that infect a particular cell type, neurons. Herpes simplex virus type 1 is a common human pathogen that causes cold sores.

Besides virus-mediated gene-delivery systems, there are several nonviral options for gene delivery. The simplest method is the direct introduction of therapeutic DNA into target cells. This approach is limited in its application because it can be used only with certain tissues and requires large amounts of DNA.

Another nonviral approach involves the creation of an artificial lipid sphere with an aqueous core. This liposome, which carries the therapeutic DNA, is capable of passing the DNA through the target cell's membrane.

Therapeutic DNA also can get inside target cells by chemically linking the DNA to a molecule that will bind to special cell receptors. Once bound to these receptors, the therapeutic DNA constructs are engulfed by the cell membrane and passed into the interior of the target cell. This delivery system tends to be less effective than other options.

Researchers also are experimenting with introducing a forty-seventh (artificial human) chromosome into target cells. This chromosome would exist autonomously alongside the standard forty-six—not affecting their workings or causing any mutations. It would be a large vector capable of carrying substantial amounts of genetic code, and scientists anticipate that, because of its construction and autonomy, the body's immune systems would not attack it. A problem with this potential method is the difficulty in delivering such a large molecule to the nucleus of a target cell.

What is the current status of gene therapy research?

The Food and Drug Administration (FDA) has not yet approved any human gene therapy product for sale. Current gene therapy is experimental and has not proven very successful in clinical trials. Little progress has been made since the first gene therapy clinical trial began in 1990. In 1999, gene therapy suffered a major setback with the death of eighteen-year-old Jesse Gelsinger. Jesse was participating in a gene therapy trial for ornithine transcarboxylase deficiency (OTCD). He died from multiple organ failures four days after starting the treatment. His death is believed to have been triggered by a severe immune response to the adenovirus carrier.

Another major blow came in January 2003, when the FDA placed a temporary halt on all gene therapy trials using retroviral vectors in blood stem cells. FDA took this action after it learned that a second child treated in a French gene therapy trial had developed a leukemia-like condition. Both this child and another who had developed a similar condition in August 2002 had been successfully treated by gene therapy for X-linked severe combined immunodeficiency disease (X-SCID), also known as "bubble baby syndrome."

FDA's Biological Response Modifiers Advisory Committee (BRMAC) met at the end of February 2003 to discuss possible measures that could allow a number of retroviral gene therapy trials for treatment of life-threatening diseases to proceed with appropriate safeguards.

In April of 2003 the FDA eased the ban on gene therapy trials using retroviral vectors in blood stem cells.

What factors have kept gene therapy from becoming an effective treatment for genetic disease?

Short-lived nature of gene therapy: Before gene therapy can become a permanent cure for any condition, the therapeutic DNA introduced into target cells must remain functional and the cells containing the therapeutic DNA must be long-lived and stable. Problems with integrating therapeutic DNA into the genome and the rapidly dividing nature of many cells prevent gene therapy from achieving any long-term benefits. Patients will have to undergo multiple rounds of gene therapy.

Immune response: Anytime a foreign object is introduced into human tissues, the immune system is designed to attack the invader. The risk of stimulating the immune system in a way that reduces gene therapy effectiveness is always a potential risk. Furthermore, the immune system's enhanced response to invaders it has seen before makes it difficult for gene therapy to be repeated in patients.

Problems with viral vectors: Viruses, while the carrier of choice in most gene therapy studies, present a variety of potential problems to the patient—toxicity, immune and inflammatory responses, and gene control and targeting issues. In addition, there is always the fear that the viral vector, once inside the patient, may recover its ability to cause disease.

Multigene disorders: Conditions or disorders that arise from mutations in a single gene are the best candidates for gene therapy. Unfortunately, some of the most commonly occurring disorders, such as heart disease, high blood pressure, Alzheimer disease, arthritis, and diabetes, are caused by the combined effects of variations in many genes. Multigene or multifactorial disorders such as these would be especially difficult to treat effectively using gene therapy.

What are some recent developments in gene therapy research?

- Results of the world's first gene therapy for inherited blindness show sight improvement. United Kingdom researchers from the

UCL Institute of Ophthalmology and Moorfields Eye Hospital NIHR Biomedical Research Centre have announced results from the world's first clinical trial to test a revolutionary gene therapy treatment for a type of inherited blindness. The results, published in the September 2008 *New England Journal of Medicine*, show that the experimental treatment is safe and can improve sight. The findings are a landmark for gene therapy technology and could have a significant impact on future treatments for eye disease.

- A combination of two tumor suppressing genes delivered in lipid-based nanoparticles drastically reduces the number and size of human lung cancer tumors in mice during trials conducted by researchers from The University of Texas M. D. Anderson Cancer Center and the University of Texas Southwestern Medical Center. (January 11, 2007)

- Researchers at the National Cancer Institute (NCI), part of the National Institutes of Health, successfully reengineer immune cells, called lymphocytes, to target and attack cancer cells in patients with advanced metastatic melanoma. This is the first time that gene therapy is used to successfully treat cancer in humans. (August 30, 2006)

- Gene therapy is effectively used to treat two adult patients for a disease affecting nonlymphocytic white blood cells called myeloid cells. Myeloid disorders are common and include a variety of bone marrow failure syndromes, such as acute myeloid leukemia. The study is the first to show that gene therapy can cure diseases of the myeloid system. (March 31, 2006)

- Gene Therapy cures deafness in guinea pigs. Each animal had been deafened by destruction of the hair cells in the cochlea that translate sound vibrations into nerve signals. A gene, called Atoh1, which stimulates the hair cells' growth, was delivered to the cochlea by an adenovirus. The genes triggered regrowth of the hair cells and many of the animals regained up to 80 percent of their original hearing thresholds. This study, which may pave the way to human trials of the gene, is the first to show that gene therapy can repair deafness in animals. (February 11, 2005)

- University of California, Los Angeles, research team gets genes into the brain using liposomes coated in a polymer call polyethylene glycol (PEG). The transfer of genes into the brain is a significant achievement because viral vectors are too big to get across the "blood-brain barrier." This method has potential for treating Parkinson disease. (March 20, 2003)

- RNA interference or gene silencing may be a new way to treat Huntington disease. Short pieces of double-stranded RNA (short, interfering RNAs or siRNAs) are used by cells to degrade RNA of a particular sequence. If an siRNA is designed to match the RNA copied from a faulty gene, then the abnormal protein product of that gene will not be produced. (March 13, 2003)

- New gene therapy approach repairs errors in messenger RNA derived from defective genes. Technique has potential to treat the blood disorder thalassemia, cystic fibrosis, and some cancers. (October 11, 2002)

- Gene therapy for treating children with X-SCID (severe combined immunodeficiency) or the "bubble boy" disease is stopped in France when the treatment causes leukemia in one of the patients. (October 3, 2002)

- Researchers at Case Western Reserve University and Copernicus Therapeutics are able to create tiny liposomes twenty-five nanometers across that can carry therapeutic DNA through pores in the nuclear membrane. (May 12, 2002)

- Sickle cell is successfully treated in mice. (March 18, 2002)

What are some of the ethical considerations for using gene therapy?

Some questions to consider:

- What is normal and what is a disability or disorder, and who decides?

- Are disabilities diseases? Do they need to be cured or prevented?

- Does searching for a cure demean the lives of individuals presently affected by disabilities?

- Is somatic gene therapy (which is done in the adult cells of persons known to have the disease) more or less ethical than germline gene therapy (which is done in egg and sperm cells and prevents the trait from being passed on to further generations)? In cases of somatic gene therapy, the procedure may have to be repeated in future generations.

- Preliminary attempts at gene therapy are exorbitantly expensive. Who will have access to these therapies? Who will pay for their use?

Part Six

Information for Parents of Children with Genetic Disorders

Chapter 64

When Your Baby Has a Birth Defect

We see happy images of and tend to hear about only healthy babies. But many babies are born with problems called birth defects. These are abnormalities of structure, function, or body chemistry that will require medical or surgical care or could have some effect on a child's development.

About 150,000 babies are born in the United States each year with birth defects, according to the March of Dimes. There is a wide range of birth defects, from mild to severe, and they can be inherited or caused by something in the environment. In many cases, the cause is unknown. Often, doctors can detect a birth defect when they do prenatal tests.

If you've just found out that your child has a birth defect, you're probably experiencing many emotions. Parents in your situation often say that they feel overwhelmed and uncertain whether they will be able to care for their child properly. Fortunately, you aren't alone—with a little effort, you'll find that there are lots of people and resources to help you.

As the parent of a child with a birth defect, it's important for you to:

- **Acknowledge your emotions:** Parents of children with birth defects experience shock, denial, grief, and even anger. Acknowledge your feelings and give yourself permission to mourn the loss of the healthy child you thought you'd have. Talk about your feelings with your spouse or partner and with other family members. You might also consider seeing a counselor. Your doctor may be able to guide you to a social worker or psychologist in the area.

- **One of the best things you can do for yourself and your child is to seek support:** Getting in touch with someone who's been through the same thing can be helpful; ask your doctor or a social worker at your hospital if they know any other parents in the area who have children with the same condition. Joining a support group may also help—consult your child's doctors or specialists for advice about finding a local or national support group.

- **Celebrate your child:** Remember to let yourself enjoy your child the same way any parent would—by cuddling or playing, watching for developmental milestones (even if they're different from those in children without birth defects), and sharing your joy with family members and friends. Many parents of kids with birth defects wonder if they should send out birth announcements. This is a personal decision—the fact that your child has a health problem doesn't mean you shouldn't be excited about the new addition to your family.

Getting Help and Information

Seek information. The amount each person would like to learn varies from parent to parent, but try to educate yourself as much and as soon as you are able. Start by asking your doctors lots of questions. Record the answers as best as you can. If you're not satisfied with the answers—or if a doctor is unable to answer your questions thoroughly —don't be afraid to seek second opinions.

Additional places to get information include:

- books written for parents of children with birth defects;

- national organizations such as the March of Dimes, the National Information Center for Children and Youth With Disabilities, or those representing a specific birth defect;

- support groups or other parents.

Keep a binder with a running list of questions and the answers you find, as well as suggestions for further reading and any materials your child's doctor gives you. In addition, keep an updated list of all health care providers and their phone numbers, as well as emergency numbers, so you're able to reach them quickly and efficiently.

Part of this process of collecting information should involve exploring options for paying for treatment and ongoing care for your child. There may be extra medical and therapeutic costs associated with caring for a child with a birth defect. In addition to health insurance, many resources are available, including nonprofit disability organizations, private foundations, Medicaid, and state and local programs. One of the hospital social workers should be able to help you learn more about these resources.

Seek early intervention. Early intervention is usually the best strategy. Designed to bring a team of experts together to assess your child's needs and establish a program of treatment, early intervention services include feeding support, identification of assistive technology that may help your child, occupational therapy, physical therapy, speech therapy, nutrition services, and social work services.

Besides identifying, evaluating, and treating your child's needs, early intervention programs will:

- tell you where you can get information about the disability;
- help you to learn how to care for your child at home;
- help you determine your payment options and tell you where you can find services for free;
- help you make important decisions about your child's care;
- provide counseling to you and your family.

Your child's doctor or a social worker at the hospital where you gave birth should be able to connect you with the early intervention program in your area.

Use a team approach. Most children with birth defects require a team of professionals to treat them. Even if your child needs to see only one specialist, that person will need to coordinate care with your primary doctor. Although some hospitals already have teams ready to deal with problems such as heart defects, cleft lip and palate, or cerebral palsy, you may find yourself having to serve as both the main point of contact between the different care providers and the coordinator of your child's appointments. As soon as you are able, get to know the different team members. Make sure they know who else will be caring for your child and that you intend to play a key role.

The Future of Birth Defects

Research into the environmental and genetic causes of birth defects is ongoing. Technology contributes to understanding and preventing defects in various ways—for example, prenatal testing is growing increasingly sophisticated.

Safer and more accurate tests include:

- results of ultrasound tests and magnetic resonance imaging (MRI), which are sometimes combined with information from blood tests to determine the risk of having a child with certain birth defects;

- maternal blood screening to determine risk of chromosomal abnormalities;

- amniocentesis and chorionic villi sampling;

- pre-conception counseling to help you understand any risks for having a child with a birth defect.

Although none of these tests can prevent birth defects, they give a clearer, safer, and more accurate diagnosis at an earlier stage of pregnancy—giving parents more time to seek advice and consider their options.

Genetics research is advancing quickly. The Human Genome Project is working on identifying all of the genes in the human body, including gene mutations that are associated with a high risk for birth defects.

Early surgery is becoming an option in the treatment of some birth defects—and can take place even while your child is still in the womb. Surgeons now operate on fetuses to repair structural defects, such as hernias of the diaphragm, spina bifida, and lung malformations. These treatments can be controversial, however, because they can cause premature labor. And it's still a bit unclear as to whether they ultimately improve the final outcome.

To get information on specific research about your child's disability, contact the national organization for that disability. Also, the March of Dimes and the National Information Center for Children and Youth With Disabilities and the National Organization for Rare Disorders, Inc. (NORD) may have information about current research.

Chapter 65

Parenting a Child with a Disability: Where to Start

If you have a child with a disability, you are not alone. Millions of parents in America are raising children with disabilities. Many resources (including fellow parents) can help you along the way. Here are some tips for parents:

- Learn as much as you can about your child's disability.
- Find programs to help your child.
- Talk to your family about how you're feeling.
- Talk to other parents of children with disabilities.
- Join a support group.
- Stick to a daily routine.
- Take it one day at a time.
- Take good care of yourself.

An important quality that you will need to nurture in your child is called "self-determination." Children who develop this quality have a sense of control over their lives and can set goals and work to attain them. Self-determination is important for all children. But researchers have found that students with disabilities who also have high levels of self-determination are more likely to be:

Reprinted from "Parenting a Child with a Disability," National Women's Health Information Center, May 15, 2008.

- employed;

- satisfied with their lives;

- living independently, or with support, outside of their family homes.

Here are some tips on helping your child become self-determined:

- As early as possible, give your child opportunities to make choices and encourage your child to express wants and wishes. For instance, these could be choices about what to wear, what to eat, and how much help with doing things your child wants from you.

- Strike a balance between being protective and supporting risk-taking. Learn to let go a little and push your child out into the world, even though it may be a little scary.

- Guide children toward solving their own problems and making their own choices. For instance, if your child has a problem at school, offer a listening ear and together brainstorm possible solutions. To the extent that your child can, let your child decide on the plan and the back-up plan.

Programs and Services

There are programs and services to help you meet your child's and your family's needs.

Early intervention services try to address the needs of children with disabilities and the needs of their families as early as possible. Often, the sooner issues are addressed, the better the outcome. Examples include nutrition counseling for parents, physical therapy for a baby with cystic fibrosis, or sign language lessons for a deaf child. Services vary by state.

Special education and related services ensure that each child is given a free public education that accommodates his or her special needs. The law requires that every student with a disability have an Individualized Education Program (IEP), which is a plan for that child's education. The IEP includes a list of the services, accommodations, and assistive technology your child will need to succeed in school. Parents of a child with a disability are an important part of the team that writes the IEP. To the extent that they can, children with disabilities should also be encouraged to take part in writing the IEP.

Parent Training and Information (PTI) centers provide parents with information about disabilities and legal rights under laws involving children with disabilities. PTIs can also tell you about resources in the community, state, and nation. PTI centers conduct workshops, conferences, and seminars for parents. And many have libraries where you can borrow books and videos. Every state has at least one PTI. Some states also have Community Parent Resource Centers (CPRCs). CPRCs do the same work as the PTIs, but they focus on reaching underserved parents of children with disabilities. Underserved parents include low-income parents, parents with limited ability to speak and write English, and parents with disabilities.

Parent to Parent is a program that provides information and one-to-one emotional support to parents of children with disabilities. Trained and experienced parents are carefully matched in one-to-one relationships with parents who are new to the program. The matches are based upon similarities in disability and family issues.

Chapter 66

Early Intervention: An Overview

Broadly speaking, early intervention services are specialized health, educational, and therapeutic services designed to meet the needs of infants and toddlers, from birth through age two, who have a developmental delay or disability, and their families. At the discretion of each state, services can also be provided to children who are considered to be at risk of developing substantial delays if services are not provided.

Sometimes it is known from the moment a child is born that early intervention services will be essential in helping the child grow and develop. Often this is so for children who are diagnosed at birth with a specific condition or who experience significant prematurity, very low birth weight, illness, or surgery soon after being born. Even before heading home from the hospital, this child's parents may be given a referral to their local early intervention office.

Some children have a relatively routine entry into the world, but may develop more slowly than others, experience setbacks, or develop in ways that seem very different from other children. For these children, a visit with a developmental pediatrician and a thorough evaluation may lead to an early intervention referral, as well. However a child comes to be referred, assessed, and determined eligible—early intervention services provide vital support so that children with developmental needs can thrive and grow.

Excerpted from "Overview of Early Intervention," National Dissemination Center for Children with Disabilities, 2008.

What areas of child development are early intervention services designed to address?

In a nutshell, early intervention is concerned with all the basic and brand new skills that babies typically develop during the first three years of life, including the following:

- physical (reaching, rolling, crawling, and walking)
- cognitive (thinking, learning, solving problems)
- communication (talking, listening, understanding)
- social/emotional (playing, feeling secure and happy)
- self-help (eating, dressing)

My child seems to be developing much slower than other children. Would he/she be eligible for early intervention services?

It is possible that your child may be eligible for early intervention, but more investigation is necessary to determine that. If you think that your child is not developing at the same pace or in the same way as most children his or her age, it is often a good idea to talk first to your child's pediatrician. Explain your concerns. Tell the doctor what you have observed with your child. Your child may have a disability or what is known as a developmental delay, or he or she may be at risk of having a disability or delay.

"Developmental delay" is a term that means an infant or child is developing slower than normal in one or more areas (Anderson, Chitwood, & Hayden, 1997). For example, he or she may not be sitting up (or walking or talking) when most children of that age are. The term "at risk" means that a child's development may be delayed unless he or she receives early intervention services.

So, if you are concerned about your child's development, you will need to have your child evaluated to find out if he or she is eligible for early intervention services. This evaluation is provided at no cost to you. There are many people who can help you with this.

Where do I go for help?

Ask your child's pediatrician to put you in touch with the early intervention system in your community or region.

Contact the pediatrics branch in a local hospital and ask where you should call to find out about early intervention services in your area.

It is very important to write down the names and phone numbers of everyone you talk to. Having this information available will be helpful to you later on.

What do I say to the early intervention contact person?

Explain that you are concerned about your child's development. Say that you think your child may need early intervention services. Explain that you would like to have your child evaluated under the Individuals with Disabilities Education Act (IDEA). Write down any information the contact person gives you.

The person may refer you to what is known as Child Find. One of Child Find's purposes is to identify children who need early intervention services. Child Find operates in every state and conducts screenings to identify children who may need early intervention services. These screenings are provided free of charge.

Each state has one agency that is in charge of the early intervention system for infants and toddlers with special needs. This agency is known as the lead agency. It may be the state education agency or another agency, such as the health department. Each state decides which agency will serve as the lead agency.

What happens next?

Once you are in contact with the early intervention system, the system will assign someone to work with you and your child through the evaluation and assessment process. This person will be your temporary service coordinator. He or she should have a background in early childhood development and ways to help young children who may have developmental delays. The service coordinator should also know the policies for early intervention programs and services in your state.

The early intervention system will need to determine if your child is eligible for early intervention services. To do this, the staff will set up and carry out a multidisciplinary evaluation and assessment of your child. Read on for more information about this process.

What is a multidisciplinary evaluation and assessment?

IDEA requires that your child receive a timely, comprehensive, multidisciplinary evaluation and assessment. The purposes of the evaluation and assessment are to determine the following things:

- The nature of your child's strengths, delays, or difficulties
- Whether your child is eligible for early intervention services

"Multidisciplinary" means that the evaluation group is made up of qualified people who have different areas of training and experience. Together, they know about children's speech and language skills, physical abilities, hearing and vision, and other important areas of development. They know how to work with children, even very young ones, to discover if a child has a problem or is developing within normal ranges. Group members may evaluate your child together or individually.

"Evaluation" refers to the procedures used by these professionals to find out if your child is eligible for early intervention services. As part of the evaluation, the team will observe your child, ask your child to do things, talk to you and your child, and use other methods to gather information. These procedures will help the team find out how your child functions in five areas of development: cognitive development, physical development, communication, social-emotional development, and adaptive development.

Following your child's evaluation, you and a team of professionals will meet and review all of the data, results, and reports. The people on the team will talk with you about whether your child meets the criteria under IDEA and state policy for having a developmental delay, a diagnosed physical or mental condition, or being at risk for having a substantial delay. If so, your child is generally found to be eligible for services.

If found eligible, he or she will then be assessed. "Assessment" refers to the procedures used throughout the time your child is in early intervention. The purpose of these ongoing procedures is to identify your child's unique strengths and needs, and determine what services are necessary to meet those needs.

With your consent, your family's needs will also be identified. This process, which is family-directed, is intended to identify the resources, priorities, and concerns of your family. It also identifies the supports and services you may need to enhance your family's capacity to meet your child's developmental needs. The family assessment is usually conducted through an interview with you, the parents.

When conducting the evaluation and assessment, team members may get information from some or all of the following:

- Doctor's reports
- Results from developmental tests and performance assessments given to your child

- Your child's medical and developmental history
- Direct observations and feedback from all members of the multidisciplinary team, including you, the parents
- Interviews with you and other family members or caretakers
- Any other important observations, records, and/or reports about your child

Who pays for the evaluation and assessment?

It depends on your state's policies or rules. Ask your local contact person or service coordinator about this. However, evaluations and assessments must be done by qualified personnel. As was said above, a multidisciplinary group of professionals will evaluate your child. The group may include a psychologist or social worker, an early interventionist or special educator, and an occupational or physical therapist. All assessments must be performed in your child's native language.

Under IDEA, evaluations and assessments are provided at no cost to parents. They are funded by state and federal money.

Who is eligible for services?

Under the IDEA, "infants and toddlers with disabilities" are defined as children from birth through age two who need early intervention services because they are experiencing developmental delays, as measured by appropriate diagnostic instruments and procedures, in one or more of the following areas:

- Cognitive development
- Physical development, including vision and hearing
- Communication development
- Social or emotional development
- Adaptive development

Also included are children from birth through age two who have a diagnosed physical or mental condition that has a high probability of resulting in developmental delay.

The term may also include, if a state chooses, children from birth through age two who are at risk of having substantial developmental delays if early intervention services are not provided. (34 Code of Federal Regulations §303.16)

My child has been found eligible for services. What's next?

If your child and family are found eligible, you and a team will meet to develop a written plan for providing early intervention services to your child and, as necessary, to your family. This plan is called the Individualized Family Service Plan, or IFSP. It is a very important document, and you, as parents, are important members of the team that develops it.

What is an Individualized Family Service Plan, or IFSP?

The IFSP is a written document that, among other things, outlines the early intervention services that your child and family will receive. One guiding principal of the IFSP is that the family is a child's greatest resource, that a young child's needs are closely tied to the needs of his or her family. The best way to support children and meet their needs is to support and build upon the individual strengths of their family. So, the IFSP is a whole family plan with the parents as major contributors in its development. Involvement of other team members will depend on what the child needs. These other team members could come from several agencies and may include medical people, therapists, child development specialists, social workers, and others.

Your child's IFSP must include the following:

- Your child's present physical, cognitive, communication, social/emotional, and adaptive development levels and needs

- Family information (with your agreement), including the resources, priorities, and concerns of you, as parents, and other family members closely involved with the child

- The major results or outcomes expected to be achieved for your child and family; the specific services your child will be receiving

- Where in the natural environment (e.g., home, community) the services will be provided (if the services will not be provided in the natural environment, the IFSP must include a statement justifying why not)

- When and where your son or daughter will receive services

- The number of days or sessions he or she will receive each service and how long each session will last

- Whether the service will be provided on a one-on-one or group basis

- Who will pay for the services

- The name of the service coordinator overseeing the implementation of the IFSP

- The steps to be taken to support your child's transition out of early intervention and into another program when the time comes

The IFSP may also identify services your family may be interested in, such as financial information or information about raising a child with a disability. The IFSP is reviewed every six months and is updated at least once a year. The IFSP must be fully explained to you, the parents, and your suggestions must be considered. You must give written consent before services can start. If you do not give your consent in writing, your child will not receive services. Each state has specific guidelines for the IFSP. Your service coordinator can explain what the IFSP guidelines are in your state.

What's included in early intervention services?

Under IDEA, early intervention services must include a multidisciplinary evaluation and assessment, a written Individualized Family Service Plan, service coordination, and specific services designed to meet the unique developmental needs of the child and family. Early intervention services may be simple or complex, depending on the child's needs. They can range from prescribing glasses for a two-year-old to developing a comprehensive approach with a variety of services and special instruction for a child, including home visits, counseling, and training for his or her family. Depending on your child's needs, his or her early intervention services may include the following:

- Family training, counseling, and home visits

- Special instruction

- Speech-language pathology services (sometimes referred to as speech therapy)

- Audiology services (hearing impairment services)

- Occupational therapy

- Physical therapy

- Psychological services; medical services (only for diagnostic or evaluation purposes)

- Health services needed to enable your child to benefit from the other services

- Social work services

- Assistive technology devices and services

- Transportation

- Nutrition services

- Service coordination services

How are early intervention services delivered?

Early intervention services may be delivered in a variety of ways and in different places. Sometimes services are provided in the child's home with the family receiving additional training. Services may also be provided in other settings, such as a clinic, a neighborhood daycare center, hospital, or the local health department. To the maximum extent appropriate, the services are to be provided in natural environments or settings. Natural environments, broadly speaking, are where the child lives, learns, and plays. Services are provided by qualified personnel and may be offered through a public or private agency.

Will I have to pay for services?

Whether or not you, as parents, will have to pay for any services for your child depends on the policies of your state. Under IDEA, the following services must be provided at no cost to families: Child Find services; evaluations and assessments; the development and review of the Individualized Family Service Plan; and service coordination.

Depending on your state's policies, you may have to pay for certain other services. You may be charged a "sliding-scale" fee, meaning the fees are based on what you earn. Check with the contact person in your area or state. Some services may be covered by your health insurance, by Medicaid, or by Indian Health Services. Every effort is made to provide services to all infants and toddlers who need help, regardless of family income. Services cannot be denied to a child just because his or her family is not able to pay for them.

What about record keeping?

As you contact different people and places, it's a good idea to keep records of people you've talked with and what was said. As time goes by, you will want to add other information to your file, such as: letters and notes (from doctors, therapists, etc.); medical records and reports; results of tests and evaluations; notes from meetings about your child; therapist(s') reports; IFSP and IEP records; your child's developmental history, including personal notes or diaries on your child's development; records of shots and vaccinations; and family medical histories.

Make sure you get copies of all written information about your child (records, reports, etc.). This will help you become an important coordinator of services and a better advocate for your child. Remember, as time goes on, you'll probably have more information to keep track of, so it's a good idea to keep it together in one place.

Chapter 67

Assistive Technology for Infants and Toddlers

Research shows that assistive technology (AT) can help young children with disabilities learn valuable skills.[1] For example, by using computers and special software, young children may improve in the following areas:

- Social skills including sharing and taking turns
- Communication skills
- Attention span
- Fine and gross motor skills
- Self-confidence and independence

In addition, by using the right type of assistive technology, some negative behaviors may decrease as a child's ability to communicate increases. Some common examples of assistive technology include wheelchairs, computers and computer software, and communication devices.

What types of assistive technology devices can infants and toddlers use?

There are two types of AT devices most commonly used by infants and toddlers—switches and augmentative communication devices.

There are many types of switches that can be used in many different ways. Switches can be used with battery-operated toys to give infants opportunities to play with them. For example, a switch could be attached directly to a stuffed pig so that every time an infant touches the toy, it wiggles and snorts. Switches can also be used to turn many things off and on. Toddlers can learn to press a switch to turn on a computer or to use cause and effect (interactive) software. Children who have severe disabilities can also use switches. For example, a switch could be placed next to an infant's head so that every time she moved her head to the left a musical mobile hanging overhead would play.

Augmentative communication devices allow children who cannot speak or who cannot yet speak to communicate with the world around them. These devices can be as simple as pointing to a photo on a picture board or they can be more complicated—for instance, pressing message buttons on a device that activate prerecorded messages such as, "I'm hungry."

Why is assistive technology important?

Many of the skills learned in life begin in infancy. AT can help infants and toddlers with disabilities learn many of these crucial skills. In fact, with assistive technology, they can usually learn the same things that nondisabled children learn at the same age, only in a different way. Communication skills at this age are especially important because most of what an infant or toddler learns is through interacting with other people, especially family members and other primary caregivers.

Sometimes parents are reluctant to begin using an AT device because they believe it will discourage their child from learning important skills. However, the opposite may be true. Research has shown that using AT devices, especially augmentative communication devices, may actually encourage a child to increase communication efforts and skills. It is important to remember that the earlier a child is taught to use an AT device, the more easily a child will accept and use it.

Assistive technology is also important because expectations for a child increase as those around them learn to say, "This is what the baby can do, with supports," instead of, "This is what the baby can't do." With assistive technology, parents learn that the dreams they had for their child don't necessarily end when he or she is diagnosed with a disability. The dreams may have to be changed a little, but they can still come true.

How can a family obtain AT devices for their infant or toddler?

There are two ways. First, infants and toddlers who have a disability are eligible for early intervention services under Part C of the federal law called the Individuals with Disabilities Education Act (IDEA). If the child meets the state eligibility criteria for early intervention services under IDEA, he or she will receive assistive technology devices and services if their Individual Family Services Program (IFSP) team decides that these services are needed to meet the child's unique needs and includes them in the IFSP.

Secondly, some infants and toddlers have delays that are not significant enough or are not yet significant enough to be eligible for IDEA early intervention services under the state's eligibility criteria. Many of these infants and toddlers may still benefit from using an AT device. In some cases, private insurance or medical assistance will pay for a device or you may choose to purchase a device directly for your child.

Many schools and communities have special lending libraries where parents can borrow toys with switches, computer software, and other devices. These libraries, such as the Tech Tots libraries sponsored by United Cerebral Palsy chapters around the country, give parents an opportunity to try various AT devices to see if they will help their child before purchasing them.

If my child is not eligible for early intervention services under IDEA, how will I know if she could still benefit from using an AT device?

Asking certain questions may help you make that decision. For example: Compared to other children her age, can my child play with toys independently? How does my child communicate—can she communicate effectively? How does my child move from place to place—can she sit, stand, or walk independently? And, can my child feed herself? If you answer "No" to these questions, then assistive technology may help. In some cases, children with behavior problems actually have a communication impairment and are frustrated that they cannot tell someone how they feel.

What is assistive technology for children who are eligible for early intervention under IDEA?

IDEA defines an AT device as any item, piece of equipment, or product system, whether purchased directly off the shelf, changed or adjusted, or customized, that is used to increase, maintain, or improve the functional capabilities of children with disabilities.

Under IDEA, assistive technology services are any services that directly help a child with a disability to choose, obtain, or use assistive technology. AT services include:

- finding and paying for the device (including purchasing, leasing or otherwise acquiring);

- selecting, designing, fitting, adapting, applying, maintaining, or customizing a device for a particular child;

- repairing or replacing a device;

- coordinating and using other therapies, interventions, or services with AT devices;

- evaluating the needs of a child with a disability, including a functional evaluation of the child in the child's customary environment;

- training or technical assistance for a child with disabilities or, if appropriate, that child's family; and

- training or technical assistance for professionals, including those providing early intervention services, or others who provide services to or are substantially involved in the major life functions of individuals with disabilities.

How does a parent request an AT evaluation under IDEA?

Generally, an AT evaluation should be included as part of the early intervention evaluation if there is reason to believe the child may need an AT device or service. However, parents may request an evaluation at any time. Parents and significant others—such as siblings or grandparents, if appropriate—should be involved in the entire process because they have valuable insights and information about the child. When parents are actively involved it is more likely that the child will get the right device and that it will be used properly.

What is the most effective way to evaluate an infant or toddler for AT devices or services?

Ideally, a multidisciplinary team will do an AT evaluation. Generally, this team will include an assistive technology specialist who understands computer hardware and software, augmentative communication devices, and other types of equipment. A member of the team should also understand how technology could be used in all areas of a child's life to support the child's early intervention outcomes. (This person should also have knowledge of infant and toddler development.) Some early intervention programs have assistive technology specialists on staff; others use a physical, occupational, or speech therapist that has received additional training. If an early intervention program does not have a technology expert, they can contract with a provider, a school district, or a community agency. Parents and early intervention providers are always vital members of the team.

Before they do the evaluation, team members should gather background information about the child's interests, abilities, and family routines. This will help to determine what type of AT devices, if any, should be used during the evaluation. Generally, the evaluation is done wherever the child is most comfortable or wherever he spends most of his time. For infants and toddlers, this could be the family home or a childcare or preschool setting. When the evaluation is done, the team should then write specific recommendations about the type of devices and services that would help the child reach the expected outcomes. Any AT devices recommended should be easy for the family and other primary caregivers, such as childcare providers, to use.

The most important thing about the evaluation is that it focuses on the child's strengths and abilities. For example, if an infant with cerebral palsy can only wiggle her left foot, then this is considered one of her strengths. Any AT devices used should build on this strength. In this case, a switch could be positioned so that every time the infant wiggled her foot a music box would play. Creativity is a must when thinking about AT for children who have significant impairments! Again, parents and other primary caretakers are great resources to tap.

Under IDEA, where can assistive technology devices and services be provided?

To the maximum extent appropriate to the child's needs, early intervention services must be provided in natural environments such as the child's home, a childcare setting, or other community settings where children without disabilities are found.

It is the responsibility of the IFSP team to determine—based on evaluations and assessments—what services are needed to meet the unique needs of the child. These services, including AT devices and services, should be included in the child's IFSP. As a part of this process, the team would discuss the environments in which AT devices and services would best meet the child's needs, including home, childcare, and other community settings.

As children move from one service to another, it is critical that everyone involved with the child know what AT devices the child is using and how to obtain and use them. For example, if a two-and-a-half-year-old child is in early intervention and will move to preschool at age three, the need for AT should be discussed at the transition planning conference. This will help to ensure that the child's AT access is continuous.

Under IDEA, who pays for assistive technology devices and services?

All early intervention services, including AT devices and services, must be provided at no cost to the family unless the state has established a system of payment for early intervention services.

What type of training can be provided under IDEA?

In general, parents, service providers, childcare providers, and others who work with infants and toddlers and their families should be trained to use the AT device. Training could include:

- basic information about the device, how to set it up, and how it works;

- how the device can be used in all parts of the child's life;

- how to know when something is wrong and how to fix minor problems;

- what to do or where to take the device if there is a major problem;

- how to change or adapt the device for a child as he grows or as her activities become more complex.

If parents and service providers are trained and comfortable with the device, then they are more likely to find creative ways to use it in all parts of the child's life. The need for training and who will provide it should be included in the child's IFSP.

References

1. Research cited in this chapter is from the Early Childhood Comprehensive Technology System (Project ECCTS) study funded by the U.S. Department of Education's Office of Special Education Programs, under IDEA's Technology, Demonstration, and Utilization and Media Services Program.

Chapter 68

A Guide to the Individualized Education Program

Basic Information about the Individualized Education Program

Each public school child who receives special education and related services must have an Individualized Education Program (IEP). Each IEP must be designed for one student and must be a truly individualized document. The IEP creates an opportunity for teachers, parents, school administrators, related services personnel, and students (when appropriate) to work together to improve educational results for children with disabilities. The IEP is the cornerstone of a quality education for each child with a disability.

To create an effective IEP, parents, teachers, other school staff—and often the student—must come together to look closely at the student's unique needs. These individuals pool knowledge, experience, and commitment to design an educational program that will help the student be involved in, and progress in, the general curriculum. The IEP guides the delivery of special education supports and services for the student with a disability. Without a doubt, writing—and implementing—an effective IEP requires teamwork.

This chapter explains the IEP process, which we consider to be one of the most critical elements to ensure effective teaching, learning, and better results for all children with disabilities. The chapter is designed to help teachers, parents, and anyone involved in the education of a child with a disability develop and carry out an IEP. The information in this chapter is based on what is required by our nation's special education law—the Individuals with Disabilities Education Act, or IDEA.

The IDEA requires certain information to be included in each child's IEP. It is useful to know, however, that states and local school systems often include additional information in IEPs in order to document that they have met certain aspects of federal or state law. The flexibility that states and school systems have to design their own IEP forms is one reason why IEP forms may look different from school system to school system or state to state. Yet each IEP is critical in the education of a child with a disability.

The Basic Special Education Process under IDEA

The writing of each student's IEP takes place within the larger picture of the special education process under IDEA. Before taking a detailed look at the IEP, it may be helpful to look briefly at how a student is identified as having a disability and needing special education and related services and, thus, an IEP.

Step 1: Child Is Identified as Possibly Needing Special Education and Related Services. The state must identify, locate, and evaluate all children with disabilities in the state who need special education and related services. To do so, states conduct "Child Find" activities. A child may be identified by "Child Find," and parents may be asked if the "Child Find" system can evaluate their child. Parents can also call the "Child Find" system and ask that their child be evaluated.

Alternatively, a school professional may ask that a child be evaluated to see if he or she has a disability. Parents may also contact the child's teacher or other school professional to ask that their child be evaluated. This request may be verbal or in writing. Parental consent is needed before the child may be evaluated. Evaluation needs to be completed within a reasonable time after the parent gives consent.

Step 2: Child Is Evaluated. The evaluation must assess the child in all areas related to the child's suspected disability. The evaluation results will be used to determine the child's eligibility for special education and related services and to make decisions about an appropriate educational program for the child. If the parents disagree with the evaluation, they have the right to take their child for an independent educational evaluation (IEE). They can ask that the school system pay for this IEE.

Step 3: Eligibility Is Decided. A group of qualified professionals and the parents look at the child's evaluation results. Together, they decide if the child is a "child with a disability," as defined by IDEA. Parents may ask for a hearing to challenge the eligibility decision.

Step 4: Child Is Found Eligible for Services. If the child is found to be a "child with a disability," as defined by IDEA, he or she is eligible for special education and related services. Within thirty calendar days after a child is determined eligible, the IEP team must meet to write an IEP for the child.

Step 5: IEP Meeting Is Scheduled. The school system schedules and conducts the IEP meeting. School staff must do the following:

- Contact the participants, including the parents
- Notify parents early enough to make sure they have an opportunity to attend
- Schedule the meeting at a time and place agreeable to parents and the school
- Tell the parents the purpose, time, and location of the meeting
- Tell the parents who will be attending
- Tell the parents that they may invite people to the meeting who have knowledge or special expertise about the child

Step 6: IEP Meeting Is Held and IEP Is Written. The IEP team gathers to talk about the child's needs and write the student's IEP. Parents and the student (when appropriate) are part of the team. If the child's placement is decided by a different group, the parents must be part of that group as well.

Before the school system may provide special education and related services to the child for the first time, the parents must give consent.

613

The child begins to receive services as soon as possible after the meeting.

If the parents do not agree with the IEP and placement, they may discuss their concerns with other members of the IEP team and try to work out an agreement. If they still disagree, parents can ask for mediation, or the school may offer mediation. Parents may file a complaint with the state education agency and may request a due process hearing, at which time mediation must be available.

Step 7: Services Are Provided. The school makes sure that the child's IEP is being carried out as it was written. Parents are given a copy of the IEP. Each of the child's teachers and service providers has access to the IEP and knows his or her specific responsibilities for carrying out the IEP. This includes the accommodations, modifications, and supports that must be provided to the child, in keeping with the IEP.

Step 8: Progress Is Measured and Reported to Parents. The child's progress toward the annual goals is measured, as stated in the IEP. His or her parents are regularly informed of their child's progress and whether that progress is enough for the child to achieve the goals by the end of the year. These progress reports must be given to parents at least as often as parents are informed of their nondisabled children's progress.

Step 9: IEP Is Reviewed. The child's IEP is reviewed by the IEP team at least once a year, or more often if the parents or school ask for a review. If necessary, the IEP is revised. Parents, as team members, must be invited to attend these meetings. Parents can make suggestions for changes, can agree or disagree with the IEP goals, and can agree or disagree with the placement.

If parents do not agree with the IEP and placement, they may discuss their concerns with other members of the IEP team and try to work out an agreement. There are several options, including additional testing, an independent evaluation, or asking for mediation (if available) or a due process hearing. They may also file a complaint with the state education agency.

Step 10: Child Is Reevaluated. At least every three years the child must be reevaluated. This evaluation is often called a "triennial." Its purpose is to find out if the child continues to be a "child with a disability," as defined by IDEA, and what the child's educational needs are. However, the child must be reevaluated more often if conditions warrant or if the child's parent or teacher asks for a new evaluation.

A Closer Look at the IEP

Clearly, the IEP is a very important document for children with disabilities and for those who are involved in educating them. Done correctly, the IEP should improve teaching, learning, and results. Each child's IEP describes, among other things, the educational program that has been designed to meet that child's unique needs. This part of the chapter looks closely at how the IEP is written and by whom, and what information it must, at a minimum, contain.

Contents of the IEP

By law, the IEP must include certain information about the child and the educational program designed to meet his or her unique needs. In a nutshell, this information is as follows.

Current Performance. The IEP must state how the child is currently doing in school (known as present levels of educational performance). This information usually comes from the evaluation results such as classroom tests and assignments, individual tests given to decide eligibility for services or during reevaluation, and observations made by parents, teachers, related service providers, and other school staff. The statement about "current performance" includes how the child's disability affects his or her involvement and progress in the general curriculum.

Annual Goals. These are goals that the child can reasonably accomplish in a year. The goals are broken down into short-term objectives or benchmarks. Goals may be academic, address social or behavioral needs, relate to physical needs, or address other educational needs. The goals must be measurable—meaning that it must be possible to measure whether the student has achieved the goals.

Special Education and Related Services. The IEP must list the special education and related services to be provided to the child or on behalf of the child. This includes supplementary aids and services that the child needs. It also includes modifications (changes) to the program or supports for school personnel—such as training or professional development—that will be provided to assist the child.

Participation with Nondisabled Children. The IEP must explain the extent (if any) to which the child will not participate with nondisabled children in the regular class and other school activities.

Participation in State and District-Wide Tests. Most states and districts give achievement tests to children in certain grades or age groups. The IEP must state what modifications in the administration of these tests the child will need. If a test is not appropriate for the child, the IEP must state why the test is not appropriate and how the child will be tested instead.

Dates and Places. The IEP must state when services will begin, how often they will be provided, where they will be provided, and how long they will last.

Transition Service Needs. Beginning when the child is age fourteen (or younger, if appropriate), the IEP must address (within the applicable parts of the IEP) the courses he or she needs to take to reach his or her post-school goals. A statement of transition services needs must also be included in each of the child's subsequent IEPs.

Needed Transition Services. Beginning when the child is age sixteen (or younger, if appropriate), the IEP must state what transition services are needed to help the child prepare for leaving school.

Age of Majority. Beginning at least one year before the child reaches the age of majority, the IEP must include a statement that the student has been told of any rights that will transfer to him or her at the age of majority. (This statement would be needed only in states that transfer rights at the age of majority.)

Measuring Progress. The IEP must state how the child's progress will be measured and how parents will be informed of that progress.

Additional State and School-System Content

States and school systems have a great deal of flexibility about the information they require in an IEP. Some states and school systems have chosen to include in the IEP additional information to document their compliance with other state and federal requirements. (Federal law requires that school districts maintain documentation to demonstrate their compliance with federal requirements.) Generally speaking, extra elements in IEPs may be included to document that the state or school district has met certain aspects of federal or state law, such as the following:

- Holding the meeting to write, review, and, if necessary, revise a child's IEP in a timely manner

- Providing parents with a copy of the procedural safeguards they have under the law

- Placing the child in the least restrictive environment

- Obtaining the parents' consent

IEP Forms in Different Places

While the law tells us what information must be included in the IEP, it does not specify what the IEP should look like. No one form or approach or appearance is required or even suggested. Each state may decide what its IEPs will look like. In some states individual school systems design their own IEP forms.

Thus, across the United States, many different IEP forms are used. What is important is that each form be as clear and as useful as possible, so that parents, educators, related service providers, administrators, and others can easily use the form to write and implement effective IEPs for their students with disabilities.

The IEP Team Members

By law, certain individuals must be involved in writing a child's Individualized Education Program. Note that an IEP team member may fill more than one of the team positions if properly qualified and designated. For example, the school system representative may also be the person who can interpret the child's evaluation results.

These people must work together as a team to write the child's IEP. A meeting to write the IEP must be held within thirty calendar days of deciding that the child is eligible for special education and related services.

Each team member brings important information to the IEP meeting. Members share their information and work together to write the child's Individualized Education Program. Each person's information adds to the team's understanding of the child and what services the child needs.

Parents are key members of the IEP team. They know their child very well and can talk about their child's strengths and needs as well as their ideas for enhancing their child's education. They can offer insight into how their child learns, what his or her interests are, and other aspects of the child that only a parent can know. They can listen to what the other team members think their child needs to work on at school and share their suggestions. They can also report on whether the skills the child is learning at school are being used at home.

Teachers are vital participants in the IEP meeting as well. At least one of the child's regular education teachers must be on the IEP team if the child is (or may be) participating in the regular education environment. The regular education teacher has a great deal to share with the team. For example, he or she might talk about any of the following:

- The general curriculum in the regular classroom

- The aids, services, or changes to the educational program that would help the child learn and achieve

- Strategies to help the child with behavior, if behavior is an issue.

The regular education teacher may also discuss with the IEP team the supports for school staff that are needed so that the child can do the following:

- Advance toward his or her annual goals

- Be involved and progress in the general curriculum

- Participate in extracurricular and other activities

- Be educated with other children, both with and without disabilities

Supports for school staff may include professional development or more training. Professional development and training are important for teachers, administrators, bus drivers, cafeteria workers, and others who provide services for children with disabilities.

The child's special education teacher contributes important information and experience about how to educate children with disabilities. Because of his or her training in special education, this teacher can talk about the following issues:

- How to modify the general curriculum to help the child learn

- The supplementary aids and services that the child may need to be successful in the regular classroom and elsewhere

- How to modify testing so that the student can show what he or she has learned

- Other aspects of individualizing instruction to meet the student's unique needs

Beyond helping to write the IEP, the special educator has responsibility for working with the student to carry out the IEP. He or she may do any of the following:

- Work with the student in a resource room or special class devoted to students receiving special education services

- Team teach with the regular education teacher

- Work with other school staff, particularly the regular education teacher, to provide expertise about addressing the child's unique needs.

Another important member of the IEP team is the individual who can interpret what the child's evaluation results mean in terms of designing appropriate instruction. The evaluation results are very useful in determining how the child is currently doing in school and what areas of need the child has. This IEP team member must be able to talk about the instructional implications of the child's evaluation results, which will help the team plan appropriate instruction to address the child's needs.

The individual representing the school system is also a valuable team member. This person knows a great deal about special education services and educating children with disabilities. He or she can talk about the necessary school resources. It is important that this individual have the authority to commit resources and be able to ensure that whatever services are set out in the IEP will actually be provided.

The IEP team may also include additional individuals with knowledge or special expertise about the child. The parent or the school system can invite these individuals to participate on the team. Parents, for example, may invite an advocate who knows the child, a professional with special expertise about the child and his or her disability, or others (such as a vocational educator who has been working with the child) who can talk about the child's strengths or needs. The school system may invite one or more individuals who can offer special expertise or knowledge about the child, such as a paraprofessional or related services professional. Because an important part of developing an IEP is considering a child's need for related services, related service professionals are often involved as IEP team members or participants. They share their special expertise about the child's needs and how their own professional services can address those needs. Depending on the child's individual needs, some related service professionals attending the IEP meeting or otherwise helping to develop the IEP might include occupational or physical therapists, adaptive physical education providers, psychologists, or speech-language pathologists.

When an IEP is being developed for a student of transition age, representatives from transition service agencies can be important participants. Whenever a purpose of meeting is to consider needed transition services, the school must invite a representative of any other agency that is likely to be responsible for providing or paying for transition services. This individual can help the team plan any transition services the student needs. He or she can also commit the resources of the agency to pay for or provide needed transition services. If he or she does not attend the meeting, then the school must take alternative steps to obtain the agency's participation in the planning of the student's transition services.

Last but not least, the student may also be a member of the IEP team. If transition service needs or transition services are going to be discussed at the meeting, the student must be invited to attend. More and more students are participating in and even leading their own IEP meetings. This allows them to have a strong voice in their own education and can teach them a great deal about self-advocacy and self-determination.

The Regular Education Teacher as Part of the IEP Team

Appendix A of the federal regulations for Part B of IDEA answers many questions about the IEP. Question 24 addresses the role of the regular education teacher on the IEP team. Here's an excerpt from the answer:

> While a regular education teacher must be a member of the IEP team if the child is, or may be, participating in the regular education environment, the teacher need not (depending upon the child's needs and the purpose of the specific IEP team

meeting) be required to participate in all decisions made as part of the meeting or to be present throughout the entire meeting or attend every meeting. For example, the regular education teacher who is a member of the IEP team must participate in discussions and decisions about how to modify the general curriculum in the regular classroom to ensure the child's involvement and progress in the general curriculum and participation in the regular education environment.

Depending upon the specific circumstances, however, it may not be necessary for the regular education teacher to participate in discussions and decisions regarding, for example, the physical therapy needs of the child, if the teacher is not responsible for implementing that portion of the child's IEP.

In determining the extent of the regular education teacher's participation at IEP meetings, public agencies and parents should discuss and try to reach agreement on whether the child's regular education teacher that is a member of the IEP team should be present at a particular IEP meeting and, if so, for what period of time. The extent to which it would be appropriate for the regular education teacher member of the IEP team to participate in IEP meetings must be decided on a case-by-case basis.

Related Services

A child may require any of the following related services in order to benefit from special education. Related services, as listed under IDEA, include (but are not limited to) the following:

- Audiology services
- Counseling services
- Early identification and assessment of disabilities in children
- Medical services
- Occupational therapy
- Orientation and mobility services
- Parent counseling and training
- Physical therapy
- Psychological services

- Recreation
- Rehabilitation counseling services
- School health services
- Social work services in schools
- Speech-language pathology services
- Transportation

If a child needs a particular related service in order to benefit from special education, the related service professional should be involved in developing the IEP. He or she may be invited by the school or parent to join the IEP team as a person "with knowledge or special expertise about the child."

Transition Services

Transition refers to activities meant to prepare students with disabilities for adult life. This can include developing postsecondary education and career goals, getting work experience while still in school, setting up linkages with adult service providers such as the vocational rehabilitation agency—whatever is appropriate for the student, given his or her interests, preferences, skills, and needs. Statements about the student's transition needs must be included in the IEP after the student reaches a certain age.

Transition Planning. This is for students beginning at age fourteen (and sometimes younger) and involves helping the student plan his or her courses of study (such as advanced placement or vocational education) so that the classes the student takes will lead to his or her post-school goals.

Transition Services. This is for students beginning at age sixteen (and sometimes younger) and involves providing the student with a coordinated set of services to help the student move from school to adult life. Services focus upon the student's needs or interests in such areas as higher education or training, employment, adult services, independent living, or taking part in the community.

Writing the IEP

To help decide what special education and related services the student needs, generally the IEP team will begin by looking at the child's evaluation results, such as classroom tests, individual tests given to establish the student's eligibility, and observations by teachers, parents, paraprofessionals, related service providers, administrators, and others. This information will help the team describe the student's "present levels of educational performance"—in other words, how the student is currently doing in school. Knowing how the student is currently performing in school will help the team develop annual goals to address those areas where the student has an identified educational need.

The IEP team must also discuss specific information about the child. This includes the following:

- The child's strengths
- The parents' ideas for enhancing their child's education
- The results of recent evaluations or reevaluations
- How the child has done on state and district-wide tests

In addition, the IEP team must consider the "special factors" described in the following text.

It is important that the discussion of what the child needs be framed around how to help the child do the following:

- Advance toward the annual goals
- Be involved in and progress in the general curriculum
- Participate in extracurricular and nonacademic activities
- Be educated with and participate with other children with disabilities and nondisabled children

Based on the preceding discussion, the IEP team will then write the child's IEP. This includes the services and supports the school will provide for the child. If the IEP team decides that a child needs a particular device or service (including an intervention, accommodation, or other program modification), the IEP team must write this information in the IEP. As an example, consider a child whose behavior interferes with learning. The IEP team would need to consider positive and effective ways to address that behavior. The team would discuss the positive behavioral interventions, strategies, and supports that the child needs in order to learn how to control or manage his or her behavior. If the team decides that the child needs a particular service (including an intervention, accommodation, or other program modification), they must include a statement to that effect in the child's IEP.

Special Factors to Consider

Depending on the needs of the child, the IEP team needs to consider what the law calls special factors. These include the following:

- If the child's behavior interferes with his or her learning or the learning of others, the IEP team will consider strategies and supports to address the child's behavior.

- If the child has limited proficiency in English, the IEP team will consider the child's language needs as these needs relate to his or her IEP.

- If the child is blind or visually impaired, the IEP team must provide for instruction in Braille or the use of Braille, unless it determines after an appropriate evaluation that the child does not need this instruction.

- If the child has communication needs, the IEP team must consider those needs.

- If the child is deaf or hard of hearing, the IEP team will consider his or her language and communication needs. This includes the child's opportunities to communicate directly with classmates and school staff in his or her usual method of communication (for example, sign language).

- The IEP team must always consider the child's need for assistive technology devices or services.

Will Parents Need an Interpreter in Order to Participate Fully?

If the parents have a limited proficiency in English or are deaf, they may need an interpreter in order to understand and be understood. In this case, the school must make reasonable efforts to arrange for an interpreter during meetings pertaining to the child's educational placement. For meetings regarding the development or review of the IEP, the school must take whatever steps are necessary to ensure that parents understand the meetings—including arranging for an interpreter. This provision should help to ensure that parents are not limited in their ability to participate in their child's education because of language or communication barriers.

Therefore, if parents need an interpreter for a meeting to discuss their child's evaluation, eligibility for special education, or IEP, they should let the school know ahead of time. Telling the school in advance allows the school to make arrangements for an interpreter so that parents can participate fully in the meeting.

Deciding Placement

In addition, the child's placement (where the IEP will be carried out) must be decided. The placement decision is made by a group of people, including the parents and others who know about the child, what the evaluation results mean, and what types of placements are appropriate. In some states, the IEP team serves as the group making the placement decision. In other states, this decision may be made by another group of people. In all cases, the parents have the right to be members of the group that decides the educational placement of the child.

Placement decisions must be made according to IDEA's least restrictive environment requirements, commonly known as LRE. These requirements state that, to the maximum extent appropriate, children with disabilities must be educated with children who do not have disabilities.

The law also clearly states that special classes, separate schools, or other removal of children with disabilities from the regular educational environment may occur only if the nature or severity of the child's disability is such that education in regular classes with the use of supplementary aids and services cannot be achieved satisfactorily.

What type of placements are there? Depending on the needs of the child, his or her IEP may be carried out in the regular class (with supplementary aids and services, as needed), in a special class (where every student in the class is receiving special education services for some or all of the day), in a special school, at home, in a hospital and institution, or in another setting. A school system may meet its obligation to ensure that the child has an appropriate placement available by doing the following:

- Providing an appropriate program for the child on its own

- Contracting with another agency to provide an appropriate program

- Utilizing some other mechanism or arrangement that is consistent with IDEA for providing or paying for an appropriate program for the child

The placement group will base its decision on the IEP and which placement option is appropriate for the child.

Can the child be educated in the regular classroom, with proper aids and supports? If the child cannot be educated in the regular classroom, even with appropriate aids and supports, then the placement group will talk about other placements for the child.

After the IEP Is Written

When the IEP has been written, parents must receive a copy at no cost to themselves. The IDEA also stresses that everyone who will be involved in implementing the IEP must have access to the document. This includes all of the following people:

- The child's regular education teacher(s)

- The child's special education teacher(s)

- The child's related service provider(s) (for example, a speech therapist)

- Any other service provider (such as a paraprofessional) who will be responsible for a part of the child's education

Each of these individuals needs to know what his or her specific responsibilities are for carrying out the child's IEP. This includes the specific accommodations, modifications, and supports that the child must receive, according to the IEP.

Parents' Permission

Before the school can provide a child with special education and related services for the first time, the child's parents must give their written permission.

Implementing the IEP

Once the IEP is written, it is time to carry it out—in other words, to provide the student with the special education and related services as listed in the IEP. This includes all supplementary aids and services and program modifications that the IEP team has identified as necessary for the student to advance appropriately toward his or her IEP goals, to be involved in and progress in the general curriculum, and to participate in other school activities. While it is beyond the scope of this chapter to discuss in detail the many issues involved in implementing a student's IEP, certain suggestions can be offered.

- Every individual involved in providing services to the student should know and understand his or her responsibilities for carrying out the IEP. This will help ensure that the student receives the services that have been planned, including the specific modifications and accommodations the IEP team has identified as necessary.

- Teamwork plays an important part in carrying out the IEP. Many professionals are likely to be involved in providing services and supports to the student. Sharing expertise and insights can help make everyone's job a lot easier and can certainly improve results for students with disabilities. Schools can encourage teamwork by giving teachers, support staff, and paraprofessionals time to plan or work together on such matters as adapting the general curriculum to address the student's unique needs. Teachers, support staff, and others providing services for children with disabilities may request training and staff development.

- Communication between home and school is also important. Parents can share information about what is happening at home and build upon what the child is learning at school. If the child is having difficulty at school, parents may be able to offer insight or help the school explore possible reasons as well as possible solutions.

- It is helpful to have someone in charge of coordinating and monitoring the services the student receives. In addition to special education, the student may be receiving any number of related services. Many people may be involved in delivering those services. Having a person in charge of overseeing that services are being delivered as planned can help ensure that the IEP is being carried out appropriately.

- The regular progress reports that the law requires will help parents and schools monitor the child's progress toward his or her annual goals. It is important to know if the child is not making the progress expected—or if he or she has progressed much faster than expected. Together, parents and school personnel can then address the child's needs as those needs become evident.

Reviewing and Revising the IEP

The IEP team must review the child's IEP at least once a year. One purpose of this review is to see whether the child is achieving his or her annual goals. The team must revise the child's individualized education program, if necessary, to address the following:

- The child's progress or lack of expected progress toward the annual goals and in the general curriculum

- Information gathered through any reevaluation of the child

- Information about the child that the parents share

- Information about the child that the school shares (for example, insights from the teacher based on his or her observation of the child or the child's class work)

- The child's anticipated needs

- Other matters

Although the IDEA requires this IEP review at least once a year, in fact the team may review and revise the IEP more often. Either the parents or the school can ask to hold an IEP meeting to revise the child's IEP. For example, the child may not be making progress toward his or her IEP goals, and his or her teacher or parents may become concerned. On the other hand, the child may have met most or all of the goals in the IEP, and new ones may need to be written. In either case, the IEP team would meet to revise the IEP.

Look at Those Factors Again!

When the IEP team is meeting to conduct a review of the child's IEP and, as necessary, to revise it, members must again consider all of the factors discussed previously. This includes the following:

- The child's strengths

- The parents' ideas for enhancing their child's education

- The results of recent evaluations or reevaluations

- How the child has done on state- and district-wide tests

The IEP team must also consider the "special factors," as listed earlier.

What If Parents Don't Agree with the IEP?

There are times when parents may not agree with the school's recommendations about their child's education. Under the law, parents have the right to challenge decisions about their child's eligibility, evaluation, placement, and the services that the school provides to the child. If parents disagree with the school's actions—or refusal to take action—in these matters, they have the right to pursue a number of options. Some of the options are as follows.

Try to Reach an Agreement. Parents can talk with school officials about their concerns and try to reach an agreement. Sometimes the agreement can be temporary. For example, the parents and school can agree to try a plan of instruction or a placement for a certain period of time and see how the student does.

Ask for Mediation. During mediation, the parents and school sit down with someone who is not involved in the disagreement and try to reach an agreement. The school may offer mediation, if it is available as an option for resolving disputes prior to due process.

Ask for Due Process. During a due process hearing, the parents and school personnel appear before an impartial hearing officer and present their sides of the story. The hearing officer decides how to solve the problem. (Note: Mediation must be available at least at the time a due process hearing is requested.)

File a Complaint with the State Education Agency. To file a complaint, generally parents write directly to the state education agency (SEA) and say what part of IDEA they believe the school has violated. The agency must resolve the complaint within sixty calendar days. An extension of that time limit is permitted only if exceptional circumstances exist with respect to the complaint.

Office of Special Education Programs Monitoring

The U.S. Department of Education's Office of Special Education Programs (OSEP) regularly monitors states to see that they are complying with IDEA. Every two years OSEP requires that states report progress toward meeting established performance goals that, at a minimum, address the performance of children on assessments, drop-out rates, and graduation rates. As part of its monitoring, the department reviews IEPs and interviews parents, students, and school staff to find out the following information:

- Whether, and how, the IEP team made the decisions reflected in the IEP

- Whether those decisions and the IEP content are based on the child's unique needs, as determined through evaluation and the IEP process

- Whether any state or local policies or practices have interfered with decisions of the IEP team about the child's educational needs and the services that the school would provide to meet those needs

- Whether the school has provided the services listed in the IEP

Updates in the Individualized Education Program with IDEA 2004

When Congress reauthorized IDEA 2004, they made significant changes to Individualized Education Programs (IEPs) in several areas, including:

- Content of IEP;
- IEP meeting attendance;
- IEPs by agreement;
- Review and revision of IEPs;
- Transition;
- Alternate means of participating in meetings.

This part of the chapter will provide you with an overview of changes in the law about IEPs and IEP meetings under IDEA 2004.

Content of IEPs

Some requirements for the contents of IEPs changed with IDEA 2004 while other requirements remained the same. Here is a summary of changes between IDEA 97 and IDEA 2004.

Present Levels of Performance. In IDEA 97, IEPs were required to include "a statement of the child's present levels of educational performance."

Under IDEA 2004, the child's IEP must include "a statement of the child's present levels of academic achievement and functional performance."

Present levels of academic achievement and functional performance are objective data from assessments.

Annual Goals. Under IDEA 97, IEPs were required to include a "statement of measurable annual goals, including benchmarks or short-term objectives." IDEA 2004 eliminated the requirements for "benchmarks and short-term objectives" in IEPs—except that the IEPs of children who take alternate assessments must include "a description of benchmarks or short-term objectives."

IDEA 2004 added new language about "academic and functional goals." IEPs must now include "a statement of measurable annual goals, including academic and functional goals."

Educational Progress. IDEA 97 required IEPs to include a statement about how the child's progress toward the annual goals would be measured, how the child's parents would be regularly informed about "their child's progress toward the annual goals," and whether the child's progress was sufficient.

Under IDEA 2004, the child's IEP must include "a description of how the child's progress toward meeting the annual goals . . . will be measured and when periodic reports on the progress the child is making toward meeting the annual goals (such as through the use of quarterly or other periodic reports, concurrent with the issuance of report cards) will be provided."

Special Education and Related Services. IDEA 2004 includes important new language about research-based instruction.

The child's IEP must include "a statement of the special education and related services and supplementary aids and services, based on peer-reviewed research to the extent practicable, to be provided to the child . . . and a statement of the program modifications or supports for school personnel."

Accommodations and Alternate Assessments. IDEA 2004 contains new language about "individual appropriate accommodations" on state and district testing and new requirements for alternate assessments.

The child's IEP must include: "a statement of any individual appropriate accommodations that are necessary to measure the academic achievement and functional performance of the child on State and districtwide assessments" and " if the IEP Team determines that the child shall take an alternate assessment on a particular State or districtwide assessment of student achievement, a statement of why (AA) the child cannot participate in the regular assessment; and (BB) the particular alternate assessment selected is appropriate for the child."

Transition. Congress made extensive changes to the legal requirements for transition. IDEA 97 required "a statement of transition services needs" (beginning at age fourteen) and "a statement of needed transition services for the child" (beginning at age sixteen). The statement of transition services needs at age fourteen was eliminated.

Under IDEA 2004, the first IEP after the child is sixteen (and updated annually) must include: "appropriate measurable postsecondary goals based upon age appropriate transition assessments related to training, education, employment, and, where appropriate, independent living skills . . . and the transition services (including courses of study) needed to assist the child in reaching these goals. (Section 1414(d)(1)(A))

When IEP Team Members May Be Excused from IEP Meetings

An IEP team member may be excused from attending an IEP meeting if the member's area of curriculum or service will not be discussed or modified and if the parent and school agree.

A member of the IEP team may also be excused if the member's area of curriculum or service will be discussed or modified, if the member submits a written report to the parent and the IEP team in advance, and if the parent provides written consent. (Section 1414(d)(1)(C))

Developing the IEP

In developing the IEP, the IEP team shall consider:

- The child's strengths;
- The parent's concerns for enhancing the child's education;
- The results of the initial evaluation or most recent evaluation;
- The child's academic, developmental, and functional needs. (Section 1414(d)(3)(A))

The IEP team shall consider special factors for children:

- Whose behavior impedes learning;
- Who have limited English proficiency;
- Who are blind or visually impaired;
- Who are deaf or hard of hearing. (Section 1414(d)(3)(B))

Educational Placements

The law about educational placements is in Section 1414(e). Parents are members of the team that decides the child's placement. The decision about placement cannot be made until after the IEP team, which includes the parent, reaches consensus about the child's needs, program, and goals.

Although the law is clear on this issue, the child's "label" often drives decisions about services and placement, leading school personnel to determine the child's placement before the IEP meeting.

These unilateral actions prevent parents from "meaningful participation" in educational decision making for their child. When Congress added this provision to the law in 1997, they sent a message to school officials that unilateral placement decisions are illegal.

Reviewing and Revising the IEP

The IEP must be reviewed at least once a year to determine if the child is achieving the annual goals. The IEP team must revise the IEP to address:

- Any lack of expected progress;
- Results of any reevaluation;
- Information provided by the parents;
- Anticipated needs. (Section 1414(d)(4)(A))

Revising IEP by Agreement, Without an IEP Meeting

IDEA 2004 changed the process by which IEPs can be amended or modified. If the parent and school agree to amend or modify the IEP, they may revise the IEP by agreement without convening an IEP meeting.

The team must create a written document that describes the changes or modifications in the IEP and note that, by agreement of the parties, an IEP meeting was not held. (Section 1414(d)(3)(D))

Alternative Ways to Participate in Meetings

School meetings do not have to be face-to-face. IEP and placement meetings, mediation meetings, and due process (IEP) resolution sessions may be convened by conference calls or videoconferences. (Section 1414(f))

Children Who Transfer: In-State and Out-of State

If a child transfers to a district in the same state, the receiving school must provide comparable services to those in the sending district's IEP until they develop and implement a new IEP. If a child transfers to another state, the receiving district must provide comparable services to those in the sending district's IEP until they complete an evaluation and create a new IEP. (Section 1414(d)(2)(C))

Multi-Year IEPs

Fifteen states may request approval to implement optional "comprehensive, multi-year IEPs" for periods of no longer than three years. IEP review dates must be based on "natural transition points."

Parents have the right to opt out of this program. The parent of a child served under a multi-year IEP can request a review of the IEP without waiting for the "natural transition point." (Section 1414(d)(5))

Chapter 69

Transition to Adulthood

Chapter Contents

635

Section 69.1

Issues to Consider as Your Child with Special Needs Transitions to Adulthood

All parents go through a rite of passage when their children turn eighteen, a time when, in most states, children are recognized as adults. These eighteen-year-old adults can now enter into contracts, live where they want, and make their own medical and educational decisions, including quitting school, if they so choose. In most cases, parents automatically lose their authority to make medical, legal, financial, and educational decisions for their children, even when those children may not be able to make informed decisions on their own behalf because they lack the capacity to do so.

This abrupt transition to legal adulthood causes concern for all parents. For parents of children with special needs, the transition can be particularly daunting because of the complex financial, medical, educational, vocational, residential, and social issues their children face, plus the need to take affirmative action to deal with them. All special needs families are different, but most must answer two critical questions when their special child is turning eighteen: Does my child have the capacity to make his or her own choices about his person and property? Will my child be self-supporting, or will he or she need government assistance to live independently?

Capacity Issues

The law presumes that children under eighteen are legally incompetent and that parents, as their natural guardians, can make all important medical and other decisions for them. The law presumes that all adults are legally competent to make their own choices whether or not they actually have the capacity to do so. For children who clearly lack the capacity to make their own choices, a guardianship may be necessary when they turn eighteen. For children with physical disabilities who have the mental capacity to make their own choices, a guardianship is not needed, though some help through the labyrinth of support services and programs may well be necessary. "Disabled" does not mean "incompetent."

For many children with special needs, the correct answer to the capacity question is not clear as they turn eighteen. For those who have the capacity to understand what they are doing, the preferred course might be to execute Powers of Attorney that name agents to make important property and healthcare decisions for them. Careful professional evaluations and parent/child discussions are needed before taking this path. This option, although preferred because it is private, swift, and relatively simple, does have one major pitfall: if a child has the capacity to name agents, he or she also has the capacity to fire them in cases of disagreement.

Government Benefit Programs for Adults with Disabilities

Parents have a duty to support their minor child, and, during childhood, their income and assets are often (but not always) "deemed" to be available to the child, thus preventing the child from qualifying for means-tested government benefit programs like Medicaid. When a child with a disability reaches the age of eighteen, the parents' income and resources are no longer deemed available to their child for Social Security purposes. When the deeming rules no longer apply, the adult child's own assets and income determine financial eligibility. Most means-tested programs have an asset limit of $2,000.

If the young adult has a disabling diagnosis that will prevent him or her from engaging in "substantial gainful employment" (that is, from working and earning a living), he or she is likely to be considered "disabled" and should be medically eligible for benefits. If the young adult is both medically and financially eligible, he or she should probably apply for Supplemental Security Income (SSI) at the local Social Security office. In most states, eligibility for SSI makes the adult child eligible for Medicaid assistance as well.

Special SSI rules apply to children living at home. It is often advisable to charge rent to help ensure maximum SSI benefits and to prevent the loss of Medicaid eligibility if SSI benefits fall below $1.00. In addition, proving the child's disability began before the age of twenty-two can have important benefits for non-means-tested benefits, like Social Security Disability, for which the child may be eligible when the qualified parent becomes disabled, retires, or dies.

Special education benefits are not means-tested, and deeming does not apply in certain waiver programs for children with disabilities. However, eligibility for special education programs ends at twenty-two, and many families are unprepared for the lack of any kind of support to fill the gap when both special education and waiver programs for children are no longer available and regular or sheltered work programs are not yet in place.

Conclusion

Each family and each child is unique. What is right for your friend's child or situation, as he or she transitions to adulthood, may not be what is right for your child. The child's ability and his or her support structure, medical needs, future residential plans, and educational challenges all need to be considered when deciding how to proceed once a special child reaches age eighteen. State-specific guardianship proceedings and government benefit programs that exist for adults with disabilities are complex and difficult to explain in a way that puts parents on notice about all possible problems in the planning process. Good advice from experienced legal practitioners who have been down this rocky path with others is essential.

Guardianship in a Nutshell

A guardianship is a technical legal proceeding in which a court names a guardian to make important decisions for a person found to be legally incompetent. State rules vary widely, and it is prudent to retain competent local counsel familiar with guardianship proceedings to ensure the best results for your child.

Section 69.2

Parent Tips for Transition Planning

Successful and meaningful transition services are the result of careful planning. This planning is driven by a young person's dreams, desires, and abilities. It builds a youth's participation in school, home, and community living.

Transition planning helps to prepare young people for their futures. It helps them to develop skills they need to go on to other education programs after high school. It builds skills to live, work, and play in the community. It helps to build independence. Youth learn important adult decision making roles when they participate in this school-based planning.

Must transition planning be part of the Individualized Education Program (IEP)?

Transition planning is required in the IEP for students by age sixteen. Many students will begin this planning at age fourteen or earlier so that they have the time to build skills they will need as adults. Parents should feel comfortable asking for transition planning to start earlier than age sixteen if they believe it is needed. Transition planning, goals, and services will be different for each student.

Transition services include instruction, community experiences, and building employment skills. They include post-school adult living objectives and, if needed, daily living skills training and functional vocational evaluations. All of these services must be provided in a manner that is sensitive to a student's cultural background and native language.

Transition services are based on a student's strengths as well as needs. They consider a young person's preferences and interests. Activities that are part of transition services must be results-oriented. This means that they are focused on building specific skills.

639

Must students be involved in transition planning?

Schools are required to invite students to participate in their IEP meetings whenever transition goals or services are considered. Transition services are a required component of IEPs for students age sixteen and older, and should be routinely discussed at IEP meetings. These services may become part of discussion and planning as early as the IEP team finds is needed for an individual student. (Some states require transition planning beginning at age fourteen.)

What if my child does not attend his or her IEP meeting?

If a youth is unable to participate in his or her IEP meeting or chooses not to attend, school personnel must take steps to ensure that the youth's preferences and interests are considered in developing the IEP.

The best transition plans are those that help youth achieve their dreams and aspirations. Youth should be included in all aspects of planning and goal setting, and encouraged to participate at IEP meetings. This participation helps keep team members focused on the young person's individual needs and desires. It also helps the youth to develop the skills for making decisions and becoming a self-advocate. Preparing a young person for his or her role in transition planning helps them to become knowledgeable members of the IEP team.

How can I be sure that the IEP meets my child's transition needs?

Transition services begin with age-appropriate transition assessments. They include student and parent interviews, interest and skill inventories, and other tools.

In order for an IEP to meet a student's transition needs, both parents and school personnel participate in the assessment. The school does this through assessments and observations. Parents do it through day-to-day knowledge and talks with their child about their goals and dreams.

Answering the following questions may help guide how parents and students prepare for and participate in an effective IEP meeting that is focused on transition planning:

- What does the young person want to do with his or her life? What are his or her dreams, aspirations, or goals? The youth's answers should be incorporated into all aspects of transition planning. If a young person is nonverbal or has difficulty communicating, parents can still use their knowledge of their child to be sure that transition planning and services reflect the youth's preferences and choices.

- What are the young person's needs, abilities, and skills? Parents should be familiar with how much assistance their child needs or does not need to accomplish tasks.

- What are the outcomes that the youth and parents want? Parents and their child should bring suggestions to the transition planning meeting. Suggestions might include the kind of services, actions, or planning they believe is needed to achieve desired goals in the transition section of the IEP.

- Will the young person attend the transition IEP conference? Parents can help by encouraging their son or daughter to attend. He or she will be invited. Together, parents and youth can prepare for the meeting. If the youth does not attend, parents may represent their desires and wishes.

- How do young people develop self-advocacy skills? Parents and school staff should encourage self-advocacy in young people. Staff should direct questions to the youth, even when it is the parents who may provide answers. It is important to encourage young people to have and state (by any means available to them) their own opinions. It is important for students to understand their disability and to ask for the accommodations they may need.

- What are the programs, services, accommodations, or modifications the young person wants or needs? Parents and their youth need to think about and be clear on what they want or need. IEP team discussions address these topics, but often parents and young people have had conversations at home that will be useful in planning.

- What kinds of accommodations will students need when they go on to higher education or employment? Parents and youth need to think what accommodations will be needed after high school and how the youth will obtain them.

- Who will be responsible for what part of the transition plan in the IEP? It is wise for parents and youth to know who is responsible for each transition goal. Each task should have a specific timeline that is included in the IEP.

- Should the educational and transition programs emphasize practical or academic goals? Does the young person need a combination of both? This will depend on the goals of each individual student.

- What are the community-based training opportunities the school provides? Parents and their child should decide how much to participate in those activities.

- If a student plans on going to college, is he or she taking the courses needed to meet college entrance requirements?

- When will the young person graduate? What kind of diploma option is the best choice?

- Are work experience classes appropriate to reach employment goals? Research suggests that youth have more successful employment outcomes after high school if they have had hands-on, work-based learning experiences as students.

- How could the educational and transition program be more integrated into the regular program?

- Who will attend the IEP meeting? Parents and the youth should become familiar with the roles and functions of team members. They should also know what community agencies might be present (vocational rehabilitation, etc.). Parents may request that a specific community agency be invited to the IEP meeting if the youth is or may be using services from that agency. Becoming familiar with adult service systems or agencies now can be helpful in making future decisions. At times parents may want a family member, friend, or advocate to go to planning meetings with them for support or to take notes.

Parents and youth will want to have a copy of the daily school schedule each quarter or semester. It is important to have information on all classes available so that their child can participate in selecting classes and the scheduling process.

A final tip: Parents will need to start thinking about their child's legal status before he or she turns eighteen. If a youth is not able to make informed decisions about major issues (medical treatment, living accommodations, financial arrangements, etc.), the family may need to learn more about guardianship or conservatorship.

The Individuals with Disabilities Education Act (IDEA) 2004 requires that students be notified at least one year in advance of the rights that will transfer to the student upon reaching the age of majority (becoming a legal adult in that state). These rights include being the responsible person for planning and agreeing or disagreeing with services in the IEP. It is important that parents understand what this means for them and their role in planning. The age of majority is eighteen in most states.

By learning as much as possible about the options available for transition planning, a parent can ensure that their young person's rights are protected while they are learning the skills needed to develop independence.

Section 69.3

Preparing for Employment

"Preparing for Employment: On the Home Front," by Sean Roy and Beth Casper. © 2006 National Center on Secondary Education and Transition (www.ncset.org). Reprinted with permission.

Young people looking for their first jobs may be overwhelmed by the process and seek help from others. Individualized Education Program (IEP) teams can help young people with disabilities develop a plan that includes employment goals. Schools can also help youth develop specific career skills by guiding students to courses needed to enter a particular field, helping students practice interviewing and asking for employment accommodations, or offering work-based learning opportunities.

Work-based learning during the school years leads to better postschool employment outcomes (Hughes, Moore, & Bailey, 1999). Volunteer experiences and unpaid internships, in addition to paid employment, can be steppingstones to future employment. Youth and their families need not rely solely on school programs to pursue such opportunities. They can do much on their own to launch the youth's career search. Recent studies demonstrate the effectiveness of using personal networks as a job search strategy (Timmons, Hamner, & Boes, 2003), and highlight the fact that families make key contributions to successful employment outcomes for individuals with disabilities (26th Institute on Rehabilitation Issues, 2000).

There are creative ways to combine community relationships, a young person's interests, and family or personal networks to help a young person effectively explore work-based learning outside of school settings. Parents may seek opportunities through co-workers, relatives, and neighbors. Moreover, parents often know their children better than professionals do and can help their sons and daughters explore their unique abilities, strengths, and interests—all of which may lead to an appropriate career path.

Many practical strategies for preparing a young adult with disabilities for employment are not difficult. These include such things as assigning chores at home, encouraging youth to volunteer in their community, or keeping an eye open for employment opportunities. Families can adopt these or other approaches within their own communities or share their ideas with the Individualized Education Program (IEP) team. The insights of family members can serve as the basis for strategies and services identified in a student's IEP transition goals. Youth can also learn to be self-advocates in seeking a good job.

Self-Determination: Youth Can Take Control

Ultimately, to be successful in the workplace, youth must develop skills that allow them to become as independent as possible. Skills such as self-knowledge, goal setting, decision making, problem solving, and self-advocacy are crucial for young people with disabilities. These skills are all considered aspects of self-determination. Research supports the idea that youth who leave high school with self-determination skills have a greater chance of achieving positive post-school outcomes than those who do not (Wehmeyer & Schwartz, 1997). Self-determined youth will also be able to exert greater control in the selection and use of adult services and supports in their postsecondary education and employment goals.

Parents can help their children develop self-determination skills by creating a supportive environment, which allows youth to take risks, test their abilities and limitations, develop their problem solving skills, and practice positive work habits and behaviors. Although parents can do much to launch their sons and daughters into the workforce, their children's future is their own. An understanding of oneself, including how one's health and disability will impact work, is key to becoming an effective self-advocate and essential to postsecondary education and employment success.

Learning about Skills, Needs, and Interests

Starting a journey toward successful employment may seem more difficult than the journey itself. Often young people blossom once they are given a chance to prove themselves, and a career path is more easily identified using the new knowledge of their skills and interests.

Learning about Themselves

Parents can help organize and clarify a young person's strengths, needs, and interests. Keep in mind a student's skills and preferences:

- **Perceptual skills:** Ability to judge where, how, and if things fit together.

- **Interpersonal skills:** Attitude, cooperation, teamwork, and communication skills. Look at how a student gets along with family, people in the community, peers, teachers, and employers.

- **Work aptitudes:** Ability to remember and follow instructions and procedures; ability to plan, organize, and improve with practice.

- **Work behaviors:** Ability to concentrate and stay on a task and ability to remain motivated.

- **Interests:** Personal goals and interests, hobbies, leisure-time activities, academics, and favorite and least-favorite subjects.

- **Cognitive skills:** Reading and math skills, concept formation, thinking style, and problem solving abilities.

- **Motor skills:** Using one's hands, eye/hand coordination, fine motor skills, and mobility (PACER, 2003).

It is also important to talk with a young person about his or her dreams. A young person should answer questions such as: What do I do well? What is hard for me? What do I like to do?

Résumé Basics: Work Experience and References

Putting Together a Résumé

Paid work experience is not the only thing that makes a job applicant's résumé appealing to an employer. Employers appreciate a young person who shows the motivation to do a good job. Youth who may be too young or not ready for a paid job can create a résumé and gain valuable experience by doing jobs around the house or neighborhood or by volunteering even for a day. Including a list of informational interviews conducted by youth in a résumé can also help document an individual's initiative as well as vocational education experiences. Parents can help youth identify the types of experiences that may be included in the youth's résumé.

Job Satisfaction and Long-Term Goals

Matching a person's strengths and interests to a job is important to ensuring long-term success and job satisfaction (Dawis, 1987; Jagger, Neukrug, & McAuliffe, 1992; Mank, 2003). Youth should explore vocations that interest them. Matching youth with jobs that suit their interests and strengths is one way to promote success in the workplace.

Combining Formal and Natural Supports

Many youth with significant disabilities use job coaches, assistive technology, and/or workplace accommodations when entering employment. These formal supports can be provided or funded by service providers from special education, county social services, waiver programs, vocational rehabilitation, or developmental disabilities systems. Formal supports can be short term or extend long into the course of an individual's employment. Parents and youth should also be aware of natural supports that may be available in the workplace. Natural supports include training, job sharing, mentoring, and flexible scheduling. An example of a natural support is when a more experienced employee helps a co-worker solve a problem. Natural supports are provided directly by the employer (not an outside agency) and may be generally available to employees who are not disabled. Natural supports are appealing to employers because they are generally low cost. They are also appealing to people with disabilities and their families because they promote normal interaction and relationships with co-workers.

Involving co-workers in support of employment is important even when an individual requires formal supports from an outside agency. Employees with disabilities who receive natural supports from co-workers are more likely to have more typical work roles, higher wages, and positive relationships with co-workers (Mank, 2003). It may require some effort to find the right situation for a person who needs extra support on the job, but once in place, a system of natural supports can increase the feelings of accomplishment and independence on the job for a person with a disability.

Using Your Personal Network

Most people have a circle of contacts within a community. Relatives, friends, co-workers, and people who own or work at the grocery stores, restaurants, or other businesses regularly patronized by a family can have potential job leads. Think outside of your close friends and acquaintances. The personal contacts of IEP team members may also lead to independent job opportunities. The vast majority of jobs are gained not by responding to an advertisement in the newspaper, but by using contacts. Using this method can also help identify safe and familiar worksite locations. Don't despair if this method does not yield results right away. Sometimes notifying friends and acquaintances will prompt them to think of you when a job opportunity arises in the future.

Unpaid Work Experience Can Lead to Paid Jobs

Building Confidence Through Volunteering

Learning on the job is the best way to develop job skills. However, young people with disabilities may need help obtaining real work experience. School guidance counselors, religious leaders, or friends may know of job shadowing, volunteer, or internship opportunities for youth. When young people feel too insecure to find volunteer work on their own, parents or other family members can help them overcome their initial anxiety by offering to volunteer together. Through experience, youth will see they have the ability to work on their own.

Summary

Youth with disabilities who participate in quality work-based learning activities have more successful post-school outcomes, including employment and further education. Real-life work experiences help a young person develop important "soft skills" such as teamwork and time management, make career decisions, network with potential employers, and develop job skills relevant to future employment. They also help youth assess the impact of their disability in an employment setting and learn what job accommodations they need in the workplace. Using their combined resources, youth, families, and IEP teams can ensure that work-based learning opportunities are a good match with a student's individual interests, strengths, and needs. These experiences not only help youth to build their résumés, but provide the foundation for a life of increased earning and self determination.

References

Dawis, R. (1987). A theory of work adjustment. In B. Bolton (Ed.), *Handbook on the measurement and evaluation in rehabilitation* (2nd ed.) (pp. 207–217). Baltimore: Paul H. Brookes.

Hughes, K. L., Moore, D. T., & Bailey, T. R. (1999). Work-based learning and academic skills. Retrieved February 23, 2006, from http://www.tc.edu/iee/PAPERS/workpap15.pdf

Jagger, L., Neukrug, E., & McAuliffe, G. (1992). Congruence between personality traits and chosen occupation as a predictor of job satisfaction for people with disabilities. *Rehabilitation Counseling Bulletin*, 36(1), 53–60.

Mank, D. (2003). A synthesis of a research series on typicalness, coworker supports, and quality outcomes in supported employment. Bloomington, IN: Indiana Institute on Disability and Community, Indiana University. Retrieved February 23, 2006, from http://www.indiana.edu/~soedean/mank.ppt

Timmons, J. C., Hamner, D., & Boes, J. (2003). Four strategies to find a good job: Advice from job seekers with disabilities. *Tools for Inclusion*, 11(2), 1–5.

Twenty-Sixth Institute on Rehabilitation Issues. (2000). *The family as a critical partner in the achievement of a successful employment outcome*. Hot Springs, AR: University of Arkansas.

Wehmeyer, M., & Schwartz, M. (1997). Self-determination and positive adult outcomes: A follow-up study of youth with mental retardation or learning disabilities. *Exceptional Children*, 63(2), 245–55.

Section 69.4

Community Services Can Aid in Independence

"Community Services: Frequently Asked Questions,"
© 2007 National Center on Secondary Education and Transition
(www.ncset.org). Reprinted with permission.

How can young adults with disabilities ensure that they will have stable and adequate income?

As with anyone else, young adults with disabilities must have money in order to live successfully and independently. While all young adults need to have opportunities for employment, many times, young adults with disabilities are not able to earn enough money to enjoy a satisfactory quality of life. This can happen for a variety of reasons, including lack of extensive direct experience, lack of opportunity, misconceptions about ability, inadequate support, and lack of knowledge about services and supports that can make this a reality.

However, the federal government, through the Social Security Administration, has several programs that can provide young adults with disabilities monetary support to help meet living expenses. While in the past, remaining eligible for such programs essentially made it impossible for persons with disabilities to also work and earn an income, there are now several options to use Social Security payments as a way to supplement a young person's paychecks. Young adults with disabilities may also be eligible for other forms of economic assistance available through federal, state, and local government to assist them with subsidized housing programs, food stamps, and vouchers.

The bottom line is that preparing for fiscal independence must happen during the transition planning process. Although not every young adult will need the programs described above or qualify for these programs, it is still essential to develop goals and steps to achieve those goals on the Individualized Education Program (IEP) in the area of financial management, fiscal responsibility, and independent living.

How can young adults with disabilities find support and assistance to live independently in the community?

A normal life passage for most young adults is to leave their family home and live independently. Although they may receive support from time to time, their ultimate goal is to have a place of their own and to manage their lives as independent adults. This process can become more complicated when the young adult has a disability. For some young adults, the disability can make it difficult to care for their personal needs or manage a household without some support. Support could include living with friends or obtaining help through a supervised living arrangement, such as a group home.

This does not change the fact that most young adults with disabilities express the same desires as their nondisabled peers—to have their own place and to live as independently as possible. This does not mean it has to be accomplished without support. The goal is to make sure it is addressed through the transition planning process, and to connect a young adult with all of the necessary resources, services, and supports before they are ready to make this move.

There are many resources and supports that can be invaluable in this area. Centers for Independent Living (CILs) are an excellent place to start. Most cities around the United States have one or more CILs that can provide assistance with locating affordable and accessible housing. CILs can also provide training to help youth with disabilities prepare for living independently. This can include things like cooking, cleaning, safety, budgeting, understanding rental contracts, how to interview landlords, and much more.

Another source of support might include programs offered through Social Security, such as Supplemental Security Income, or SSI. SSI provides eligible recipients with a monthly check to support their daily living needs, such as rent, a car or transportation costs, food, and other necessities.

A third program that can support independent living is Medical Assistance, which may provide funding to pay for durable medical equipment or for personal assistants that provide help with personal care or household management tasks in the individual's home.

What helps young adults to build friendships and relationships in which they feel valued?

Young adults with disabilities really want the same things as any other young adult—a social or peer group to be a part of, a place where they feel they belong and are valued, friends to have fun with, and social activities to enjoy. High school provides many opportunities to build friendships and to get involved in activities that provide a forum for friendships to be built. However, it is a common scenario to find that few young adults with disabilities are involved in school clubs and organizations such as student council, the school newspaper, the homecoming committee, and sports. When young adults with disabilities are developing their transition plan, involvement in these types of activities is essential to include as goals on their plan. Academics and employment experience are only a part of what contributes to an individual's quality of life.

As young adults graduate or leave school, it may become difficult for them to maintain existing relationships or to build new friendships. Connecting young adults with disabilities to community organizations and opportunities that match their interests before they leave high school is one way to ensure that relationships continue to be built and to grow. There are a wide variety of community organizations youth can become involved with; everything from those focused on health and fitness such as the YMCA/YWCA, to political parties, volunteer opportunities, and hobby groups.

Young adults with disabilities also need frequent opportunities to engage in other typical activities for their age, such as attending parties or going shopping. While many young adults with disabilities only need occasional encouragement and support in maintaining their social networks, other young adults may need ongoing and direct assistance to maintain and build upon social contacts. Such assistance can be afforded by a paid support person, or by supportive family members and friends who make a conscious effort to include the young adult with the disability in activities, and in assisting them with contacting others.

What considerations are important in ensuring that young adults with disabilities have access to appropriate healthcare?

Young adults with disabilities are exposed to all the health and safety perils of anyone in our society, as well as additional ones that may be specific to their disabilities. Youth with disabilities need access to general practitioners and healthcare coordinators who will take the time to learn about their disabilities and how those disabilities fit into the context of their overall physical and emotional health.

Young adults with disabilities also occasionally need access to specialized healthcare provided by specialized healthcare professionals.

Finally, these young adults need healthcare insurance that is capable of meeting any needs that may arise. This may be available through an employer-sponsored health plan or Medicaid, a federally sponsored health insurance program, or some combination of the two.

What transportation options are typically available for young adults with disabilities?

Transportation is a critical issue for young adults with disabilities if they are to be employed and maintain active lives in their communities. It is always important to consider whether the young adult is interested and able to drive a car or van. Centers for Independent Living or vocational rehabilitation agencies should be aware of local programs that assess an individual's ability to drive, recommend adapted equipment, and provide driving instruction, especially for persons with disabilities.

According to the Americans with Disabilities Act, all modes of public transportation, such as buses, trains, and subways, must now be accessible to people with disabilities. Youth and young adults with disabilities may benefit from training and an opportunity to practice safely using such systems. Young adults who have disabilities that would cause them to be especially vulnerable in using public transportation may be eligible for other transportation options supported through the local transit authority or government social service agency.

Chapter 70

Estate Planning for Families of Children with Special Needs

Chapter Contents

653

Section 70.1

Securing Your Family's Financial Future

"Securing Your Family's Financial Future," by Joanne M. Gruszkos, December 2008, reprinted with permission from www.eparent.com. © 2008 EP Global Communications. All rights reserved.

You've now accepted the reality of the diagnosis. You've navigated a bewildering maze of medical specialists and insurers. You've learned a new language of tests, assessments, and therapies. You've taken on grinding battles with school districts. And, finally, you have created an environment in which your child with a disability or other special need can live productively and happily.

Now, ask yourself this one important question: If something happened to you, your spouse, and/or other caregiver whom you depend on tomorrow, what would happen to your child and the world you've created for him or her?

Who would take care of your child? Do those people know that you're expecting them to take over? Would they know what to do? Would they be up to the task? Would they understand your child's special personality? Would they be aware of your hopes, dreams, and plans for your child? Would they have the financial means to support your child in the manner that you would want? Would they be equipped to balance the needs of your other children as well?

If those questions feel overwhelming, it's OK, because they are. That's why many dedicated and caring parents understandably postpone, do very little or nothing at all in the area of creating a life care plan or preparing financially for the future. The challenges of the present are often so monumental as to discourage any thought of the future. Yet addressing these questions is a critical step in care giving, not only for your child with special needs but for other family members and yourself as well.

Take comfort. With knowledgeable help, you can create a life care plan to put your family on sound financial footing today and prepare your family for a secure future tomorrow.

You're not alone in facing this need. Nearly 7 percent of the population in this country has at least one physical, mental or emotional disability, according to the U.S. Census.[1] Many of these Americans require lifelong support and, furthermore, are outliving their parents thanks to improved care and advances in medical technology. As a result, parents and caregivers are increasingly faced with the prospect of providing support—even after they have died—to their loved ones with a disability.

Getting started is not as hard as you might think. Here are a few first steps to help you get going.

Get help: This isn't a "do-it-yourself" job. Preparing a life care plan for the financial future and security of your family and child requires specialized expertise and working with a financial professional who specializes in special needs is a wise move. In securing a financial services professional, make sure the person you work with is qualified, experienced, and involved in the area of special needs.

Build a team: It is important that the family seek out advisors who embrace the team planning approach to ensure proper coordination of all efforts. Besides a financial professional, you will need an attorney (preferably one who is experienced in special needs planning), a certified public accountant (CPA), and others, such as social workers and medical professionals, all working together. A financial professional should be able to refer you to qualified professionals and will welcome working closely with them on your behalf. If the financial professional you're considering resists working closely with these other professionals, you might consider looking for a new financial professional.

Write a letter of intent: Although not a legal document, a letter of intent provides you with an opportunity to put in writing important information such as your child's routines, important contact information, medical issues, your preference for how the child should be schooled, your desire for raising your child within the traditions of a specific religion, and other such matters. Preparing this letter can be a clarifying and edifying process that causes parents to crystallize their intentions and verbalize their sentiments, leaving little to interpretation for the future caregiver. The letter is a "living" document that you will update frequently to reflect changing information or preferences. Financial professionals who specialize in special needs usually have sample letters of intent they can provide to get you started.

Pick a successor caregiver: Many families simply assume a child's aunt or uncle or sibling will step in as a primary caregiver should anything happen to the parents, but assuming so without verifying is a dangerous proposition. Sometimes family members do not feel emotionally or psychologically equipped for the task. Sometimes they might be prepared for one aspect of the job (e.g., providing daily care) but not for other aspects of the job (e.g., managing finances). In fact, families sometimes split duties among two or more people. So, for example, one trusted person could become the primary caregiver to your child while a second trusted person could manage money. Whichever decision you make, decide carefully. Be certain that the person or people you choose can do the very difficult work before them.

Consider a special needs trust: Many parents may be unaware that if their child were to inherit as little as $2,000 in assets they could be disqualified from many governmental programs, such as Medicaid or Supplemental Security income. A special needs trust, if properly structured, is a mechanism that provides for the child without jeopardizing his or her benefits. For example, a trust can be funded by a donor—usually a parent, sibling, or guardian—and the trustee can manage assets in the best interest of the trust's beneficiary, in this case the child. Because the assets are owned by the trust, the child still remains eligible for government programs. A trust can fund a wide range of supplemental needs, such as transportation, equipment, education, and rehabilitation, to name a few. There are many ways to fund a trust account; one common one is life insurance.

Write—or rewrite—your wills: Assuming you create a special needs trust, write or rewrite your wills to ensure that they coordinate with the trust and your other planning documents. The wills will dictate how you want your estate to be distributed, and by coordinating with the trust, you will avoid unintentionally harming your child's eligibility for governmental programs.

One final piece of advice: Don't forget yourself or others in your family. As parents who spend every waking hour—and many of the hours you're supposed to be sleeping, too—worrying about or caring for a child with a disability, it often is possible to overlook your own financial needs, such as retirement, and/or those of your other children. All of these needs are related and can impact each other. For example, if you are under-prepared for retirement and, as a result, begin pulling retirement income out of the resources you intend to be part of your estate, you will undermine your best-laid plans.

A truly effective life care plan will address not only the needs of your child with disabilities, but also the needs of the whole family, securing your and their financial futures.

Notes

1. U.S. Census Bureau, 2004 American Community Survey.

Section 70.2

Supplemental Needs Trusts: Some Frequently Asked Questions

Why Use a Supplemental Needs Trust?

To Preserve Governmental Benefits and Protect Assets . . .

A supplemental needs trust (sometimes called a special needs trust) is a specialized legal document designed to benefit an individual who has a disability. A supplemental needs trust is most often a "stand alone" document, but it can form part of a last will and testament. Supplemental needs trusts have been in use for many years, and were given an "official" legal status by the United States Congress in 1993.

A supplemental needs trust enables a person under a physical or mental disability, or an individual with a chronic or acquired illness, to have, held in trust for his or her benefit, an unlimited amount of assets. In a properly drafted supplemental needs trust, those assets are not considered countable assets for purposes of qualification for certain governmental benefits.

Such benefits may include Supplemental Security Income (SSI), Medicaid, vocational rehabilitation, subsidized housing, and other benefits based upon need. For purposes of a supplemental needs trust, an individual is considered impoverished if his or her personal assets are less than $2,000.00.

A supplemental needs trust provides for supplemental and extra care over and above that which the government provides.

Supplemental needs trusts had been used for years based upon case law. In 1993, Congress created an exception under the amendments to the Omnibus Budget and Reconciliation Act (OBRA-93) which specifically authorized the use of supplemental needs trusts for the benefit of individuals who are under the age of sixty-five years and disabled according to Social Security standards. The Social Security Operations Manual authorizes the use of supplemental needs trusts to hold noncountable assets.

Each supplemental needs trust is its own "entity" with its own federal identification number (employer identification number) issued by the Internal Revenue Service. The trust is not registered under either the grantor's or the beneficiary's Social Security numbers.

According to Congress a supplemental needs trust must be irrevocable. A properly drafted trust will include provisions for trust termination or dissolution under certain circumstances, and will include explicit directions for amendment when necessary.

My Family Is Wealthy and We're Not Too Concerned about Governmental Benefits. Why Bother Creating a Supplemental Needs Trust?

To Protect Your Disabled Family Member . . .

Other types of spendthrift or family trusts aren't appropriate for special needs persons because they don't address the specific needs of the disabled beneficiary or his future lifestyle. Even in situations where a family may have significant resources to help a disabled family member a supplemental needs trust should be established to address these issues.

Monies placed in the trust remain noncountable assets and allow the beneficiary to qualify for available benefits and programs. Why sacrifice services that might be available to your relative now and in the future?

Just as importantly, Trust funds are not subject to creditors or seizure. Therefore, if the disabled beneficiary should ever be sued in a personal injury or other type of lawsuit, the beneficiary is not a "deep pocket" because moneys placed in the trust are not subject to a judgment.

If Having Money Causes Problems for My Disabled Daughter, Why Can't I Just Leave That Money to Her Brother So That He Can Look After Her?

Leaving Money to Others Can Create Serious Problems . . .

"Disinheritance" was commonly used before the use of supplemental needs trusts was officially recognized by Congress.

Disinheritance as a means of providing for a disabled or ill person puts the assets at risk. A nondisabled sibling holding assets for the benefit of a disabled sibling could be subject to such liabilities such as judgments from automobile accidents, a bankruptcy, or a divorce.

Asset transfers, particularly of the beneficiary's own funds, other than to supplemental needs trusts are usually considered "transfers for purposes of benefit qualification," and are subject to a thirty-six- to sixty-month "look back" period, which in effect means that the disabled beneficiary might not be eligible to receive benefits for up to five years after the date of transfer. Transfers to supplemental needs trusts are exempt from this "look back" and do not cause a disqualification.

In such circumstances, the assets meant to benefit the disabled or chronically ill person could go to pay the judgment creditors or the estranged spouse of the nondisabled sibling. Using a supplemental needs trust guarantees that the funds will be held only for the benefit of the person under the disability or chronic illness, and not for any other purpose whatsoever.

What Must a Supplemental Needs Trust Say?

Supplemental Needs Trusts Need Special Language . . .

At a bare minimum, the trust should state that it is intended to provide "supplemental and extra care" over and above that which the government provides.

The trust must state that it is not intended to be a basic support trust. It should not contain an estate tax provision called a "Crummey clause."

A properly drafted supplemental needs trust should reference the Social Security Operations Manual and the relevant portions from within the manual that authorize the creation of the trust. It must contain the required language regarding payback to Medicaid.

The trust should also have language explaining the exception to the Omnibus Budget and Reconciliation Act (OBRA-93) provisions which authorize the creation of the trust, and a copy of the relevant provisions from the United States Code (USC).

When Should I Create a Supplemental Needs Trust?

A Supplemental Needs Trust Is a Valuable Estate Planning and Investment Tool . . .

A supplemental needs trust can be established at any time before the beneficiary's sixty-fifth birthday. It is very common to create a supplemental needs trust early in a child's life as a long-term means for holding assets to benefit the disabled family member. This is particularly true of parents who wish to leave funds for a child's benefit after the parents' death. The supplemental needs trust is the estate-planning tool of choice for those parents. As a part of estate planning, the costs of the creation of the trust are tax deductible.

Additionally, the disabled or chronically ill individual may at some time during his or her lifetime come into funds from third-party sources, such as a personal injury settlement or a bequest from relatives or friends, Social Security back payments, insurance proceeds, or the like.

Is There an Obligation to Repay Medicaid, or Other State and Federal Funding Sources?

There May Be Repayment Obligations in Some Situations . . .

A properly drafted trust will address the issue concerning paybacks to Medicaid or other such sources. The United States Congress mandates that repayment language must be included in all supplemental needs trusts, whether repayment is required or not.

The amendments to the Omnibus Budget and Reconciliation Act of 1993 (OBRA-93) require that a payback be made to Medicaid, but only under certain specific circumstances.

A supplemental needs trust that is funded by parents or other third-party sources will not be required to pay back Medicaid.

A trust which is funded by a personal injury settlement that is properly court-ordered into the trust will not be required to pay back Medicaid.

The only assets within the trust that are subject to the repayment obligation are those assets which originally belonged to the disabled individual him- or herself that are transferred into the trust.

Examples of assets which would belong to the disabled individual in the first place could be such assets as earnings from a job, savings, certain Social Security back payments, personal injury recoveries which are not court-ordered into the trust, and the like.

The disabled individual's estate then might be liable for an amount equal to the Medicaid used during the lifetime of the disabled or chronically ill individual.

It is not uncommon for a trustee or a disabled individual to ask a court to direct certain assets into the trust. In that event, those assets may not be subject to the repayment provision of OBRA-93.

Can Any Lawyer Create a Supplemental Needs Trust?

Just as Most Podiatrists Aren't Neurosurgeons . . .

A family or person that wishes to benefit an individual under a disability or chronic illness will be well advised to utilize the services of an attorney that specializes in special needs issues.

A supplemental needs trust can very easily be "invaded" by governmental benefit sources, and the trust can be easily invalidated if the proper language is not utilized throughout the trust.

A poorly written trust can cause a loss of benefits, a loss of savings, or other financial and legal hardships for the beneficiary or the trustee, some quite severe, including civil litigation or criminal prosecution in some extraordinary circumstances.

Using a law firm that specializes in special needs issues assures you that the attorney is familiar with the benefits systems, the proper creation of the trust, and ultimately the defense of the trust in the event that it should be challenged by a court, the Social Security Administration, Medicaid, or the like.

My Sister Is Disabled. Can I Set Up a Trust for Her?

Yes, But . . .

The United States Code section that authorizes supplemental needs trusts states that "a parent, grandparent, or guardian" is authorized to establish a supplemental needs trust. Siblings, caregivers, or friends are not mentioned at all. However, the law does not forbid siblings and others from setting up supplemental needs trusts. The law does not specify whether the "guardian" mentioned must be court-appointed or can be a "guardian-in-fact," such as a concerned sibling. And it does permit an interested third party (such as a sibling) to establish the trust under certain circumstances. A well-written supplemental needs trust established by someone other than a parent, grandparent, or legal guardian should include a citation to this law for the sake of clarity.

In addition, the courts in most states have recognized the right of a sibling, friend, or caregiver to establish a trust, and case law supports the idea.

Benefits providers and agencies often create "red herring" difficulties around this issue. Be cautious, and make sure you work with a lawyer familiar with this problem and that the trust is properly drafted.

I Have Twins with Down Syndrome. Can I Use One Trust for Both of Them?

Just as Your Children Are Exceptional So Are Their Trusts . . .

Each disabled individual must have his or her own trust document. The law requires that each supplemental needs trust contain specific examples of what constitutes supplemental care for the beneficiary. No one's needs, not even twins, are absolutely identical. This is particularly the case as people get older and their abilities change.

I'm Very Confused. I Heard a Lawyer Say Something about Having Two Separate Trusts.

It Really Isn't Necessary . . .

This confusion stems from the Social Security regulations, which make a distinction between "first party" (or self-funded) supplemental needs trusts that contain the beneficiary's own money and "third party" funded trusts that contain money from other sources. "First party" money is usually subject to the Medicaid repayment requirements. Therefore, many lawyers insist on creating separate trusts. This costs more and is often confusing to the trustee.

A well-drafted supplemental needs trust should be able to hold money from both "first party" and "third party" sources. Funds from the different sources can be held and managed in the trust in separate accounts.

I Heard That a Pooled Trust Does Not Have to Repay Medicaid. Why Bother Using a Supplemental Needs Trust?

Pooled Trusts Aren't For Everybody . . .

"Pooled" or cooperative master trusts are a special form of supplemental needs trust which can be established by not-for-profit organizations or groups on behalf of their membership (for example, a group home may create one for its residents). While it is true that cooperative master trusts are exempt from the Medicaid repayment rules, the money that is placed in a cooperative master trust is used generally to address the needs of all the members of the group, not just the specific needs of your disabled family member.

Once you place your money in the pool it usually cannot be withdrawn or returned to you. You cannot direct where the trust avails will go if your family member leaves the group for any reason. Your money remains in the pool to assist future members.

You do not have control over how the money is spent. As a result, your family member may not get all the services he or she needs or might want. Management of pooled trusts is often given over to accountants, professional trustees, financial planners, or financial institutions. Due to their relative rarity, cooperative master trusts are frequently mismanaged and many have failed, leaving the group members without funds.

Medicaid has implemented recent rule changes in some jurisdictions that specifically state that funds placed in cooperative master trusts *are* subject to the thirty-six- to-sixty-month asset transfer "look back" period under certain specific circumstances; hence, transferring funds to a cooperative master trust *may* disqualify a beneficiary from benefits for up to five years.

Cooperative master trusts can work well if you find one that is properly written and supervised and if you are willing to relinquish control of your assets to others. If this is an option that appeals to you, you are well advised to seek out a group that you know well and trust, can serve your special needs, and which has an established track record of successful trust management.

I'm My Son's Trustee. That Makes Me His Guardian, Right?

Not Right . . .

Parents often assume that because they are their children's caregivers that they are also their lifetime guardians. This is not correct.

Every person over the age of eighteen is presumed to have the legal rights of an adult, no matter what their abilities.

In order to be someone's guardian a parent or sibling must go to court and petition to become responsible for that person. They must demonstrate to the court that the disabled person is unable to act responsibly on their own behalf.

Merely setting up a trust, becoming a trustee, becoming a power of attorney, or being someone's representative payee for Social Security purposes does not make you a guardian even if you may have effective control of the disabled person's finances and provide for all their needs.

There are several types of guardianship. If you feel one is necessary consult an attorney familiar with guardianship law to determine which is proper for your circumstances.

Part Seven

Additional Help
and Information

Chapter 71

Glossary of Terms Related to Human Genetics

additive genetic effects: When the combined effects of alleles at different loci are equal to the sum of their individual effects.

allele: Alternative form of a genetic locus; a single allele for each locus is inherited from each parent (e.g., at a locus for eye color the allele might result in blue or brown eyes).

amino acid: Any of a class of 20 molecules that are combined to form proteins in living things. The sequence of amino acids in a protein and hence protein function are determined by the genetic code.

amplification: An increase in the number of copies of a specific deoxyribonucleic acid (DNA) fragment; can be in vivo or in vitro.

anticipation: Each generation of offspring has increased severity of a genetic disorder; e.g., a grandchild may have earlier onset and more severe symptoms than the parent, who had earlier onset than the grandparent.

apoptosis: Programmed cell death, the body's normal method of disposing of damaged, unwanted, or unneeded cells.

Excerpted from "Genome Glossary," Human Genome Project Information, April 26, 2007.

autosomal dominant: A gene on one of the non-sex chromosomes that is always expressed, even if only one copy is present. The chance of passing the gene to offspring is 50 percent for each pregnancy.

autosome: A chromosome not involved in sex determination. The diploid human genome consists of a total of forty-six chromosomes: twenty-two pairs of autosomes, and one pair of sex chromosomes (the X and Y chromosomes).

base: One of the molecules that form DNA and ribonucleic acid (RNA) molecules.

base sequence: The order of nucleotide bases in a DNA molecule; determines structure of proteins encoded by that DNA.

birth defect: Any harmful trait, physical or biochemical, present at birth, whether a result of a genetic mutation or some other nongenetic factor.

cancer: Diseases in which abnormal cells divide and grow unchecked. Cancer can spread from its original site to other parts of the body and can be fatal.

candidate gene: A gene located in a chromosome region suspected of being involved in a disease.

carrier: An individual who possesses an unexpressed, recessive trait.

cell: The basic unit of any living organism that carries on the biochemical processes of life.

chromosomal deletion: The loss of part of a chromosome's DNA.

chromosomal inversion: Chromosome segments that have been turned 180 degrees. The gene sequence for the segment is reversed with respect to the rest of the chromosome.

chromosome: The self-replicating genetic structure of cells containing the cellular DNA that bears in its nucleotide sequence the linear array of genes.

chromosome region p: A designation for the short arm of a chromosome.

chromosome region q: A designation for the long arm of a chromosome.

codominance: Situation in which two different alleles for a genetic trait are both expressed.

complex trait: Trait that has a genetic component that does not follow strict Mendelian inheritance. May involve the interaction of two or more genes or gene-environment interactions.

congenital: Any trait present at birth, whether the result of a genetic or nongenetic factor.

crossing over: The breaking during meiosis of one maternal and one paternal chromosome, the exchange of corresponding sections of DNA, and the rejoining of the chromosomes. This process can result in an exchange of alleles between chromosomes.

deletion: A loss of part of the DNA from a chromosome; can lead to a disease or abnormality.

diploid: A full set of genetic material consisting of paired chromosomes, one from each parental set. Most animal cells except the gametes have a diploid set of chromosomes. The diploid human genome has forty-six chromosomes.

disease-associated genes: Alleles carrying particular DNA sequences associated with the presence of disease.

DNA (deoxyribonucleic acid): The molecule that encodes genetic information. DNA is a double-stranded molecule held together by weak bonds between base pairs of nucleotides. The four nucleotides in DNA contain the bases adenine (A), guanine (G), cytosine (C), and thymine (T). In nature, base pairs form only between A and T and between G and C; thus the base sequence of each single strand can be deduced from that of its partner.

DNA sequence: The relative order of base pairs, whether in a DNA fragment, gene, chromosome, or an entire genome.

dominant: An allele that is almost always expressed, even if only one copy is present.

embryonic stem cells: An embryonic cell that can replicate indefinitely, transform into other types of cells, and serve as a continuous source of new cells.

exogenous DNA: DNA originating outside an organism that has been introduced into the organism.

669

forensics: The use of DNA for identification. Some examples of DNA use are to establish paternity in child support cases, establish the presence of a suspect at a crime scene, and identify accident victims.

fraternal twin: Siblings born at the same time as the result of fertilization of two ova by two sperm. They share the same genetic relationship to each other as any other siblings.

full gene sequence: The complete order of bases in a gene. This order determines which protein a gene will produce.

gamete: Mature male or female reproductive cell (sperm or ovum) with a haploid set of chromosomes (twenty-three for humans).

gene: The fundamental physical and functional unit of heredity. A gene is an ordered sequence of nucleotides located in a particular position on a particular chromosome that encodes a specific functional product (i.e., a protein or RNA molecule).

gene amplification: Repeated copying of a piece of DNA; a characteristic of tumor cells.

gene expression: The process by which a gene's coded information is converted into the structures present and operating in the cell.

gene family: Group of closely related genes that make similar products.

gene mapping: Determination of the relative positions of genes on a DNA molecule (chromosome or plasmid) and of the distance, in linkage units or physical units, between them.

gene therapy: An experimental procedure aimed at replacing, manipulating, or supplementing nonfunctional or misfunctioning genes with healthy genes.

gene transfer: Incorporation of new DNA into an organism's cells, usually by a vector such as a modified virus. Used in gene therapy.

genetic counseling: Provides patients and their families with education and information about genetic-related conditions and helps them make informed decisions.

genetic discrimination: Prejudice against those who have or are likely to develop an inherited disorder.

genetic engineering: Altering the genetic material of cells or organisms to enable them to make new substances or perform new functions.

genetic marker: A gene or other identifiable portion of DNA whose inheritance can be followed.

genetic predisposition: Susceptibility to a genetic disease. May or may not result in actual development of the disease.

genetic screening: Testing a group of people to identify individuals at high risk of having or passing on a specific genetic disorder.

genetic testing: Analyzing an individual's genetic material to determine predisposition to a particular health condition or to confirm a diagnosis of genetic disease.

genetics: The study of inheritance patterns of specific traits.

genome: All the genetic material in the chromosomes of a particular organism; its size is generally given as its total number of base pairs.

genomics: The study of genes and their function.

genotype: The genetic constitution of an organism, as distinguished from its physical appearance (its phenotype).

germ cell: Sperm and egg cells and their precursors. Germ cells are haploid and have only one set of chromosomes (twenty-three in all), while all other cells have two copies (forty-six in all).

germ line: The continuation of a set of genetic information from one generation to the next.

haploid: A single set of chromosomes (half the full set of genetic material) present in the egg and sperm cells of animals and in the egg and pollen cells of plants. Human beings have twenty-three chromosomes in their reproductive cells.

hemizygous: Having only one copy of a particular gene. For example, in humans, males are hemizygous for genes found on the Y chromosome.

hereditary cancer: Cancer that occurs due to the inheritance of an altered gene within a family.

homology: Similarity in DNA or protein sequences between individuals of the same species or among different species.

homozygote: An organism that has two identical alleles of a gene.

identical twin: Twins produced by the division of a single zygote; both have identical genotypes.

imprinting: A phenomenon in which the disease phenotype depends on which parent passed on the disease gene. For instance, both Prader-Willi and Angelman syndromes are inherited when the same part of chromosome 15 is missing. When the father's complement of 15 is missing, the child has Prader-Willi, but when the mother's complement of 15 is missing, the child has Angelman syndrome.

in vitro: Studies performed outside a living organism such as in a laboratory.

in vivo: Studies carried out in living organisms.

inherit: In genetics, to receive genetic material from parents through biological processes.

insertion: A chromosome abnormality in which a piece of DNA is incorporated into a gene and thereby disrupts the gene's normal function.

interference: One crossover event inhibits the chances of another crossover event. Also known as positive interference. Negative interference increases the chance of a second crossover.

karyotype: A photomicrograph of an individual's chromosomes arranged in a standard format showing the number, size, and shape of each chromosome type; used in low-resolution physical mapping to correlate gross chromosomal abnormalities with the characteristics of specific diseases.

linkage: The proximity of two or more markers (e.g., genes, RFLP markers) on a chromosome; the closer the markers, the lower the probability that they will be separated during DNA repair or replication processes, and hence the greater the probability that they will be inherited together.

locus: The position on a chromosome of a gene or other chromosome marker; also, the DNA at that position.

Mendelian inheritance: One method in which genetic traits are passed from parents to offspring. Named for Gregor Mendel, who first studied and recognized the existence of genes and this method of inheritance.

mitochondrial DNA: The genetic material found in mitochondria, the organelles that generate energy for the cell. Not inherited in the same fashion as nucleic DNA.

mitosis: The process of nuclear division in cells that produces daughter cells that are genetically identical to each other and to the parent cell.

monogenic disorder: A disorder caused by mutation of a single gene.

monosomy: Possessing only one copy of a particular chromosome instead of the normal two copies.

mutagen: An agent that causes a permanent genetic change in a cell. Does not include changes occurring during normal genetic recombination.

mutation: Any heritable change in DNA sequence.

oligogenic: A phenotypic trait produced by two or more genes working together.

oligonucleotide: A molecule usually composed of twenty-five or fewer nucleotides; used as a DNA synthesis primer.

oncogene: A gene, one or more forms of which is associated with cancer. Many oncogenes are involved, directly or indirectly, in controlling the rate of cell growth.

penetrance: The probability of a gene or genetic trait being expressed. "Complete" penetrance means the gene or genes for a trait are expressed in all the population who have the genes. "Incomplete" penetrance means the genetic trait is expressed in only part of the population.

pharmacogenomics: The study of the interaction of an individual's genetic makeup and response to a drug.

phenotype: The physical characteristics of an organism or the presence of a disease that may or may not be genetic.

polygenic disorder: Genetic disorder resulting from the combined action of alleles of more than one gene (e.g., heart disease, diabetes, and some cancers). Although such disorders are inherited, they depend on the simultaneous presence of several alleles; thus the hereditary patterns usually are more complex than those of single-gene disorders.

protein: A large molecule composed of one or more chains of amino acids in a specific order; the order is determined by the base sequence of nucleotides in the gene that codes for the protein. Proteins are required for the structure, function, and regulation of the body's cells, tissues, and organs; and each protein has unique functions. Examples are hormones, enzymes, and antibodies.

proteomics: The study of the full set of proteins encoded by a genome.

pseudogene: A sequence of DNA similar to a gene but nonfunctional; probably the remnant of a once-functional gene that accumulated mutations.

recessive gene: A gene which will be expressed only if there are two identical copies or, for a male, if one copy is present on the X chromosome.

reciprocal translocation: When a pair of chromosomes exchange exactly the same length and area of DNA. Results in a shuffling of genes.

regulatory region or sequence: A DNA base sequence that controls gene expression.

repetitive DNA: Sequences of varying lengths that occur in multiple copies in the genome; it represents much of the human genome.

retroviral infection: The presence of retroviral vectors, such as some viruses, which use their recombinant DNA to insert their genetic material into the chromosomes of the host's cells. The virus is then propagated by the host cell.

RNA (ribonucleic acid): A chemical found in the nucleus and cytoplasm of cells; it plays an important role in protein synthesis and other chemical activities of the cell. The structure of RNA is similar to that of DNA. There are several classes of RNA molecules, including messenger RNA, transfer RNA, ribosomal RNA, and other small RNAs, each serving a different purpose.

sex chromosome: The X or Y chromosome in human beings that determines the sex of an individual. Females have two X chromosomes in diploid cells; males have an X and a Y chromosome. The sex chromosomes comprise the twenty-third chromosome pair in a karyotype.

sex-linked: Traits or diseases associated with the X or Y chromosome; generally seen in males.

single nucleotide polymorphism: DNA sequence variations that occur when a single nucleotide (A, T, C, or G) in the genome sequence is altered.

single-gene disorder: Hereditary disorder caused by a mutant allele of a single gene.

stem cell: Undifferentiated, primitive cells in the bone marrow that have the ability both to multiply and to differentiate into specific blood cells.

substitution: In genetics, a type of mutation due to replacement of one nucleotide in a DNA sequence by another nucleotide or replacement of one amino acid in a protein by another amino acid.

suppressor gene: A gene that can suppress the action of another gene.

syndrome: The group or recognizable pattern of symptoms or abnormalities that indicate a particular trait or disease.

transformation: A process by which the genetic material carried by an individual cell is altered by incorporation of exogenous DNA into its genome.

translocation: A mutation in which a large segment of one chromosome breaks off and attaches to another chromosome.

trisomy: Possessing three copies of a particular chromosome instead of the normal two copies.

X chromosome: One of the two sex chromosomes, X and Y.

Y chromosome: One of the two sex chromosomes, X and Y.

Chapter 72

Heritable Disorders: A Directory of Resources for Patients and Families

General

Genetic Alliance
4301 Connecticut Avenue NW
Suite 404
Washington, DC 20008-2369
Toll-Free: 800-336-GENE (4363)
Phone: 202-966-5557
Fax: 202-966-8553
Website: http://
www.geneticalliance.org
E-mail: info@geneticalliance.org

Genetic Science Learning Center
15 North 2030 East
Salt Lake City, Utah 84112-5330
Phone: 801-585-3470
Fax: 801-585-9557
Website: http://
learn.genetics.utah.edu

Hereditary Disease Foundation
3960 Broadway, 6th Floor
New York, NY 10032
Phone: 212-928-2121
Fax: 212-928-2172
Website: http://
www.hdfoundation.org
E-mail:
curehd@hdfoundation.org

March of Dimes
National Headquarters
1275 Mamaroneck Avenue
White Plains, NY 10605
Phone: 914-997-4488
Fax: 914-428-8203
Website: http://
www.marchofdimes.com

The information in this chapter was compiled from various sources deemed accurate. All contact information was verified and updated in June 2009. Inclusion does not imply endorsement. This list is intended to serve as a starting point for information gathering; it is not comprehensive.

Mount Sinai Center for Jewish Genetic Diseases, Inc.
Mount Sinai Medical Center
Fifth Avenue at 100th Street
New York, NY 10029
Phone: 212-659-6774
Website: http://www.mssm.edu/jewish_genetics

National Heart, Lung, and Blood Institute (NHBLI)
National Institutes of Health, DHHS
P.O. Box 30105
Bethesda, MD 20824-0105
Phone: 301-592-8573
TTY: 240-629-3255
Fax: 301-592-8563
Website: http://www.nhlbi.nih.gov
E-mail: nhlbiinfo@nhlbi.nih.gov

National Institute of Neurological Disorders and Stroke (NINDS)
NIH Neurological Institute
P.O. Box 5801
Bethesda, MD 20824
Toll-Free: 800-352-9424
Phone: 301-496-5751
TTY: 301-468-5981
Website: http://www.ninds.nih.gov

National Institute on Deafness and Other Communication Disorders (NIDCD)
National Institutes of Health
31 Center Drive, MSC 2320
Bethesda, MD USA 20892-2320
Website: http://www.nidcd.nih.gov
E-mail: nidcdinfo@nidcd.nih.gov

National Organization for Rare Disorders (NORD)
P.O. Box 1968
55 Kenosia Avenue
Danbury, CT 06813-1968
Toll-Free: 800-999-NORD (6673)
Phone: 203-744-0100
TDD: 203-797-9590
Fax: 203-798-2291
Website: http://www.rarediseases.org
E-mail: orphan@rarediseases.org

Alpha-1 Antitrypsin Deficiency

Alpha-1 Association
2937 SW 27 Avenue
Suite 106
Miami, FL 33133
Toll-Free: 800-521-3025
Phone: 305-648-0088
Fax: 305-648-0089
Website: http://www.alpha1.org
E-mail: info@alpha1.org

Alpha-1 Foundation
2937 SW 27th Avenue
Suite 302
Miami, Florida 33133
Phone: 305-567-9888
Toll-Free: 877-228-7321
Fax: 305-567-1317
Website: http://www.alphaone.org
E-mail: info@alphaone.org

Amyotrophic Lateral Sclerosis

ALS Association
27001 Agoura Road, Suite 250
Calabasas Hills, CA 91301-5104
Toll-Free: 800-782-4747
Phone: 818-880-9007
Fax: 818-880-9006
Website: http://www.alsa.org
E-mail: advocacy@alsa-national.org

ALS Therapy Development Institute
215 First Street
Cambridge, MA 02142
Phone: 617-441-7200
Fax: 617-441-7299
Website: http://www.als.net
E-mail: info@als.net

Les Turner ALS Foundation
5550 W. Touhy Avenue
Suite 302
Skokie, IL 60077-3254
Toll-Free: 888-ALS-1107
Phone: 847-679-3311
Fax: 847-679-9109
Website: http://www.lesturnerals.org
E-mail: info@lesturnerals.org

Project ALS
900 Broadway, Suite 901
New York, NY 10003
Toll-Free: 800-603-0270
Phone: 212-420-7382
Fax: 212-420-7387
Website: http://www.projectals.org
E-mail: info@projectals.org

Angelman Syndrome

Angelman Syndrome Foundation
4255 Westbrook Drive
Suite 219
Aurora, IL 60504
Toll-Free: 800-432-6435
Phone: 630-978-4245
Fax: 630-978-7408
Website: http://www.angelman.org
E-mail: info@angelman.org

The Arc of the United States
1010 Wayne Avenue
Suite 650
Silver Spring, MD 20910
Toll-Free: 800-433-5255
Phone: 301-565-3842
Fax: 301-565-3843 or -5342
Website: http://www.thearc.org
E-mail: Info@thearc.org

Blood and Blood Clotting Disorders

American Hemochromatosis Society, Inc.
4044 West Lake Mary Boulevard
104, PMB 416
Lake Mary, FL 32746–2012
Toll-Free: 888-655-IRON (4766)
Phone: 407-829-4488
Fax: 407-333-1284
Website: http://www.americanhs.org
E-mail: mail@americanhs.org

American Sickle Cell Anemia Association
10300 Carnegie Avenue
Cleveland, OH 44106
Phone: 216-229-8600
Fax: 216-229-4500
Website: http://www.ascaa.org

Iron Disorders Institute
2722 Wade Hampton Blvd.
Suite A
Greenville, SC 29615
Toll Free: 888-565-IRON (4766)
Phone: 864-292-1175
Fax: 864-292-1878
Website: http://
www.irondisorders.org

National Hemophilia Foundation
116 West 32nd Street
11th Floor
New York, NY 10001
Phone: 212-328-3700
Fax: 212-328-3777
Website: http://
www.hemophilia.org

Sickle Cell Disease Association of America, Inc.
231 East Baltimore Street
Suite 800
Baltimore, MD 21202
Toll-Free: 800-421-8453
Phone: 410-528-1555
Fax: 410-528-1495
Website: http://
www.sicklecelldisease.org
E-mail:
scdaa@sicklecelldisease.org

Sickle Cell Society
54 Station Road
London, NW10 4UA
United Kingdom
Phone: 020 8961 7795
Fax: 020 8961 8346
Website: http://
www.sicklecellsociety.org
E-mail: info@sicklecellsociety
.org

World Federation of Hemophilia
1425 René Lévesque Blvd. W.
Suite 1010
Montréal, Québec
H3G 1T7 Canada
Phone: 514-875-7944
Fax: 514-875-8916
Website: http://www.wfh.org
E-mail: wfh@wfh.org

CHARGE Syndrome

CHARGE Syndrome Foundation, Inc.
141 Middle Neck Rd.
Sands Point, NY 11050
Toll-Free: 800-442-7604
Phone: 516-684-4720
Fax: 516-883-9060
Website: http://
www.chargesyndrome.org

Connective Tissue Disorders

American Academy of Orthopaedic Surgeons (AAOS)

6300 North River Road
Rosemont, IL 60018-4262
Toll Free: 800-824-BONE (2663)
Phone: 847-823-7186
Fax: 847-823-8125
Website: http://www.aaos.org
E-mail: pemr@aaos.org

Coalition for Heritable Disorders of Connective Tissue

4301 Connecticut Ave, NW
Suite 404
Washington, DC 20008
Phone: 202-362-9599
Fax: 202-966-8553
Website: http://www.chdct.org
E-mail: chdct@pxe.org

Dystrophic Epidermolysis Bullosa Research Association of America, Inc. (DebRA)

16 East 41st Street, 3rd Floor
New York, NY 10017
Toll-Free: 866-DEBRA76
(866-332-7276)
Phone: 212-868-1573
Fax: 212-868-9296
Website: http://www.debra.org
E-mail: staff@debra.org

Ehlers-Danlos National Foundation (EDNF)

3200 Wilshire Blvd., Suite 1601
South Tower
Los Angeles, CA 90010
Phone: 213-368-3800
Fax: 213-427-0057
Website: http://www.ednf.org
E-mail: staff@ednf.org

Genetic Alliance

4301 Connecticut Avenue, NW
Suite 404
Washington, DC 20008-2369
Toll-Free: 800-336-GENE (4363)
Phone: 202-966-5557
Fax: 202-966-8553
Website: http://
www.geneticalliance.org

National Association for Pseudoxanthoma Elasticum, Inc. (NAPE)

8760 Manchester Road
St. Louis, MO 63144-2724
Phone: 314-962-0100
Fax: 314-962-0100
Website: http://www.pxenape.org
E-mail:
napestlouis@sbcglobal.net

National Institute of Arthritis and Musculoskeletal and Skin Diseases (NIAMS)
Information Clearinghouse
National Institutes of Health
1 AMS Circle
Bethesda, MD 20892-3675
Toll Free: 877-22-NIAMS
(226-4267)
Phone: 301-495-4484
Fax: 301-718-6366
TTY: 301–565–2966
Website: http://
www.niams.nih.gov
E-mail:
NIAMSinfo@mail.nih.gov

National Marfan Foundation (NMF)
22 Manhasset Avenue
Port Washington, NY 11050-2023
Toll-Free: 800-8-MARFAN
(800-862-7326)
Phone: 516-883-8712
Fax: 516-883-8040
Website: http://www.marfan.org
E-mail: staff@marfan.org

Osteogenesis Imperfecta Foundation
804 West Diamond Ave.
Suite 210
Gaithersburg, MD 20878
Toll-Free: 800-981-2663
Phone: 301-947-0083
Fax: 301-947-0456
Website: http://www.oif.org
E-mail: bonelink@oif.org

PXE International
4301 Connecticut Avenue NW
Suite 404
Washington, DC 20008-2369
Phone: 202-362-9599
Fax: 202-966-8553
Website: http://www.pxe.org
E-mail: info@pxe.org

Cystic Fibrosis

Cystic Fibrosis Foundation
National Headquarters
6931 Arlington Road
Bethesda, Maryland 20814
Toll-Free: 800-FIGHT CF
(344-4823)
Phone: 301-951-4422
Fax: 301-951-6378
Website: http://www.cff.org
E-mail: info@cff.org

Down Syndrome

Down Syndrome Research and Treatment Foundation
755 Page Mill Road, Suite A-200
Palo Alto, CA 94304-1005
Phone: 650-468-1668
Fax: 650-617-1601
Website: http://www.dsrtf.org
E-mail: dsrtf@dsrtf.org

National Association for Down Syndrome
P.O. Box 206
Wilmette, IL 60091
Phone: 630-325-9112
Website: http://www.nads.org
E-mail: info@nads.org

National Down Syndrome Society
666 Broadway, 8th Floor
New York, New York 10012
Toll-Free: 800-221-4602
Website: http://www.ndss.org
E-mail: info@ndss.org

Endocrine Disorders

Congenital Adrenal Hyperplasia Education and Support Network
Website: www
.congenitaladrenalhyperplasia
.org

Congenital Adrenal Hyperplasia Research, Education and Support Foundation (CARES)
2414 Morris Avenue
Suite 110
Union, NJ 07083
Toll-Free: 866-227-3737
Phone: 973-912-3895
Fax: 973-912-8990
Website:
www.caresfoundation.org
E-mail:
contact@caresfoundation.org

National Adrenal Diseases Foundation (NADF)
505 Northern Boulevard
Great Neck, NY 11021
Phone: 516-487-4992
Website: http://www.nadf.us
E-mail: nadfmail@aol.com

Fragile X Syndrome

FRAXA Research Foundation
45 Pleasant Street
Newburyport, MA 01950
Phone: 978-462-1866
Fax: 978-463-9985
Website: http://www.fraxa.org
E-mail: info@fraxa.org

National Fragile X Foundation
P.O. Box 37
Walnut Creek, California 94597
Toll-free: 800-688-8765
Phone: 925-938-9300
Fax: 925-938-9315
Website: http://www.nfxf.org

Growth Disorders

Human Growth Foundation
997 Glen Cove Avenue, Suite 5
Glen Head, NY 11545
Toll-Free: 800-451-6434
Fax: 516-671-4055
Website: http://www.hgfound.org
E-mail: hgf1@hgfound.org

Madisons Foundation
P.O. Box 241956
Los Angeles, CA 90024
Phone: 310-264-0826
Fax: 310-264-4766
Website: http://
www.madisonsfoundation.org
E-mail:
getinfo@madisonsfoundation.org

MAGIC Foundation
6645 W. North Avenue
Oak Park, IL 60302
Toll-Free: 800-362-4423
(800-3-MAGIC-3)
Phone: 708-383-0808
Fax: 708-383-0899
Website: http://
www.magicfoundation.org

Heart Rhythm Disorders

American Heart Association
National Center
7272 Greenville Avenue
Dallas, TX 75231
Toll-Free: 800-AHA-USA-1
(242-8721)
Website: http://
www.americanheart.org

**Cardiac Arrhythmias
Research and Education
Foundation (C.A.R.E.
Foundation, Inc.)**
427 Fulton Street
P.O. Box 69
Seymour, WI 54165
Toll-Free: 800-404-9500
Phone: 920-833-7000
Fax: 920-833-7005
Website: http://www.longqt.org
E-mail:
care@CAREforhearts.org

**Congenital Heart
Information Network
(C.H.I.N.)**
101 N Washington Avenue
Suite 1A
Margate City NJ 08402-1195
Phone: 609-822-1572
Fax: 609-822-1574
Website: http://tchin.org
E-mail: mb@tchin.org

Heart Rhythm Society
1400 K Street, NW, Suite 500
Washington, DC 20005
Phone: 202-464-3400
Fax: 202-464-3401
Website: http://www.hrsonline.org
E-mail: info@hrsonline.org

Huntington Disease

**Huntington's Disease
Society of America**
National Office
505 Eighth Avenue, Suite 902
New York, NY 10018
Toll-Free: 800-345-HDSA (4372)
Phone: 212-242-1968
Fax: 212-239-3430
Website: http://www.hdsa.org

**Huntington Society of
Canada**
151 Frederick Street, Suite 400
Kitchener, ON N2H 2M2
Canada
Toll-Free: 800-998-7398
Phone: 519-749-7063
Fax: 519-749-8965
Website: http://
www.huntingtonsociety.ca
E-mail: info@huntingtonsociety.ca

Inborn Errors of Metabolism

American Liver Foundation
75 Maiden Lane, Suite 603
New York, NY 10038
Toll-Free: 800-GO-LIVER
(800-465-4837)
Phone: 212-668-1000
Fax: 212-483-8179
Website: http://
www.liverfoundation.org

CLIMB (Children Living with Inherited Metabolic Diseases)
176 Nantwich Road
Crewe, CW2 6BG
Cheshire, UK
Phone: 0800 652 3181 or
0845 241 2172 (or 73, 74)
Website: http://
www.CLIMB.org.uk
E-mail: info.svcs@climb.org.uk

Maple Syrup Urine Disease Family Support Group
24806 SR119
Goshen, IN 46526
Phone: 219-862-2992
Fax: 219-862-2012
Website: http://www
.msud-support.org

National Coalition for PKU & Allied Disorders
P.O. Box 1244
Mansfield, MA 02048
Phone: 877-996-2723

National Urea Cycle Disorders Foundation
Toll-Free: 800-38-NUCDF
(800-386-8233)
Website: http://www.nucdf.org
E-mail: info@nucdf.org

Kidney and Urinary System Disorders

American Association of Kidney Patients
3505 East Frontage Road
Suite 315
Tampa, FL 33607
Toll-Free: 800–749–2257
Phone: 813–636–8100
Fax: 813-636-8122
Website: www.aakp.org
E-mail: info@aakp.org

Cystinuria Support Network
Website: http://
www.cystinuria.com

International Cystinuria Foundation
P.O. Box 271004
Fort Collins, CO 80527-1004
Website: http://
www.cystinuria.org

National Kidney Foundation
30 East 33rd Street
New York, NY 10016
Toll-Free: 800–622–9010
Phone: 212–889–2210
Website: www.kidney.org

Polycystic Kidney Disease Foundation

9221 Ward Parkway, Suite 400
Kansas City, MO 64114–3367
Toll-Free: 800–PKD–CURE
(753–2873)
Phone: 816–931–2600
Fax: 816-931-8655
Website: www.pkdcure.org
E-mail: pkdcure@pkdcure.org

Klinefelter Syndrome

American Association for Klinefelter Syndrome Information and Support (AAKSIS)

c/o Roberta Rappaport
2945 W. Farwell Ave.
Chicago, IL 60645-2925
Toll-Free: 888-466-KSIS
(888-466-5747)
Website: http://www.aaksis.org
E-mail: KSinfo@aaksis.org

Klinefelter Syndrome and Associates, Inc.

11 Keats Court
Coto de Caza, CA 92679
Toll-Free: 888-999-9428
Phone: 949-858-9428 x41
Website: http://www.genetic.org

Leukodystrophies

Hunter's Hope Foundation

P.O. Box 643
Orchard Park, NY 14127
Toll-Free: 877-984-HOPE
(877-984-4673)
Phone: 716-667-1200
Fax: 716-667-1212
Website: http://
www.huntershope.org
E-mail: info@huntershope.org

National Tay-Sachs and Allied Diseases Association

2001 Beacon Street, Suite 204
Brighton, MA 02135
Toll-Free: 800-90-NTSAD
(800-906-8723)
Phone: 617-277-4463
Fax: 617-277-0134
Website: http://www.ntsad.org
E-mail: info@ntsad.org

United Leukodystrophy Foundation

2304 Highland Drive
Sycamore, IL 60178
Toll-Free: 800-728-5483
Phone: 815-895-3211
Fax: 815-895-2432
Website: http://www.ulf.org
E-mail: office@ulf.org

Lipid Storage Diseases

Ara Parseghian Medical Research Foundation (For Niemann-Pick Type C Disease)
3530 East Campo Abierto
Suite 105
Tucson, AZ 85718-3327
Phone: 520-577-5106
Fax: 520-577-5212
Website: http://
www.parseghian.org
E-mail: victory@parseghian.org

Batten Disease Support and Research Association
166 Humphries Drive
Reynoldsburg, OH 43068
Toll-Free: 800-448-4570
Phone: 740-927-4298
Fax: 740-927-7683
Website: http://www.bdsra.org
E-mail: bdsra1@bdsra.org

Children's Brain Disease Foundation
Parnassus Heights Medical
Building, Suite 900
San Francisco, CA 94117
Phone: 415-665-3003
Fax: 415-665-3003
E-mail: jrider6022@aol.com

Children's Gaucher Research Fund
P.O. Box 2123
Granite Bay, CA 95746-2123
Phone: 916-797-3700
Fax: 916-797-3707
Website: http://
www.childrensgaucher.org
E-mail:
research@childrensgaucher.org

Fabry Support and Information Group
108 NE 2nd Street, Suite C
P.O. Box 510
Concordia, MO 64020-0510
Phone: 660-463-1355
Fax: 660-463-1356
Website: http://www.fabry.org
E-mail: info@fabry.org

Hide and Seek Foundation for Lysosomal Storage Disease Research
6475 East Pacific Coast Highway
Suite 466
Long Beach, CA 90803
Toll-Free: 888-858-7894
Phone: 818-762-8621
Toll-Free Fax: 866-215-8850
Fax: 818-762-2502
Website: http://
www.hideandseek.org
E-mail: info@hideandseek.org

Nathan's Battle Foundation (For Batten Disease Research)
459 South State Road 135
Greenwood, IN 46142
Phone: 317-888-7396
Fax: 317-888-0504
Website: http://
www.nathansbattle.com
E-mail: pmilto@indy.net

National Gaucher Foundation
2227 Idlewood Road, Suite 12
Tucker, GA 30084
Toll-Free: 800-504-3189
Fax: 770-934-2911
Website: http://
www.gaucherdisease.org
E-mail: ngf@gaucherdisease.org

National Niemann-Pick Disease Foundation, Inc.
P.O. Box 49
401 Madison Avenue, Suite B
Ft. Atkinson, WI 53538
Toll-Free: 877-CURE-NPC
(287-3672)
Phone: 920-563-0930
Fax: 920-563-0931
Website: http://www.nnpdf.org
E-mail: nnpdf@idcnet.org

National Tay-Sachs and Allied Diseases Association
2001 Beacon Street, Suite 204
Brighton, MA 02135
Toll-Free: 800-90-NTSAD
(906-8723)
Phone: 617-277-4463
Fax: 617-277-0134
Website: http://www.ntsad.org
E-mail: info@ntsad.org

Mitochondrial Disease

United Mitochondrial Disease Foundation
8085 Saltsburg Road, Suite 201
Pittsburgh, PA 15239
Toll Free: 888-317-UMDF (8633)
Phone: 412-793-8077
Fax: 412-793-6477
Website: http://www.umdf.org
E-mail: info@umdf.org

Neurofibromatosis

Acoustic Neuroma Association
600 Peachtree Parkway
Suite 108
Cumming, GA 30041
Toll-Free: 877-200-8211
Phone: 770-205-8211
Toll-Free Fax: 877-202-0239
Fax: 770-205-0239
Website: http://www.anausa.org
E-mail: info@anausa.org

Children's Tumor Foundation

95 Pine Street, 16th Floor
New York, NY 10005
Toll-Free: 800-323-7938
Phone: 212-344-6633
Fax: 212-747-0004
Website: http://www.ctf.org
E-mail: info@ctf.org

International Radio Surgery Association (IRSA)

3002 N Second Street
Harrisburg, PA 17110
Phone: 717-260-9808
Fax: 717-260-9809
Website: http://www.irsa.org
E-mail: office1@irsa.org

National Cancer Institute (NCI)

National Institutes of Health, DHHS
6116 Executive Boulevard
Suite 3036A, MSC 8322
Bethesda, MD 20892-8322
Toll-Free: 800-4-CANCER (422-6237)
TTY: 800-332-8615
Website: http://cancer.gov
E-mail: cancergovstaff@mail.nih.gov

Neurofibromatosis, Inc. (NF Inc.)

P.O. Box 66884
Chicago, IL 60666
Toll-Free: 800-942-6825
Phone: 630-627-1115
Website: http://www.nfinc.org
E-mail: nfinfo@nfinc.org

Neuromuscular Disorders

Charcot-Marie-Tooth Association (CMTA)

2700 Chestnut Parkway
Chester, PA 19013-4867
Toll-Free: 800-606-CMTA (2682)
Phone: 610-499-9264
Fax: 610-499-9267
Website: http://www.charcot-marie-tooth.org
E-mail: info@charcot-marie-tooth.org

Dystonia Medical Research Foundation

National Headquarters
1 East Wacker Drive, Suite 2810
Chicago, IL 60601-1905
Toll-Free: 800-377-DYST (3978)
Phone: 312-755-0198
Fax: 312-803-0138
Website: http://www.dystonia-foundation.org
E-mail: dystonia@dystonia-foundation.org

Facioscapulohumeral Muscular Dystrophy (FSH) Society

3 Westwood Road
Lexington, MA 02420
Phone: 781-275-7781 or 781-860-0501
Fax: 781-860-0599
Website: http://www.fshsociety.org
E-mail: info@fshsociety.org

Families of Spinal Muscular Atrophy
P.O. Box 196
14047 Petronella Drive, Suite 107
Libertyville, IL 60048-0196
Toll-Free: 800-886-1762
Phone: 847-367-7620
Fax: 847-367-7623
Website: http://www.curesma.org
E-mail: info@fsma.org

Friedreich's Ataxia Research Alliance (FARA)
P.O. Box 1537
Springfield, VA 22151
Phone: 703-426-1576
Fax: 703-425-0643
Website: http://www.CureFA.org
E-mail: fara@CureFA.org

Hereditary Neuropathy Foundation Inc.
1751 2nd Avenue, Suite 103
New York, NY 10128
Toll Free: 877-463-1287
Phone: 212-722-8396
Fax: 917-591-2758
Website: http://www.hnf-cure.org
E-mail: info@hnf-cure.org

International Myotonic Dystrophy Organization
P.O. Box 1121
Sunland, CA 91041-1121
Toll-Free: 866-679-7954
Phone: 760-918-0377
Fax: 760-444-2716
Website: http://
www.myotonicdystrophy.org
E-mail:
info@myotonicdystrophy.org

Muscular Dystrophy Association
National Headquarters
3300 East Sunrise Drive
Tucson, AZ 85718-3208
Toll-Free: 800-344-4863
Toll-Free: 800-572-1717 (Connects callers to their local MDA)
Phone: 520-529-2000
Fax: 520-529-5300
Website: http://www.mda.org
E-mail: mda@mdausa.org

Muscular Dystrophy Family Foundation
3951 North Meridian Street
Suite 100
Indianapolis, IN 46208-4062
Toll-Free: 800-544-1213
Phone: 317-923-MDFF (6333)
Fax: 317-923-6334
Website: http://www.mdff.org
E-mail: mdff@mdff.org

National Ataxia Foundation (NAF)
2600 Fernbrook Lane North
Suite 119
Minneapolis, MN 55447-4752
Phone: 763-553-0020
Fax: 763-553-0167
Website: http://www.ataxia.org
E-mail: naf@ataxia.org

Neuropathy Association, Inc.
60 East 42nd Street, Suite 942
New York, NY 10165-0999
Phone: 212-692-0662
Fax: 212-692-0668
Website: http://
www.neuropathy.org
E-mail: info@neuropathy.org

Spastic Paraplegia Foundation, Inc.
7700 Leesburg Pike, Suite 123
Falls Church, VA 22043
Toll-Free: 877-SPF-GIVE
(773-4483)
Website: http://sp-foundation.org

Spinal Muscular Atrophy Foundation
888 Seventh Avenue, Suite 400
New York, NY 10019
Toll-Free: 877-FUND-SMA
(877-386-3762)
Phone: 646-253-7100
Fax: 212-247-3079
Website: http://
www.smafoundation.org
E-mail: info@smafoundation.org

Worldwide Education & Awareness for Movement Disorders (WE MOVE)
204 West 84th Street
New York, NY 10024
Phone: 212-875-8312
Fax: 212-875-8389
Website: http://www.wemove.org
E-mail: wemove@wemove.org

Phenylketonuria

Children's PKU Network
3790 Via De La Valle, Suite 120
Del Mar, CA 92014
Toll-Free: 800-377-6677
Phone: 858-509-0767
Fax: 858-509-0768
Website: http://
www.pkunetwork.org
E-mail: pkunetwork@aol.com

Porphyria

American Porphyria Foundation
4900 Woodway, Suite 780
Houston, TX 77056–1837
Toll-Free: 866-APF-3635
(273-3635)
Phone: 713-266-9617
Fax: 713-840-9552
Website: http://
www.porphyriafoundation.com
E-mail: porphyrus@aol.com

Iron Disorders Institute
2722 Wade Hampton Boulevard
Suite A
Greenville, SC 29615
Toll-Free: 888-565-IRON (4766)
Phone: 864-292-1175
Fax: 864-292-1878
Website: www.irondisorders.org
E-mail: PatientServices@
irondisorders.org

Prader-Willi Syndrome

Foundation for Prader-Willi Research
209 Pennsylvania Avenue, SE
Suite 229 D
Washington, DC 20003
Phone: 202-547-7117
Fax: 202-547-7119
Website: http://www.fpwr.org

Prader-Willi Syndrome Association

8588 Potter Park Drive
Suite 500
Sarasota, FL 34238
Toll-Free: 800-926-4797
Phone: 941-312-0400
Fax: 941-312-0142
Website: www.pwsausa.org

Rett Syndrome

International Rett Syndrome Foundation

4600 Devitt Drive
Cincinnati, OH 45246
Toll-Free: 800-818-RETT (7388)
Phone: 513-874-3020
Fax: 513-874-2520
Website: http://
www.rettsyndrome.org
E-mail:
admin@rettsyndrome.org

Smith-Magenis Syndrome

Parents and Researchers Interested in Smith-Magenis Syndrome (PRISMS)

21800 Town Center Plaza
Suite #266A-633
Sterling, VA 20164
Phone: 972-231-0035
Fax: 972-499-1832
Website: http://www.prisms.org
E-mail: info@prisms.org

Sotos Syndrome

Sotos Syndrome Support Association

P.O. Box 4626
Wheaton, IL 60189
Toll-Free: 888-246-SSSA (7772)
Website: http://www.well.com/
user/sssa
E-mail: info@sotossyndrome.org

Tourette Syndrome

Tourette Syndrome Association, Inc. (TSA)

42-40 Bell Boulevard, Suite 205
Bayside, NY 11361-2820
Toll-Free: 888-4-TOURET
(486-8738)
Phone: 718-224-2999
Fax: 718-279-9596
Website: http://tsa-usa.org
E-mail: ts@tsa-usa.org

Tourette Syndrome Foundation of Canada

#206, 194 Jarvis Street
Toronto, Ontario
Canada M5B 2B7
Toll Free: 800-361-3120
Phone: 416-861-8398
Fax: 416-861-2472
Website: http://www.tourette.ca
E-mail: tsfc@tourette.ca

Tuberous Sclerosis

Tuberous Sclerosis Alliance
801 Roeder Road, Suite 750
Silver Spring, MD 20910-4467
Toll-Free: 800-225-6827
Phone: 301-562-9890
Fax: 301-562-9870
Website: http://
www.tsalliance.org
E-mail: info@tsalliance.org

Tuberous Sclerosis Association
P.O. Box 12979
Barnt Green
Birmingham B45 5AN
England
Phone: +44 (0)121 445 6970
Website: http://
www.tuberous-sclerosis.org

Turner Syndrome

Turner Unit
National Institutes of Health
National Institute of Child
Health and Human Development
Developmental Endocrinology
Branch, Section on Women's
Health
10 Center Dr. CRC 1-3330
Bethesda, MD 20892-1103
Toll-Free: 888-437-4338
Phone: 301-496-7731
Website: http://
turners.nichd.nih.gov
E-mail: Bakalov@mail.nih.gov
(for Turner Syndrome questions)

Turner Syndrome Society of the United States
10960 Millridge North Drive
#214A
Houston, TX 77070
Toll-Free: 800-365-9944
Phone: 832-912-6006
Fax: 832-912-6446
Website: http://
www.turnersyndrome.org

Williams Syndrome

Williams Syndrome Association
P.O. Box 297
Clawson, MI 48017-0297
Toll-Free: 800-806-1871
Phone: 248-244-2229
Fax: 248-244-2230
Website: http://
www.williams-syndrome.org
E-mail: info@williams-syndrome.org

Wilson Disease

American Liver Foundation
75 Maiden Lane, Suite 603
New York, NY 10038–4810
Toll-Free: 800-GO-LIVER
(465–4837)
Phone: 212–668–1000
Fax: 212–483–8179
Website:
www.liverfoundation.org
E-mail: info@liverfoundation.org

***Wilson's Disease
Association International***
1802 Brookside Drive
Wooster, OH 44691
Toll-Free: 888–264–1450
Phone: 330–264–1450
Website:
www.wilsonsdisease.org
E-mail: info@wilsonsdisease.org

Index

Index

Page numbers followed by 'n' indicate a footnote. Page numbers in *italics* indicate a table or illustration.

A

697

Health Reference Series
Complete Catalog
List price $93 per volume. School and library price $84 per volume.

Adolescent Health Sourcebook, 2nd Edition

Basic Consumer Health Information about the Physical, Mental, and Emotional Growth and Development of Adolescents, Including Medical Care, Nutritional and Physical Activity Requirements, Puberty, Sexual Activity, Acne, Tanning, Body Piercing, Common Physical Illnesses and Disorders, Eating Disorders, Attention Deficit Hyperactivity Disorder, Depression, Bullying, Hazing, and Adolescent Injuries Related to Sports, Driving, and Work

Along with Substance Abuse Information about Nicotine, Alcohol, and Drug Use, a Glossary, and Directory of Additional Resources

Edited by Joyce Brennfleck Shannon. 655 pages. 2007. 978-0-7808-0943-7.

"A particularly good resource for both parents and teens. The concise presentation of the material in brief and well-organized chapters creates an easy volume to browse."
—*School Library Journal*, Jun '07

"I don't believe there are any other books written in such easy to understand language that encompass such a breadth of topics. This is a complete revision of the book and is an excellent resource for parents and teens."
—*Doody's Review Service*, 2007

Adult Health Concerns Sourcebook

Basic Consumer Health Information about Medical and Mental Concerns of Adults, Including Facts about Choosing Healthcare Providers, Navigating Insurance Options, Maintaining Wellness, Preventing Cancer, Heart Disease, Stroke, Diabetes, and Osteoporosis, and Understanding Aging-Related Health Concerns, Including Menopause, Cognitive Changes, and Changes in the Coronary and Vascular Systems

Along with Tips on Caring for Aging Parents and Dealing with Health-Related Work and Travel Issues, a Glossary, and a Directory of Resources for Additional Help and Information

Edited by Sandra J. Judd. 648 pages. 2008. 978-0-7808-0999-4.

"Provides a thorough list of topics that are important to adult health and for caregivers."
—*CHOICE*, Nov '08

"Written in easy-to-understand language . . . the content is well-organized and is intended to aid adults in making health care-related decisions."
—*AORN Journal*, Dec '08

AIDS Sourcebook, 4th Edition

Basic Consumer Health Information about Human Immunodeficiency Virus (HIV) and Acquired Immunodeficiency Syndrome (AIDS), Featuring Updated Statistics and Facts about Risks, Prevention, Screening, Diagnosis, Treatments, Side Effects, and Complications, and Including a Section about the Impact of HIV/AIDS on the Health of Women, Children, and Adolescents

Along with Tips on Managing Life with AIDS, Reports on Current Research Initiatives and Clinical Trials, a Glossary of Related Terms, and Resource Directories for Further Help and Information

Edited by Ivy L. Alexander. 680 pages. 2008. 978-0-7808-0997-0.

SEE ALSO Contagious Diseases Sourcebook, 2nd Edition

Alcoholism Sourcebook, 2nd Edition

Basic Consumer Health Information about Alcohol Use, Abuse, and Dependence, Featuring Facts about the Physical, Mental, and Social Health Effects of Alcohol Addiction, Including Alcoholic Liver Disease, Pancreatic Disease, Cardiovascular Disease, Neurological Disorders, and the Effects of Drinking during Pregnancy

Along with Information about Alcohol Treatment, Medications, and Recovery Programs, in Addition to Tips for Reducing the Prevalence of Underage Drinking, Statistics about Alcohol Use, a Glossary of Related Terms, and Directories of Resources for More Help and Information

Edited by Amy L. Sutton. 625 pages. 2007. 978-0-7808-0942-0.

"A comprehensive look at the adverse effects of alcohol on people of all ages . . . It serves to whet the reader's appetite to continue learning using other resources. It is practical, easy to read, and enlightening, and is the first book a lay person should consult to learn about alcoholism."
—*Doody's Review Service, 2007*

"Should be a basic acquisition for any serious public or college-level library including health reference titles for general-interest readers."
—*California Bookwatch, Feb '07*

SEE ALSO *Drug Abuse Sourcebook, 2nd Edition*

Allergies Sourcebook, 3rd Edition

Basic Consumer Health Information about Allergic Disorders, Such as Anaphylaxis, Hives, Eczema, Rhinitis, Sinusitis, and Conjunctivitis, and Their Triggers, Including Pollen, Mold, Dust Mites, Animal Dander, Insects, Chemicals, Food, Food Additives, and Medications

Along with Advice about the Diagnosis and Treatment of Allergy Symptoms, a Glossary of Related Terms, a Directory of Resources for Help and Information, and Suggestions for Additional Reading

Edited by Amy L. Sutton. 588 pages. 2007. 978-0-7808-0950-5.

SEE ALSO *Asthma Sourcebook, 2nd Edition*

Alzheimer Disease Sourcebook, 4th Edition

Basic Consumer Health Information about Alzheimer Disease, Other Dementias, and Related Disorders, Including Multi-Infarct Dementia, Dementia with Lewy Bodies, Fronto-temporal Dementia (Pick Disease), Wernicke-Korsakoff Syndrome (Alcohol-Related Dementia), AIDS Dementia Complex, Huntington Disease, Creutzfeldt-Jacob Disease, and Delirium

Along with Information about Coping with Memory Loss and Forgetfulness, Maintaining

Skills, and Long-Term Planning for People with Dementia, and Suggestions Addressing Common Caregiver Concerns, Updated Information about Current Research Efforts, a Glossary of Related Terms, and Directories of Sources for Additional Help and Information

Edited by Karen Bellenir. 603 pages. 2008. 978-0-7808-1001-3.

"An invaluable resource for persons who have received a diagnosis, for caregivers, and for family members dealing with this insidious disease. It is recommended for public, community college, and ready-reference sections in academic libraries."
—*ARBAonline, Jul '08*

SEE ALSO *Brain Disorders Sourcebook, 2nd Edition*

Arthritis Sourcebook, 2nd Edition

Basic Consumer Health Information about Osteoarthritis, Rheumatoid Arthritis, Other Rheumatic Disorders, Infectious Forms of Arthritis, and Diseases with Symptoms Linked to Arthritis, Featuring Facts about Diagnosis, Pain Management, and Surgical Therapies

Along with Coping Strategies, Research Updates, a Glossary, and Resources for Additional Help and Information

Edited by Amy L. Sutton. 567 pages. 2004. 978-0-7808-0667-2.

"This easy-to-read volume is recommended for consumer health collections within public or academic libraries."
—*E-Streams, May '05*

"As expected, this updated edition continues the excellent reputation of this series in providing sound, usable health information. . . . Highly recommended."
—*American Reference Books Annual, 2005*

Asthma Sourcebook, 2nd Edition

Basic Consumer Health Information about the Causes, Symptoms, Diagnosis, and Treatment of Asthma in Infants, Children, Teenagers, and Adults, Including Facts about Different Types of Asthma, Common Co-Occurring Conditions, Asthma Management Plans, Triggers, Medications, and Medication Delivery Devices

Along with Asthma Statistics, Research Up-dates, a Glossary, a Directory of Asthma-Related Resources, and More

Edited by Karen Bellenir. 581 pages. 2006. 978-0-7808-0866-9.

Attention Deficit Disorder Sourcebook

Basic Consumer Health Information about Attention Deficit/Hyperactivity Disorder in Children and Adults, Including Facts about Causes, Symptoms, Diagnostic Criteria, and Treatment Options Such as Medications, Behavior Therapy, Coaching, and Homeopathy

Along with Reports on Current Research Initiatives, Legal Issues, and Government Regulations, and Featuring a Glossary of Related Terms, Internet Resources, and a List of Additional Reading Material

Edited by Dawn D. Matthews. 447 pages. 2002. 978-0-7808-0624-5.

"Recommended reference source."
—Booklist, Jan '03

SEE ALSO *Learning Disabilities Sourcebook, 3rd Edition*

Autism and Pervasive Developmental Disorders Sourcebook

Basic Consumer Health Information about Autism Spectrum and Pervasive Developmental Disorders, Such as Classical Autism, Asperger Syndrome, Rett Syndrome, and Childhood Disintegrative Disorder, Including Information about Related Genetic Disorders and Medical Problems and Facts about Causes, Screening Methods, Diagnostic Criteria, Treatments and Interventions, and Family and Education Issues

Along with a Glossary of Related Terms, Tips for Evaluating the Validity of Health Claims, and a Directory of Resources for Additional Help and Information

Edited by Sandra J. Judd. 603 pages. 2007. 978-0-7808-0953-6.

"Recommended for public libraries"
—SciTech Book News, Mar '08

SEE ALSO *Learning Disabilities Sourcebook, 3rd Edition*

Back and Neck Disorders Sourcebook, 2nd Edition

Basic Consumer Health Information about Spinal Pain, Spinal Cord Injuries, and Related Disorders, Such as Degenerative Disk Disease, Osteoarthritis, Scoliosis, Sciatica, Spina Bifida, and Spinal Stenosis, and Featuring Facts about Maintaining Spinal Health, Self-Care, Pain Management, Rehabilitative Care, Chiropractic Care, Spinal Surgeries, and Complementary Therapies

Along with Suggestions for Preventing Back and Neck Pain, a Glossary of Related Terms, and a Directory of Resources

Edited by Amy L. Sutton. 607 pages. 2004. 978-0-7808-0738-9.

"Recommended. ...An easy to use, comprehensive medical reference book."
—E-Streams, Sep '05

"For anyone who has back or neck problems, this book is ideal. Its easy-to-understand language and variety of topics makes this sourcebook a worthwhile read. The price...is reasonable for the amount of information contained in the book"
—Occupational Therapy in Health Care, 2007

Blood and Circulatory Disorders Sourcebook, 2nd Edition

Basic Consumer Health Information about the Blood and Circulatory System and Related Disorders, Such as Anemia and Other Hemoglobin Diseases, Cancer of the Blood and Associated Bone Marrow Disorders, Clotting and Bleeding Problems, and Conditions That Affect the Veins, Blood Vessels, and Arteries, Including Facts about the Donation and Transplantation of Bone Marrow, Stem Cells, and Blood and Tips for Keeping the Blood and Circulatory System Healthy

Along with a Glossary of Related Terms and Resources for Additional Help and Information

Edited by Amy L. Sutton. 634 pages. 2005. 978-0-7808-0746-4.

"Highly recommended pick for basic consumer health reference holdings at all levels."
—The Bookwatch, Aug '05

Brain Disorders Sourcebook, 2nd Edition

Basic Consumer Health Information about Acquired and Traumatic Brain Injuries, Infections of the Brain, Epilepsy and Seizure Disorders, Cerebral Palsy, and Degenerative Neurological Disorders, Including Amyotrophic Lateral Sclerosis (ALS), Dementias, Multiple Sclerosis, and More

Along with Information on the Brain's Structure and Function, Treatment and Rehabilitation Options, Reports on Current Research Initiatives, a Glossary of Terms Related to Brain Disorders and Injuries, and a Directory of Sources for Further Help and Information

Edited by Sandra J. Judd. 600 pages. 2005. 978-0-7808-0744-0.

"This easy-to-read volume provides up-to-date health information... Recommended for consumer health collections within public or academic libraries."

—*E-Streams, Feb '06*

SEE ALSO *Alzheimer Disease Sourcebook, 4th Edition*

Breast Cancer Sourcebook, 3rd Edition

Basic Consumer Health Information about Breast Health and Breast Cancer, Including Facts about Environmental, Genetic, and Other Risk Factors, Prevention Efforts, Screening and Diagnostic Methods, Surgical Treatment Options and Other Care Choices, Complementary and Alternative Therapies, and Post-Treatment Concerns

Along with Statistical Data, News about Research Advances, a Glossary of Related Terms, and Directories of Resources for Additional Information and Support

Edited by Karen Bellenir. 606 pages. 2009. 978-0-7808-1030-3.

SEE ALSO *Cancer Sourcebook for Women, 3rd Edition, Women's Health Concerns Sourcebook, 3rd Edition*

Breastfeeding Sourcebook

Basic Consumer Health Information about the Benefits of Breastmilk, Preparing to Breastfeed, Breastfeeding as a Baby Grows,

Nutrition, and More, Including Information on Special Situations and Concerns Such as Mastitis, Illness, Medications, Allergies, Multiple Births, Prematurity, Special Needs, and Adoption

Along with a Glossary and Resources for Additional Help and Information

Edited by Jenni Lynn Colson. 367 pages. 2002. 978-0-7808-0332-9.

SEE ALSO *Pregnancy and Birth Sourcebook, 2nd Edition*

Burns Sourcebook

Basic Consumer Health Information about Various Types of Burns and Scalds, Including Flame, Heat, Cold, Electrical, Chemical, and Sun Burns

Along with Information on Short-Term and Long-Term Treatments, Tissue Reconstruction, Plastic Surgery, Prevention Suggestions, and First Aid

Edited by Allan R. Cook. 604 pages. 1999. 978-0-7808-0204-9.

"This is an exceptional addition to the series and is highly recommended for all consumer health collections, hospital libraries, and academic medical centers."

—*E-Streams, Mar '00*

"This key reference guide is an invaluable addition to all health care and public libraries in confronting this ongoing health issue."

—*American Reference Books Annual, 2000*

SEE ALSO *Dermatological Disorders Sourcebook, 2nd Edition*

Cancer Sourcebook, 5th Edition

Basic Consumer Health Information about Major Forms and Stages of Cancer, Featuring Facts about Head and Neck Cancers, Lung Cancers, Gastrointestinal Cancers, Genitourinary Cancers, Lymphomas, Blood Cell Cancers, Endocrine Cancers, Skin Cancers, Bone Cancers, Metastatic Cancers, and More

Along with Facts about Cancer Treatments, Cancer Risks and Prevention, a Glossary of Related Terms, Statistical Data, and a Directory of Resources for Additional Information

Edited by Karen Bellenir. 1105 pages. 2007. 978-0-7808-0947-5.

"The 5th, updated edition of *Cancer Sourcebook* should be in every public and health lending library collection... An unparalleled discussion essential for any health collections considering an all-in-one basic general reference."

—*California Bookwatch, Aug '07*

SEE ALSO *Breast Cancer Sourcebook, 3rd Edition, Cancer Sourcebook for Women, 3rd Edition, Cancer Survivorship Sourcebook, Leukemia Sourcebook*

▪

Cancer Sourcebook for Women, 3rd Edition

Basic Consumer Health Information about Leading Causes of Cancer in Women, Featuring Facts about Gynecologic Cancers and Related Concerns, Such as Breast Cancer, Cervical Cancer, Endometrial Cancer, Uterine Sarcoma, Vaginal Cancer, Vulvar Cancer, and Common Non-Cancerous Gynecologic Conditions, in Addition to Facts about Lung Cancer, Colorectal Cancer, and Thyroid Cancer in Women

Along with Information about Cancer Risk Factors, Screening and Prevention, Treatment Options, and Tips on Coping with Life after Cancer Treatment, a Glossary of Cancer Terms, and a Directory of Resources for Additional Help and Information

Edited by Amy L. Sutton. 687 pages. 2006. 978-0-7808-0867-6.

"This excellent book provides the general public with information compiled in a way that will help them to gain the knowledge they need. 4 Stars!"

—*Doody's Review Service, Dec '06*

"An indispensable reference for health consumers and cancer patients. Recommended for public libraries and academic libraries with a medical department."

—*E-Streams, Sep '08*

▪

Cancer Survivorship Sourcebook

Basic Consumer Health Information about the Physical, Educational, Emotional, Social, and Financial Needs of Cancer Patients from Diagnosis, through Cancer Treatment, and Beyond, Including Facts about Researching Specific Types of Cancer and Learning about Clinical Trials and Treatment Options, and

Featuring Tips for Coping with the Side Effects of Cancer Treatments and Adjusting to Life after Cancer Treatment Concludes

Along with Suggestions for Caregivers, Friends, and Family Members of Cancer Patients, a Glossary of Cancer Care Terms, and Directories of Related Resources

Edited by Karen Bellenir. 633 pages. 2007. 978-0-7808-0985-7.

"Well organized and comprehensive in coverage, the book speaks to issues encountered both during and after cancer treatment. Recommended for consumer health and public libraries."

—*Library Journal, Aug 1 '07*

"*Cancer Survivorship Sourcebook* will be useful to anyone who has a friend or loved one with a cancer diagnosis."

—*American Reference Books Annual, 2008*

SEE ALSO *Cancer Sourcebook, 5th Edition*

▪

Cardiovascular Diseases and Disorders Sourcebook, 3rd Edition

Basic Consumer Health Information about Heart and Vascular Diseases and Disorders, Such as Angina, Heart Attacks, Arrhythmias, Cardiomyopathy, Valve Disease, Atherosclerosis, and Aneurysms, with Information about Managing Cardiovascular Risk Factors and Maintaining Heart Health, Medications and Procedures Used to Treat Cardiovascular Disorders, and Concerns of Special Significance to Women

Along with Reports on Current Research Initiatives, a Glossary of Related Medical Terms, and a Directory of Sources for Further Help and Information

Edited by Sandra J. Judd. 687 pages. 2005. 978-0-7808-0739-6.

"This updated sourcebook is still the best first stop for comprehensive introductory information on cardiovascular diseases."

—*American Reference Books Annual, 2006*

"Recommended for public libraries and libraries supporting health care professionals."

—*E-Streams, Sep '05*

▪

Caregiving Sourcebook

Basic Consumer Health Information for Caregivers, Including a Profile of Caregivers, Caregiving Responsibilities and Concerns, Tips for Specific Conditions, Care Environments, and the Effects of Caregiving

Along with Facts about Legal Issues, Financial Information, and Future Planning, a Glossary, and a Listing of Additional Resources

Edited by Joyce Brennfleck Shannon. 583 pages. 2001. 978-0-7808-0331-2.

"Essential for most collections."
—Library Journal, Apr 1 '02

"An ideal addition to the reference collection of any public library. Health sciences information professionals may also want to acquire the *Caregiving Sourcebook* for their hospital or academic library for use as a ready reference tool by health care workers interested in aging and caregiving."
—E-Streams, Jan '02

Child Abuse Sourcebook, 2nd Edition

Basic Consumer Health Information about the Physical, Sexual, and Emotional Abuse of Children, Neglect, Münchhausen Syndrome by Proxy (MSBP), and Shaken Baby Syndrome, and Featuring Facts about Withholding Medical Care, Corporal Punishment, Child Maltreatment in Youth Sports, and Parental Substance Abuse

Along with Information about Child Protective Services, Foster Care, Adoption, Parenting Challenges, Abuse Prevention Programs, and Intervention, Treatment, and Recovery Guidelines, a Glossary of Related Terms, and Resources for Additional Help and Information

Edited by Joyce Brennfleck Shannon. 600 pages. 2009. 978-0-7808-1037-2.

SEE ALSO Domestic Violence Sourcebook, 3rd Edition

Childhood Diseases and Disorders Sourcebook, 2nd Edition

Basic Consumer Health Information about the Physical, Mental, and Developmental Health of Pre-Adolescent Children, Including Facts about Infectious Diseases, Asthma, Allergies, Diabetes, and Other Acute and Chronic Conditions Affecting the Gastrointestinal Tract, Ears, Nose, Throat, Liver, Kidneys, Heart, Blood, Brain, Muscles, Bones, and Skin

Along with Reports on Recommended Childhood Vaccinations, Wellness Guidelines, a Glossary of Related Medical Terms, and a List of Resources for Parents

Edited by Sandra J. Judd. 694 pages. 2009. 978-0-7808-1031-0.

SEE ALSO Healthy Children Sourcebook

Colds, Flu and Other Common Ailments Sourcebook

Basic Consumer Health Information about Common Ailments and Injuries, Including Colds, Coughs, the Flu, Sinus Problems, Headaches, Fever, Nausea and Vomiting, Menstrual Cramps, Diarrhea, Constipation, Hemorrhoids, Back Pain, Dandruff, Dry and Itchy Skin, Cuts, Scrapes, Sprains, Bruises, and More

Along with Information about Prevention, Self-Care, Choosing a Doctor, Over-the-Counter Medications, Folk Remedies, and Alternative Therapies, and Including a Glossary of Important Terms and a Directory of Resources for Further Help and Information

Edited by Chad T. Kimball. 622 pages. 2001. 978-0-7808-0435-7.

"A good starting point for research on common illnesses. It will be a useful addition to public and consumer health library collections."
—American Reference Books Annual, 2002

"Will prove valuable to any library seeking to maintain a current, comprehensive reference collection of health resources. . . Excellent reference."
—The Bookwatch, Aug '01

Communication Disorders Sourcebook

Basic Information about Deafness and Hearing Loss, Speech and Language Disorders, Voice Disorders, Balance and Vestibular Disorders, and Disorders of Smell, Taste, and Touch

Edited by Linda M. Ross. 533 pages. 1996. 978-0-7808-0077-9.

"This is skillfully edited and is a welcome resource for the layperson. It should be found in every public and medical library."
—*Booklist Health Sciences Supplement, Oct '97*

Complementary and Alternative Medicine Sourcebook, 3rd Edition

Basic Consumer Health Information about Complementary and Alternative Medical Therapies, Including Acupuncture, Ayurveda, Traditional Chinese Medicine, Herbal Medicine, Homeopathy, Naturopathy, Biofeedback, Hypnotherapy, Yoga, Art Therapy, Aromatherapy, Clinical Nutrition, Vitamin and Mineral Supplements, Chiropractic, Massage, Reflexology, Crystal Therapy, Therapeutic Touch, and More

Along with Facts about Alternative and Complementary Treatments for Specific Conditions Such as Cancer, Diabetes, Osteoarthritis, Chronic Pain, Menopause, Gastrointestinal Disorders, Headaches, and Mental Illness, a Glossary, and a Resource List for Additional Help and Information

Edited by Sandra J. Judd. 630 pages. 2006. 978-0-7808-0864-5.

"A 'must' reference for any serious healthcare collection. Public library holdings, too, will welcome it as a popular reference."
—*California Bookwatch, Oct '06*

"Both basic and informative at the same time. . . a useful resource for health care professionals as well as consumers interested in learning more information about CAM therapies."
—*AORN Journal, Jan '08*

"A quality, indexed, referenced guideline for many alternative practices that are quite popular around the world...It is neatly organized to find facts quickly, is peer-reviewed, and stays current with the most recent advances."
—*Journal of Dental Hygiene, Jul '07*

Congenital Disorders Sourcebook, 2nd Edition

Basic Consumer Health Information about Nonhereditary Birth Defects and Disorders Related to Prematurity, Gestational Injuries, Congenital Infections, and Birth Complications, Including Heart Defects, Hydrocephalus, Spina Bifida, Cleft Lip and Palate, Cerebral Palsy, and More

Along with Facts about the Prevention of Birth Defects, Fetal Surgery and Other Treatment Options, Research Initiatives, a Glossary of Related Terms, and Resources for Additional Information and Support

Edited by Sandra J. Judd. 619 pages. 2007. 978-0-7808-0945-1.

"Congenital Disorders Sourcebook provides an excellent, non-technical overview of many aspects of pregnancy with the focus on congenital disorders."
—*American Reference Books Annual, 2008*

"An excellent readable reference aimed at the lay public for difficult to understand medical problems. An excellent starting point for the interested parent or family member who may then be motivated to seek more information."
—*Doody's Review Service, 2007*

SEE ALSO *Pregnancy and Birth Sourcebook, 2nd Edition*

Contagious Diseases Sourcebook, 2nd Edition

Basic Consumer Health Information about Diseases Spread from Person to Person through Direct Physical Contact, Airborne Transmissions, Sexual Contact, or Contact with Blood or Other Body Fluids, Including Pneumococcal, Staphylococcal, and Streptococcal Diseases, Colds, Influenza, Lice, Measles, Mumps, Tuberculosis, and Others

Along with Facts about Self-Care and Over-the-Counter Medications, Antibiotics and Drug Resistance, Disease Prevention, Vaccines, and Bioterrorism, a Glossary, and a Directory of Resources for More Information

Edited by Joyce Brennfleck Shannon. 600 pages. 2009. 978-0-7808-1075-4.

SEE ALSO *AIDS Sourcebook, 4th Edition, Hepatitis Sourcebook*

Cosmetic and Reconstructive Surgery Sourcebook, 2nd Edition

Basic Consumer Information about Plastic Surgery and Non-Surgical Appearance-Enhancing Procedures, Including Facts about Botulinum Toxin, Collagen Replacement, Dermabrasion,

Chemical Peels, Eyelid Surgery, Nose Reshaping, Lip Augmentation, Liposuction, Breast Enlargement and Reduction, Tummy Tucking, and Other Skin, Hair, Facial, and Body Shaping Procedures

Along with Information about Reconstructive Procedures for Congenital Disorders, Disfiguring Diseases, Burns, and Traumatic Injuries, a Glossary of Related Terms, and a Directory of Additional Resources

Edited by Karen Bellenir. 483 pages. 2007. 978-0-7808-0951-2.

"A practical guide for health care consumers and health care workers. . . . This easy-to-read reference guide would be useful for novice and veteran health care consumers, surgical technology students, nursing students, and perioperative nurses new to plastic and reconstructive surgery. It also may be helpful for medical-surgical nurses as a guide for patient teaching in their practices."

—AORN Journal, Aug '08

SEE ALSO Surgery Sourcebook, 2nd Edition

Death and Dying Sourcebook, 2nd Edition

Basic Consumer Health Information about End-of-Life Care and Related Perspectives and Ethical Issues, Including End-of-Life Symptoms and Treatments, Pain Management, Quality-of-Life Concerns, the Use of Life Support, Patients' Rights and Privacy Issues, Advance Directives, Physician-Assisted Suicide, Caregiving, Organ and Tissue Donation, Autopsies, Funeral Arrangements, and Grief

Along with Statistical Data, Information about the Leading Causes of Death, a Glossary, and Directories of Support Groups and Other Resources

Edited by Joyce Brennfleck Shannon. 626 pages. 2006. 978-0-7808-0871-3.

Dental Care and Oral Health Sourcebook, 3rd Edition

Basic Consumer Health Information about Dental Care and Oral Health Throughout the Lifespan, Including Facts about Cavities, Bad Breath, Cold and Canker Sores, Dry Mouth,

Toothaches, Gum Disease, Malocclusion, Temporomandibular Joint and Muscle Disorders, Oral Cancers, and Dental Emergencies

Along with Information about Mouth Hygiene, Crowns, Bridges, Implants, and Fillings, Surgical, Orthodontic, and Cosmetic Dental Procedures, Pain Management, Health Conditions that Impact Oral Care, a Glossary of Related Terms, and a Directory of Additional Resources

Edited by Amy L. Sutton. 619 pages. 2008. 978-0-7808-1032-7.

Depression Sourcebook, 2nd Edition

Basic Consumer Health Information about Unipolar Depression, Bipolar Disorder, Dysthymia, Seasonal Affective Disorder, Postpartum Depression, and Other Depressive Disorders, Including Facts about Populations at Special Risk, Coexisting Medical Conditions, Symptoms, Treatment Options, and Suicide Prevention

Along with Statistical Data, a Glossary of Related Terms, and a Directory of Resources for Additional Help and Information

Edited by Sandra J. Judd. 646 pages. 2008. 978-0-7808-1003-7.

"Recommended for public libraries."
—ARBAonline, Nov '08

SEE ALSO Mental Health Disorders Sourcebook, 4th Edition

Dermatological Disorders Sourcebook, 2nd Edition

Basic Consumer Health Information about Conditions and Disorders Affecting the Skin, Hair, and Nails, Such as Acne, Rosacea, Rashes, Dermatitis, Pigmentation Disorders, Birthmarks, Skin Cancer, Skin Injuries, Psoriasis, Scleroderma, and Hair Loss, Including Facts about Medications and Treatments for Dermatological Disorders and Tips for Maintaining Healthy Skin, Hair, and Nails

Along with Information about How Aging Affects the Skin, a Glossary of Related Terms, and a Directory of Resources for Additional Help and Information

Edited by Amy L. Sutton. 617 pages. 2006. 978-0-7808-0795-2.

"Helpfully brings together. . . sources in one convenient place, saving the user hours of research time."
—*American Reference Books Annual, 2006*

SEE ALSO *Burns Sourcebook*

Diabetes Sourcebook, 4th Edition

Basic Consumer Health Information about Type 1 and Type 2 Diabetes Mellitus, Gestational Diabetes, Monogenic Forms of Diabetes, and Insulin Resistance, with Guidelines for Lifestyle Modifications and the Medical Management of Diabetes, Including Facts about Insulin, Insulin Delivery Devices, Oral Diabetes Medications, Self-Monitoring of Blood Glucose, Meal Planning, Physical Activity Recommendations, Foot Care, and Treatment Options for People with Kidney Failure

Along with a Section about Diabetes Complications and Co-Occurring Conditions, a Glossary of Related Terms, and Directories of Resources for Additional Help and Information

Edited by Karen Bellenir. 627 pages. 2008. 978-0-7808-1005-1.

"Completely and comprehensively covering almost everything a student or physician would need to know.... well worth the investment."
—*Internet Bookwatch, Dec '08*

SEE ALSO *Endocrine and Metabolic Disorders Sourcebook, 2nd Edition*

Diet and Nutrition Sourcebook, 3rd Edition

Basic Consumer Health Information about Dietary Guidelines and the Food Guidance System, Recommended Daily Nutrient Intakes, Serving Proportions, Weight Control, Vitamins and Supplements, Nutrition Issues for Different Life Stages and Lifestyles, and the Needs of People with Specific Medical Concerns, Including Cancer, Celiac Disease, Diabetes, Eating Disorders, Food Allergies, and Cardiovascular Disease

Along with Facts about Federal Nutrition Support Programs, a Glossary of Nutrition and Dietary Terms, and Directories of Additional Resources for More Information about Nutrition

Edited by Joyce Brennfleck Shannon. 605 pages. 2006. 978-0-7808-0800-3.

"A valuable resource tool for any individual."
—*Journal of Dental Hygiene, Apr '07*

"From different recommended eating habits to reduce disease and common ailments to nutrition advice for those with specific conditions, *Diet and Nutrition Sourcebook* is especially important because so much is changing in this area, and so rapidly."
—*California Bookwatch, Jun '06*

SEE ALSO *Digestive Diseases and Disorders Sourcebook, Eating Disorders Sourcebook, 2nd Edition, Gastrointestinal Diseases and Disorders Sourcebook, 2nd Edition, Vegetarian Sourcebook*

Digestive Diseases and Disorders Sourcebook

Basic Consumer Health Information about Diseases and Disorders that Impact the Upper and Lower Digestive System, Including Celiac Disease, Constipation, Crohn's Disease, Cyclic Vomiting Syndrome, Diarrhea, Diverticulosis and Diverticulitis, Gallstones, Heartburn, Hemorrhoids, Hernias, Indigestion (Dyspepsia), Irritable Bowel Syndrome, Lactose Intolerance, Ulcers, and More

Along with Information about Medications and Other Treatments, Tips for Maintaining a Healthy Digestive Tract, a Glossary, and Directory of Digestive Diseases Organizations

Edited by Karen Bellenir. 323 pages. 2000. 978-0-7808-0327-5.

"An excellent addition to all public or patient-research libraries."
—*American Reference Books Annual, 2001*

"Recommended reference source."
—*Booklist, May '00*

SEE ALSO *Diet and Nutrition Sourcebook, 3rd Edition, Gastrointestinal Diseases and Disorders Sourcebook, 2nd Edition*

Disabilities Sourcebook

Basic Consumer Health Information about Physical and Psychiatric Disabilities, Including Descriptions of Major Causes of Disability, Assistive and Adaptive Aids, Workplace Issues, and Accessibility Concerns

Along with Information about the Americans with Disabilities Act, a Glossary, and Resources for Additional Help and Information

Edited by Dawn D. Matthews. 602 pages. 2000. 978-0-7808-0389-3.

"A must for libraries with a consumer health section."
—American Reference Books Annual, 2002

"A much needed addition to the Omnigraphics *Health Reference Series*. A current reference work to provide people with disabilities, their families, caregivers or those who work with them, a broad range of information in one volume, has not been available until now. . . . It is recommended for all public and academic library reference collections."
—E-Streams, May '01

"An excellent source book in easy-to-read format covering many current topics; highly recommended for all libraries."
—CHOICE, Jan '01

Disease Management Sourcebook

Basic Consumer Health Information about Coping with Chronic and Serious Illnesses, Navigating the Health Care System, Communicating with Health Care Providers, Assessing Health Care Quality, and Making Informed Health Care Decisions, Including Facts about Second Opinions, Hospitalization, Surgery, and Medications

Along with a Section about Children with Chronic Conditions, Information about Legal, Financial, and Insurance Issues, a Glossary of Related Terms, and Directories of Additional Resources

Edited by Joyce Brennfleck Shannon. 621 pages. 2008. 978-0-7808-1002-0.

"Consumers need to know how to manage their health care the same way they manage anything else in their lives. The text is very readable and is written for the layperson and consumer. The cost is not prohibitive. This book should be in all collections of health care libraries and public libraries."
—ARBAonline, Jul '08

"The information is very current, and the selection of font and layout make the book easy to read. A hardback that will stand up to much usage, this is an excellent resource for

consumers. . . . Recommended. General readers."
—CHOICE, Nov '08

"Intended for lay readers, this resource clarifies the many confusing and overwhelming details associated with chronic disease care. Meticulous and clearly explained, the book even includes diagrams intended to ease comprehension of over-the-counter medication labels. An essential guide to navigating the health-care rapids."
—Library Journal, Aug '08

Domestic Violence Sourcebook, 3rd Edition

Basic Consumer Health Information about Warning Signs, Risk Factors, and Health Consequences of Intimate Partner Violence, Sexual Violence and Rape, Stalking, Human Trafficking, Child Maltreatment, Teen Dating Violence, and Elder Abuse

Along with Facts about Victims and Perpetrators, Strategies for Violence Prevention, and Emergency Interventions, Safety Plans, and Financial and Legal Tips for Victims, a Glossary of Related Terms, and Directories of Resources for Additional Information and Support

Edited by Joyce Brennfleck Shannon. 600 pages. 2009. 978-0-7808-1038-9.

SEE ALSO Child Abuse Sourcebook, 2nd Edition

Drug Abuse Sourcebook, 2nd Edition

Basic Consumer Health Information about Illicit Substances of Abuse and the Misuse of Prescription and Over-the-Counter Medications, Including Depressants, Hallucinogens, Inhalants, Marijuana, Stimulants, and Anabolic Steroids

Along with Facts about Related Health Risks, Treatment Programs, Prevention Programs, a Glossary of Abuse and Addiction Terms, a Glossary of Drug-Related Street Terms, and a Directory of Resources for More Information

Edited by Catherine Ginther. 581 pages. 2004. 978-0-7808-0740-2.

"Commendable for organizing useful, normally scattered government and association-produced data into a logical sequence."
—American Reference Books Annual, 2006

"An excellent library reference."
—*The Bookwatch, May '05*

SEE ALSO *Alcoholism Sourcebook, 2nd Edition*

Ear, Nose, and Throat Disorders Sourcebook, 2nd Edition

Basic Consumer Health Information about Disorders of the Ears, Hearing Loss, Vestibular Disorders, Nasal and Sinus Problems, Throat and Vocal Cord Disorders, and Otolaryngologic Cancers, Including Facts about Ear Infections and Injuries, Genetic and Congenital Deafness, Sensorineural Hearing Disorders, Tinnitus, Vertigo, Ménière Disease, Rhinitis, Sinusitis, Snoring, Sore Throats, Hoarseness, and More

Along with Reports on Current Research Initiatives, a Glossary of Related Medical Terms, and a Directory of Sources for Further Help and Information

Edited by Sandra J. Judd. 631 pages. 2007. 978-0-7808-0872-0.

"A resource book for the general public that provides comprehensive coverage of basic up-to-date medical information about the causes, symptoms, diagnosis, and treatment of diseases and disorders that affect the ears, nose, sinuses, throat, and voice. . . . The majority of information is presented in question and answer format, much like questions a patient might ask of a health care provider. An extensive index facilitates the reader's ability to easily access information on any specific topic."
—*Journal of Dental Hygiene, Oct '07*

"A handy compilation of information on common and some not so common ailments of the ears, nose, and throat."
—*Doody's Review Service, 2007*

Eating Disorders Sourcebook, 2nd Edition

Basic Consumer Health Information about Anorexia Nervosa, Bulimia, Binge Eating, Compulsive Exercise, Female Athlete Triad, and Other Eating Disorders, Including Facts about Body Image and Other Cultural and Age-Related Risk Factors, Prevention Efforts, Adverse Health Effects, Treatment Options, and the Recovery Process

Along with Guidelines for Healthy Weight Control, a Glossary, and Directories of Additional Resources

Edited by Joyce Brennfleck Shannon. 557 pages. 2007. 978-0-7808-0948-2.

"Recommended for the reference collection of large public libraries."
—*American Reference Books Annual, 2008*

"A basic health reference any health or general library needs."
—*Internet Bookwatch, Jun '07*

SEE ALSO *Diet and Nutrition Sourcebook, 3rd Edition, Mental Health Disorders Sourcebook, 4th Edition*

Emergency Medical Services Sourcebook

Basic Consumer Health Information about Preventing, Preparing for, and Managing Emergency Situations, When and Who to Call for Help, What to Expect in the Emergency Room, the Emergency Medical Team, Patient Issues, and Current Topics in Emergency Medicine

Along with Statistical Data, a Glossary, and Sources of Additional Help and Information

Edited by Jenni Lynn Colson. 472 pages. 2002. 978-0-7808-0420-3.

"Handy and convenient for home, public, school, and college libraries. Recommended."
—*CHOICE, Apr '03*

"This reference can provide the consumer with answers to most questions about emergency care in the United States, or it will direct them to a resource where the answer can be found."
—*American Reference Books Annual, 2003*

SEE ALSO *Injury and Trauma Sourcebook*

Endocrine and Metabolic Disorders Sourcebook, 2nd Edition

Basic Consumer Health Information about Hormonal and Metabolic Disorders that Affect the Body's Growth, Development, and Functioning, Including Disorders of the Pancreas, Ovaries and Testes, and Pituitary, Thyroid, Parathyroid, and Adrenal Glands, with Facts about Growth Disorders, Addison Disease, Cushing Syndrome, Conn Syndrome, Diabetic Disorders, Multiple Endocrine Neoplasia, Inborn Errors of Metabolism, and More

Along with Information about Endocrine Functioning, Diagnostic and Screening Tests, a Glossary of Related Terms, and Directories of Additional Resources

Edited by Joyce Brennfleck Shannon. 597 pages. 2007. 978-0-7808-0952-9.

SEE ALSO Diabetes Sourcebook, 4th Edition

Environmental Health Sourcebook, 2nd Edition

Basic Consumer Health Information about the Environment and Its Effect on Human Health, Including the Effects of Air Pollution, Water Pollution, Hazardous Chemicals, Food Hazards, Radiation Hazards, Biological Agents, Household Hazards, Such as Radon, Asbestos, Carbon Monoxide, and Mold, and Information about Associated Diseases and Disorders, Including Cancer, Allergies, Respiratory Problems, and Skin Disorders

Along with Information about Environmental Concerns for Specific Populations, a Glossary of Related Terms, and Resources for Further Help and Information

Edited by Dawn D. Matthews. 650 pages. 2003. 978-0-7808-0632-0.

"Recommended for teenage and adult students and readers, and for public and academic libraries, as well as any library focusing on consumer health."
—E-Streams, May '04

"This recently updated edition continues the level of quality and the reputation of the numerous other volumes in Omnigraphics' **Health Reference Series.**"
—American Reference Books Annual, 2004

Ethnic Diseases Sourcebook

Basic Consumer Health Information for Ethnic and Racial Minority Groups in the United States, Including General Health Indicators and Behaviors, Ethnic Diseases, Genetic Testing, the Impact of Chronic Diseases, Women's Health, Mental Health Issues, and Preventive Health Care Services

Along with a Glossary and a Listing of Additional Resources

Edited by Joyce Brennfleck Shannon. 648 pages. 2001. 978-0-7808-0336-7.

"Not many books have been written on this topic to date, and the Ethnic Diseases Sourcebook is a strong addition to the list. It will be an important introductory resource for health consumers, students, health care personnel, and social scientists. It is recommended for public, academic, and large hospital libraries."
—American Reference Books Annual, 2002

"Will prove valuable to any library seeking to maintain a current, comprehensive reference collection of health resources. . . . An excellent source of health information about genetic disorders which affect particular ethnic and racial minorities in the U.S."
—The Bookwatch, Aug '01

Eye Care Sourcebook, 3rd Edition

Basic Consumer Health Information about Eye Care and Eye Disorders, Including Facts about the Diagnosis, Prevention, and Treatment of Refractive Disorders, Cataracts, Glaucoma, Macular Degeneration, and Problems Affecting the Cornea, Retina, and Lacrimal Glands

Along with Advice about Preventing Eye Injuries and Tips for Living with Low Vision or Blindness, a Glossary of Related Terms, and Directories of Resources for More Help and Information

Edited by Amy L. Sutton. 646 pages. 2008. 978-0-7808-1000-6.

Family Planning Sourcebook

Basic Consumer Health Information about Planning for Pregnancy and Contraception, Including Traditional Methods, Barrier Methods, Hormonal Methods, Permanent Methods, Future Methods, Emergency Contraception, and Birth Control Choices for Women at Each Stage of Life

Along with Statistics, a Glossary, and Sources of Additional Information

Edited by Amy Marcaccio Keyzer. 503 pages. 2001. 978-0-7808-0379-4.

"Recommended for public, health, and undergraduate libraries as part of the circulating collection."
—E-Streams, Mar '02

"Will prove valuable to any library seeking to maintain a current, comprehensive reference collection of health resources. . . . Excellent reference."

—The Bookwatch, Aug '01

SEE ALSO *Pregnancy and Birth Sourcebook, 2nd Edition*

Fitness and Exercise Sourcebook, 3rd Edition

Basic Consumer Health Information about the Physical and Mental Benefits of Fitness, Including Cardiorespiratory Endurance, Muscular Strength, Muscular Endurance, and Flexibility, with Facts about Sports Nutrition and Exercise-Related Injuries and Tips about Physical Activity and Exercises for People of All Ages and for People with Health Concerns

Along with Advice on Selecting and Using Exercise Equipment, Maintaining Exercise Motivation, a Glossary of Related Terms, and a Directory of Resources for More Help and Information

Edited by Amy L. Sutton. 635 pages. 2007. 978-0-7808-0946-8.

"Updates the consumer information on the physical and mental benefits of physical activity throughout the lifespan offered in earlier editions. . . . Recommended. All readers; all levels."

—CHOICE, Oct '07

"An exceptionally well-rounded coverage perfect for any concerned about developing and understanding a fitness program."

—California Bookwatch, Jun '07

SEE ALSO *Sports Injuries Sourcebook, 3rd Edition*

Food Safety Sourcebook

Basic Consumer Health Information about the Safe Handling of Meat, Poultry, Seafood, Eggs, Fruit Juices, and Other Food Items, and Facts about Pesticides, Drinking Water, Food Safety Overseas, and the Onset, Duration, and Symptoms of Foodborne Illnesses, Including Types of Pathogenic Bacteria, Parasitic Protozoa, Worms, Viruses, and Natural Toxins

Along with the Role of the Consumer, the Food Handler, and the Government in Food Safety; a Glossary, and Resources for Additional Help and Information

Edited by Dawn D. Matthews. 327 pages. 1999. 978-0-7808-0326-8.

"Recommended reference source."

—Booklist, May '00

"This book takes the complex issues of food safety and foodborne pathogens and presents them in an easily understood manner. [It does] an excellent job of covering a large and often confusing topic."

— American Reference Books Annual, 2000

Forensic Medicine Sourcebook

Basic Consumer Information for the Layperson about Forensic Medicine, Including Crime Scene Investigation, Evidence Collection and Analysis, Expert Testimony, Computer-Aided Criminal Identification, Digital Imaging in the Courtroom, DNA Profiling, Accident Reconstruction, Autopsies, Ballistics, Drugs and Explosives Detection, Latent Fingerprints, Product Tampering, and Questioned Document Examination

Along with Statistical Data, a Glossary of Forensics Terminology, and Listings of Sources for Further Help and Information

Edited by Annemarie S. Muth. 574 pages. 1999. 978-0-7808-0232-2.

"Given the expected widespread interest in its content and its easy to read style, this book is recommended for most public and all college and university libraries."

—E-Streams, Feb '01

"A wealth of information, useful statistics, references are up-to-date and extremely complete. This wonderful collection of data will help students who are interested in a career in any type of forensic field. It is a great resource for attorneys who need information about types of expert witnesses needed in a particular case. It also offers useful information for fiction and nonfiction writers whose work involves a crime. A fascinating compilation. All levels."

—CHOICE, Jan '00

"There are several items that make this book attractive to consumers who are seeking certain forensic data. . . . This is a useful current

source for those seeking general forensic medical answers."
—*American Reference Books Annual, 2000*

Gastrointestinal Diseases and Disorders Sourcebook, 2nd Edition

Basic Consumer Health Information about the Upper and Lower Gastrointestinal (GI) Tract, Including the Esophagus, Stomach, Intestines, Rectum, Liver, and Pancreas, with Facts about Gastroesophageal Reflux Disease, Gastritis, Hernias, Ulcers, Celiac Disease, Diverticulitis, Irritable Bowel Syndrome, Hemorrhoids, Gastrointestinal Cancers, and Other Diseases and Disorders Related to the Digestive Process

Along with Information about Commonly Used Diagnostic and Surgical Procedures, Statistics, Reports on Current Research Initiatives and Clinical Trials, a Glossary, and Resources for Additional Help and Information

Edited by Sandra J. Judd. 654 pages. 2006. 978-0-7808-0798-3.

"The text is designed for the general reader seeking information on prevention, disease warning signs, diagnostic and therapeutic questions. . . . It is an excellent resource for the general reader to conveniently locate credible, coordinated and indexed information. . . . The sourcebook will prove very helpful for patients, caregivers and should be available in every physician waiting room."
—*Doody's Review Service, 2006*

SEE ALSO *Diet and Nutrition Sourcebook, 3rd Edition, Digestive Diseases and Disorders Sourcebook*

Genetic Disorders Sourcebook, 4th Edition

Basic Consumer Health Information about Hereditary Diseases and Disorders, Including Facts about the Human Genome, Genetic Inheritance Patterns, Disorders Associated with Specific Genes, Such as Sickle Cell Disease, Hemophilia, and Cystic Fibrosis, Chromosome Disorders, Such as Down Syndrome, Fragile X Syndrome, and Turner Syndrome, and Complex Diseases and Disorders Resulting from the Interaction of Environmental and Genetic Factors, Such as Allergies, Cancer, and Obesity

Along with Facts about Genetic Testing, Suggestions for Parents of Children with Special Needs, Reports on Current Research Initiatives, a Glossary of Genetic Terminology, and Resources for Additional Help and Information

Edited by Sandra J. Judd. 600 pages. 2009. 978-0-7808-1076-1.

Head Trauma Sourcebook

Basic Information for the Layperson about Open-Head and Closed-Head Injuries, Treatment Advances, Recovery, and Rehabilitation

Along with Reports on Current Research Initiatives

Edited by Karen Bellenir. 414 pages. 1997. 978-0-7808-0208-7.

Headache Sourcebook

Basic Consumer Health Information about Migraine, Tension, Cluster, Rebound and Other Types of Headaches, with Facts about the Cause and Prevention of Headaches, the Effects of Stress and the Environment, Headaches during Pregnancy and Menopause, and Childhood Headaches

Along with a Glossary and Other Resources for Additional Help and Information

Edited by Dawn D. Matthews. 342 pages. 2002. 978-0-7808-0337-4.

"Highly recommended for academic and medical reference collections."
—*Library Bookwatch, Sep '02*

SEE ALSO *Pain Sourcebook, 3rd Edition*

Healthy Aging Sourcebook

Basic Consumer Health Information about Maintaining Health through the Aging Process, Including Advice on Nutrition, Exercise, and Sleep, Help in Making Decisions about Midlife Issues and Retirement, and Guidance Concerning Practical and Informed Choices in Health Consumerism

Along with Data Concerning the Theories of Aging, Different Experiences in Aging by Minority Groups, and Facts about Aging Now and Aging in the Future; and Featuring a Glossary, a Guide to Consumer Help, Additional Suggested Reading, and Practical Resource Directory

Edited by Jenifer Swanson. 537 pages. 1999. 978-0-7808-0390-9.

"Recommended reference source."
— *Booklist, Feb '00*

SEE ALSO Physical and Mental Issues in Aging Sourcebook

Healthy Children Sourcebook

Basic Consumer Health Information about the Physical and Mental Development of Children between the Ages of 3 and 12, Including Routine Health Care, Preventative Health Services, Safety and First Aid, Healthy Sleep, Dental Care, Nutrition, and Fitness, and Featuring Parenting Tips on Such Topics as Bedwetting, Choosing Day Care, Monitoring TV and Other Media, and Establishing a Foundation for Substance Abuse Prevention

Along with a Glossary of Commonly Used Pediatric Terms and Resources for Additional Help and Information.

Edited by Chad T. Kimball. 624 pages. 2003. 978-0-7808-0247-6.

"Should be required reading for parents and teachers."
— *E-Streams, Jun '04*

"It is hard to imagine that any other single resource exists that would provide such a comprehensive guide of timely information on health promotion and disease prevention for children aged 3 to 12."
— *American Reference Books Annual, 2004*

"This easy-to-read volume is a tremendous resource."
— *AORN Journal, May '05*

SEE ALSO Childhood Diseases and Disorders Sourcebook, 2nd Edition

Healthy Heart Sourcebook for Women

Basic Consumer Health Information about Cardiac Issues Specific to Women, Including Facts about Major Risk Factors and Prevention, Treatment and Control Strategies, and Important Dietary Issues

Along with a Special Section Regarding the Pros and Cons of Hormone Replacement Therapy and Its Impact on Heart Health, and Additional Help, Including Recipes, a Glossary, and a Directory of Resources

Edited by Dawn D. Matthews. 321 pages. 2000. 978-0-7808-0329-9.

"A good reference source and recommended for all public, academic, medical, and hospital libraries."
— *Medical Reference Services Quarterly, Summer '01*

"Contains very important information about coronary artery disease that all women should know. The information is current and presented in an easy-to-read format. The book will make a good addition to any library."
— *American Medical Writers Association Journal, Summer '00*

SEE ALSO Cardiovascular Diseases and Disorders Sourcebook, 3rd Edition, Women's Health Concerns Sourcebook, 3rd Edition

Hepatitis Sourcebook

Basic Consumer Health Information about Hepatitis A, Hepatitis B, Hepatitis C, and Other Forms of Hepatitis, Including Autoimmune Hepatitis, Alcoholic Hepatitis, Nonalcoholic Steatohepatitis, and Toxic Hepatitis, with Facts about Risk Factors, Screening Methods, Diagnostic Tests, and Treatment Options

Along with Information on Liver Health, Tips for People Living with Chronic Hepatitis, Reports on Current Research Initiatives, a Glossary of Terms Related to Hepatitis, and a Directory of Sources for Further Help and Information

Edited by Sandra J. Judd. 570 pages. 2006. 978-0-7808-0749-5.

"The breadth of information found in this one book would not be readily found in another source. Highly recommended."
— *American Reference Books Annual, 2006*

SEE ALSO Contagious Diseases Sourcebook

Household Safety Sourcebook

Basic Consumer Health Information about Household Safety, Including Information about Poisons, Chemicals, Fire, and Water Hazards in the Home

Along with Advice about the Safe Use of Home Maintenance Equipment, Choosing Toys and Nursery Furniture, Holiday and Recreation Safety, a Glossary, and Resources for Further Help and Information

Edited by Dawn D. Matthews. 587 pages. 2002. 978-0-7808-0338-1.

"As a sourcebook on household safety this book meets its mark. It is encyclopedic in scope and covers a wide range of safety issues that are commonly seen in the home."
—*E-Streams, Jul '02*

Hypertension Sourcebook

Basic Consumer Health Information about the Causes, Diagnosis, and Treatment of High Blood Pressure, with Facts about Consequences, Complications, and Co-Occurring Disorders, Such as Coronary Heart Disease, Diabetes, Stroke, Kidney Disease, and Hypertensive Retinopathy, and Issues in Blood Pressure Control, Including Dietary Choices, Stress Management, and Medications

Along with Reports on Current Research Initiatives and Clinical Trials, a Glossary, and Resources for Additional Help and Information

Edited by Dawn D. Matthews and Karen Bellenir. 588 pages. 2004. 978-0-7808-0674-0.

"Academic, public, and medical libraries will want to add the *Hypertension Sourcebook* to their collections."
—*E-Streams, Aug '05*

"The strength of this source is the wide range of information given about hypertension."
—*American Reference Books Annual, 2005*

SEE ALSO Stroke Sourcebook, 2nd Edition

Immune System Disorders Sourcebook, 2nd Edition

Basic Consumer Health Information about Disorders of the Immune System, Including Immune System Function and Response, Diagnosis of Immune Disorders, Information about Inherited Immune Disease, Acquired Immune Disease, and Autoimmune Diseases, Including Primary Immune Deficiency, Acquired Immunodeficiency Syndrome (AIDS), Lupus, Multiple Sclerosis, Type 1 Diabetes, Rheumatoid Arthritis, and Graves' Disease

Along with Treatments, Tips for Coping with Immune Disorders, a Glossary, and a Directory of Additional Resources

Edited by Joyce Brennfleck Shannon. 643 pages. 2005. 978-0-7808-0748-8.

"Highly recommended for academic and public libraries."
—*American Reference Books Annual, 2006*

"The updated second edition is a 'must' for any consumer health library seeking a solid resource covering the treatments, symptoms, and options for immune disorder sufferers. . . . An excellent guide."
—*MBR Bookwatch, Jan '06*

SEE ALSO AIDS Sourcebook, 4th Edition, Arthritis Sourcebook, 2nd Edition

Infant and Toddler Health Sourcebook

Basic Consumer Health Information about the Physical and Mental Development of Newborns, Infants, and Toddlers, Including Neonatal Concerns, Nutrition Recommendations, Immunization Schedules, Common Pediatric Disorders, Assessments and Milestones, Safety Tips, and Advice for Parents and Other Caregivers

Along with a Glossary of Terms and Resource Listings for Additional Help

Edited by Jenifer Swanson. 570 pages. 2000. 978-0-7808-0246-9.

"As a reference for the general public, this would be useful in any library."
—*E-Streams, May '01*

"Recommended reference source."
—*Booklist, Feb '01*

Infectious Diseases Sourcebook

Basic Consumer Health Information about Non-Contagious Bacterial, Viral, Prion, Fungal, and Parasitic Diseases Spread by Food and Water, Insects and Animals, or Environmental Contact, Including Botulism, E. Coli, Encephalitis, Legionnaires' Disease, Lyme Disease, Malaria, Plague, Rabies, Salmonella, Tetanus, and Others, and Facts about Newly Emerging Diseases, Such as Hantavirus, Mad Cow Disease, Monkeypox, and West Nile Virus

Along with Information about Preventing Disease Transmission, the Threat of Bioterrorism, and Current Research Initiatives, with a Glossary and Directory of Resources for More Information

Edited by Karen Bellenir. 610 pages. 2004. 978-0-7808-0675-7.

"This reference continues the excellent tradition of the *Health Reference Series* in consolidating a wealth of information on a selected topic into a format that is easy to use and accessible to the general public."
—*American Reference Books Annual, 2005*

"Recommended for public and academic libraries."
—*E-Streams, Jan '05*

Injury and Trauma Sourcebook

Basic Consumer Health Information about the Impact of Injury, the Diagnosis and Treatment of Common and Traumatic Injuries, Emergency Care, and Specific Injuries Related to Home, Community, Workplace, Transportation, and Recreation

Along with Guidelines for Injury Prevention, a Glossary, and a Directory of Additional Resources

Edited by Joyce Brennfleck Shannon. 675 pages. 2002. 978-0-7808-0421-0.

"Practitioners should be aware of guides such as this in order to facilitate their use by patients and their families."
—*Doody's Health Sciences Book Review Journal, Sep-Oct '02*

"Recommended reference source."
—*Booklist, Sep '02*

"Highly recommended for academic and medical reference collections."
—*Library Bookwatch, Sep '02*

SEE ALSO *Emergency Medical Services Sourcebook, Sports Injuries Sourcebook, 3rd Edition*

Learning Disabilities Sourcebook, 3rd Edition

Basic Consumer Health Information about Dyslexia, Auditory and Visual Processing Disorders, Communication Disorders, Dyscalculia, Dysgraphia, and Other Conditions That Impede Learning, Including Attention Deficit/Hyperactivity Disorder, Autism Spectrum Disorders, Hearing and Visual Impairments, Chromosome-Based Disorders, and Brain Injury

Along with Facts about Brain Function, Assessment, Therapy and Remediation, Accommodations, Assistive Technology, Legal Protections, and Tips about Family Life, School Transitions, and Employment Strategies, a Glossary of Related Terms, and Directories of Additional Resources

Edited by Joyce Brennfleck Shannon. 613 pages. 2009. 978-0-7808-1039-6.

SEE ALSO *Attention Deficit Disorder Sourcebook, Autism and Pervasive Developmental Disorders Sourcebook*

Leukemia Sourcebook

Basic Consumer Health Information about Adult and Childhood Leukemias, Including Acute Lymphocytic Leukemia (ALL), Chronic Lymphocytic Leukemia (CLL), Acute Myelogenous Leukemia (AML), Chronic Myelogenous Leukemia (CML), and Hairy Cell Leukemia, and Treatments Such as Chemotherapy, Radiation Therapy, Peripheral Blood Stem Cell and Marrow Transplantation, and Immunotherapy

Along with Tips for Life During and After Treatment, a Glossary, and Directories of Additional Resources

Edited by Joyce Brennfleck Shannon. 564 pages. 2003. 978-0-7808-0627-6.

"Unlike other medical books for the layperson, . . . the language does not talk down to the reader. . . . This volume is highly recommended for all libraries."
—*American Reference Books Annual, 2004*

"A fine title which ranges from diagnosis to alternative treatments, staging, and tips for life during and after diagnosis."
—*The Bookwatch, Dec '03*

SEE ALSO *Cancer Sourcebook, 5th Edition*

Liver Disorders Sourcebook

Basic Consumer Health Information about the Liver and How It Works; Liver Diseases, Including Cancer, Cirrhosis, Hepatitis, and Toxic and Drug Related Diseases; Tips for Maintaining a Healthy Liver; Laboratory Tests, Radiology Tests, and Facts about Liver Transplantation

Along with a Section on Support Groups, a Glossary, and Resource Listings

Edited by Joyce Brennfleck Shannon. 580 pages. 2000. 978-0-7808-0383-1.

"This title is recommended for health sciences and public libraries with consumer health collections."
—E-Streams, Oct '00

"Recommended reference source."
—Booklist, Jun '00

SEE ALSO Gastrointestinal Diseases and Disorders Sourcebook, 2nd Edition, Hepatitis Sourcebook

Lung Disorders Sourcebook

Basic Consumer Health Information about Emphysema, Pneumonia, Tuberculosis, Asthma, Cystic Fibrosis, and Other Lung Disorders, Including Facts about Diagnostic Procedures, Treatment Strategies, Disease Prevention Efforts, and Such Risk Factors as Smoking, Air Pollution, and Exposure to Asbestos, Radon, and Other Agents

Along with a Glossary and Resources for Additional Help and Information

Edited by Dawn D. Matthews. 657 pages. 2002. 978-0-7808-0339-8.

"Highly recommended for academic and medical reference collections."
—Library Bookwatch, Sep '02

SEE ALSO Respiratory Disorders Sourcebook, 2nd Edition

Medical Tests Sourcebook, 3rd Edition

Basic Consumer Health Information about X-Rays, Blood Tests, Stool and Urine Tests, Biopsies, Mammography, Endoscopic Procedures, Ultrasound Exams, Computed Tomography, Magnetic Resonance Imaging (MRI), Nuclear Medicine, Genetic Testing, Home-Use Tests, and More

Along with Facts about Preventive Care and Screening Test Guidelines, Screening and Assessment Tests Associated with Such Specific Concerns as Cancer, Heart Disease, Allergies, Diabetes, Thyroid Disfunction, and Infertility, a Glossary of Related Terms, and a Directory of Resources for Additional Help and Information

Edited by Karen Bellenir. 627 pages. 2008. 978-0-7808-1040-2

"This volume has a wide scope that makes it useful . . . Can be a valuable reference guide."
—ARBAonline, Nov '08

Men's Health Concerns Sourcebook, 3rd Edition

Basic Consumer Health Information about Wellness in Men and Gender-Related Differences in Health, With Facts about Heart Disease, Cancer, Traumatic Injury, and Other Leading Causes of Death in Men, Reproductive Concerns, Sexual Dysfunction, Disorders of the Prostate, Penis, and Testes, Sex-Linked Genetic Disorders, and Other Medical and Mental Concerns of Men

Along with Statistical Data, a Glossary of Related Terms, and a Directory of Resources for Additional Information

Edited by Sandra J. Judd. 600 pages. 2009. 978-0-7808-1033-4.

SEE ALSO Prostate and Urological Disorders Sourcebook

Mental Health Disorders Sourcebook, 4th Edition

Basic Consumer Health Information about the Causes and Symptoms of Mental Health Problems, Including Depression, Bipolar Disorder, Anxiety Disorders, Posttraumatic Stress Disorder, Obsessive-Compulsive Disorder, Eating Disorders, Addictions, and Personality and Psychotic Disorders

Along with Information about Medications and Treatments, Mental Health Concerns in Children, Adolescents, and Adults, Tips on Living with Mental Health Disorders, a Glossary of Related Terms, and a Directory of Resources for Additional Help and Information

Edited by Amy L. Sutton. 600 pages. 2009. 978-0-7808-1041-9.

SEE ALSO Depression Sourcebook, 2nd Edition, Stress-Related Disorders Sourcebook, 2nd Edition

Mental Retardation Sourcebook

Basic Consumer Health Information about Mental Retardation and Its Causes, Including

Down Syndrome, Fetal Alcohol Syndrome, Fragile X Syndrome, Genetic Conditions, Injury, and Environmental Sources

Along with Preventive Strategies, Parenting Issues, Educational Implications, Health Care Needs, Employment and Economic Matters, Legal Issues, a Glossary, and a Resource Listing for Additional Help and Information

Edited by Joyce Brennfleck Shannon. 627 pages. 2000. 978-0-7808-0377-0.

"Public libraries will find the book useful for reference and as a beginning research point for students, parents, and caregivers."
—American Reference Books Annual, 2001

"The strength of this work is that it compiles many basic fact sheets and addresses for further information in one volume. It is intended and suitable for the general public."
—E-Streams, Nov '00

"An invaluable overview."
—Reviewer's Bookwatch, Jul '00

Movement Disorders Sourcebook, 2nd Edition

Basic Consumer Health Information about the Symptoms and Causes of Movement Disorders, Including Parkinson Disease, Amyotrophic Lateral Sclerosis, Cerebral Palsy, Muscular Dystrophy, Multiple Sclerosis, Myasthenia, Myoclonus, Spina Bifida, Dystonia, Essential Tremor, Choreatic Disorders, Huntington Disease, Tourette Syndrome, and Other Disorders That Cause Slowed, Absent, or Excessive Movements

Along with Information about Surgical and Nonsurgical Interventions, Physical Therapies, Strategies for Independent Living, a Glossary of Related Terms, and a Directory of Resources for Additional Help and Information

Edited by Amy L. Sutton. 600 pages. 2009. 978-0-7808-1034-1.

SEE ALSO Multiple Sclerosis Sourcebook, Muscular Dystrophy Sourcebook

Multiple Sclerosis Sourcebook

Basic Consumer Health Information about Multiple Sclerosis (MS) and Its Effects on Mobility, Vision, Bladder Function, Speech,

Swallowing, and Cognition, Including Facts about Risk Factors, Causes, Diagnostic Procedures, Pain Management, Drug Treatments, and Physical and Occupational Therapies

Along with Guidelines for Nutrition and Exercise, Tips on Choosing Assistive Equipment, Information about Disability, Work, Financial, and Legal Issues, a Glossary of Related Terms, and a Directory of Additional Resources

Edited by Joyce Brennfleck Shannon. 553 pages. 2007. 978-0-7808-0998-7.

SEE ALSO Movement Disorders Sourcebook, 2nd Edition

Muscular Dystrophy Sourcebook

Basic Consumer Health Information about Congenital, Childhood-Onset, and Adult-Onset Forms of Muscular Dystrophy, Such as Duchenne, Becker, Emery-Dreifuss, Distal, Limb-Girdle, Facioscapulohumeral (FSHD), Myotonic, and Ophthalmoplegic Muscular Dystrophies, Including Facts about Diagnostic Tests, Medical and Physical Therapies, Management of Co-Occurring Conditions, and Parenting Guidelines

Along with Practical Tips for Home Care, a Glossary, and Directories of Additional Resources

Edited by Joyce Brennfleck Shannon. 552 pages. 2004. 978-0-7808-0676-4.

"This book is highly recommended for public and academic libraries as well as health care offices that support the information needs of patients and their families."
—E-Streams, Apr '05

"Excellent reference."
—The Bookwatch, Jan '05

SEE ALSO Movement Disorders Sourcebook, 2nd Edition

Obesity Sourcebook

Basic Consumer Health Information about Diseases and Other Problems Associated with Obesity, and Including Facts about Risk Factors, Prevention Issues, and Management Approaches

Along with Statistical and Demographic Data, Information about Special Populations,

Research Updates, a Glossary, and Source Listings for Further Help and Information

Edited by Wilma Caldwell and Chad T. Kimball. 360 pages. 2001. 978-0-7808-0333-6.

"The book synthesizes the reliable medical literature on obesity into one easy-to-read and useful resource for the general public."
—American Reference Books Annual, 2002

"Well suited for the health reference collection of a public library or an academic health science library that serves the general population."
—E-Streams, Sep '01

Osteoporosis Sourcebook

Basic Consumer Health Information about Primary and Secondary Osteoporosis and Juvenile Osteoporosis and Related Conditions, Including Fibrous Dysplasia, Gaucher Disease, Hyperthyroidism, Hypophosphatasia, Myeloma, Osteopetrosis, Osteogenesis Imperfecta, and Paget's Disease

Along with Information about Risk Factors, Treatments, Traditional and Non-Traditional Pain Management, a Glossary of Related Terms, and a Directory of Resources

Edited by Allan R. Cook. 568 pages. 2001. 978-0-7808-0239-1.

"This resource is recommended as a great reference source for public, health, and academic libraries, and is another triumph for the editors of Omnigraphics."
—American Reference Books Annual, 2002

"Will prove valuable to any library seeking to maintain a current, comprehensive reference collection of health resources. . . . From prevention to treatment and associated conditions, this provides an excellent survey."
—The Bookwatch, Aug '01

SEE ALSO Healthy Aging Sourcebook, Women's Health Concerns Sourcebook, 3rd Edition

Pain Sourcebook, 3rd Edition

Basic Consumer Health Information about Acute and Chronic Pain, Including Nerve Pain, Bone Pain, Muscle Pain, Cancer Pain, and Disorders Characterized by Pain, Such as Arthritis, Temporomandibular Muscle and Joint (TMJ) Disorder, Carpal Tunnel Syndrome, Headaches, Heartburn, Sciatica, and Shingles, and Facts about Diagnostic Tests and Treatment Options for Pain, Including Over-the-Counter and Prescription Drugs, Physical Rehabilitation, Injection and Infusion Therapies, Implantable Technologies, and Complementary Medicine

Along with Tips for Living with Pain, a Glossary of Related Terms, and a Directory of Additional Resources

Edited by Joyce Brennfleck Shannon. 644 pages. 2008. 978-0-7808-1006-8.

"Excellent for ready-reference users and can be used for beginning students in health fields . . . appropriate for the consumer health collection in both public and academic libraries."
—ARBAonline, Nov '08

Pediatric Cancer Sourcebook

Basic Consumer Health Information about Leukemias, Brain Tumors, Sarcomas, Lymphomas, and Other Cancers in Infants, Children, and Adolescents, Including Descriptions of Cancers, Treatments, and Coping Strategies

Along with Suggestions for Parents, Caregivers, and Concerned Relatives, a Glossary of Cancer Terms, and Resource Listings

Edited by Edward J. Prucha. 575 pages. 1999. 978-0-7808-0245-2.

"An excellent source of information. Recommended for public, hospital, and health science libraries with consumer health collections."
—E-Streams, Jun '00

"A valuable addition to all libraries specializing in health services and many public libraries."
—American Reference Books Annual, 2000

SEE ALSO Childhood Diseases and Disorders Sourcebook, 2nd Edition, Healthy Children Sourcebook

Physical and Mental Issues in Aging Sourcebook

Basic Consumer Health Information on Physical and Mental Disorders Associated with the Aging Process, Including Concerns about Cardiovascular Disease, Pulmonary Disease, Oral Health, Digestive Disorders, Musculoskeletal and Skin Disorders, Metabolic

Changes, Sexual and Reproductive Issues, and Changes in Vision, Hearing, and Other Senses

Along with Data about Longevity and Causes of Death, Information on Acute and Chronic Pain, Descriptions of Mental Concerns, a Glossary of Terms, and Resource Listings for Additional Help

Edited by Jenifer Swanson. 660 pages. 1999. 978-0-7808-0233-9.

"This is a treasure of health information for the layperson."
—CHOICE Health Sciences Supplement, May '00

"Recommended for public libraries."
—American Reference Books Annual, 2000

SEE ALSO Healthy Aging Sourcebook

Podiatry Sourcebook, 2nd Edition

Basic Consumer Health Information about Disorders, Diseases, and Deformities that Affect the Foot and Ankle, Including Sprains, Corns, Calluses, Bunions, Plantar Warts, Plantar Fasciitis, Neuromas, Clubfoot, Flat Feet, Achilles Tendonitis, and Much More

Along with Information about Selecting a Foot Care Specialist, Foot Fitness, Shoes and Socks, Diagnostic Tests and Corrective Procedures, Financial Assistance for Corrective Devices, a Glossary of Related Terms, and a Directory of Resources for Additional Help and Information

Edited by Ivy L. Alexander. 516 pages. 2007. 978-0-7808-0944-4.

"An excellent resource. . . . Although there have been various types of 'foot books' published in the past, none are as comprehensive as this one. 5 Stars (out of 5)!"
—Doody's Review Service, 2007

"Perfect for both health libraries and general-interest lending collections."
—Internet Bookwatch, Jul '07

Pregnancy and Birth Sourcebook, 3rd Edition

Basic Consumer Health Information about Pregnancy and Fetal Development, Including Facts about Fertility and Conception, Physical and Emotional Changes during Pregnancy, Prenatal Care and Diagnostic Tests, High-Risk Pregnancies and Complications, Labor, Delivery, and the Postpartum Period

Along with Tips on Maintaining Health and Wellness during Pregnancy and Caring for Newborn Infants, a Glossary of Related Terms, and Directories of Resources for Additional Help and Information

Edited by Amy L. Sutton. 600 pages. 2009. 978-0-7808-1074-7.

SEE ALSO Breastfeeding Sourcebook, Congenital Disorders Sourcebook, 2nd Edition, Family Planning Sourcebook, Women's Health Concerns Sourcebook, 3rd Edition

Prostate and Urological Disorders Sourcebook

Basic Consumer Health Information about Urogenital and Sexual Disorders in Men, Including Prostate and Other Andrological Cancers, Prostatitis, Benign Prostatic Hyperplasia, Testicular and Penile Trauma, Cryptorchidism, Peyronie Disease, Erectile Dysfunction, and Male Factor Infertility, and Facts about Commonly Used Tests and Procedures, Such as Prostatectomy, Vasectomy, Vasectomy Reversal, Penile Implants, and Semen Analysis

Along with a Glossary of Andrological Terms and a Directory of Resources for Additional Information

Edited by Karen Bellenir. 604 pages. 2006. 978-0-7808-0797-6.

"Certain to be a popular pick among library reference holdings. . . . No prior knowledge is assumed for any of the conditions or terms herein, making it a most accessible general-interest reference."
—California Bookwatch, Apr '06

SEE ALSO Men's Health Concerns Sourcebook, 3rd Edition, Urinary Tract and Kidney Diseases and Disorders Sourcebook, 2nd Edition

Prostate Cancer Sourcebook

Basic Consumer Health Information about Prostate Cancer, Including Information about the Associated Risk Factors, Detection, Diagnosis, and Treatment of Prostate Cancer

Along with Information on Non-Malignant Prostate Conditions, and Featuring a Section

749

Listing Support and Treatment Centers and a Glossary of Related Terms

Edited by Dawn D. Matthews. 340 pages. 2001. 978-0-7808-0324-4.

"Recommended reference source."
—*Booklist, Jan '02*

"A valuable resource for health care consumers seeking information on the subject. . . . All text is written in a clear, easy-to-understand language that avoids technical jargon. Any library that collects consumer health resources would strengthen their collection with the addition of the *Prostate Cancer Sourcebook*."
—*American Reference Books Annual, 2002*

SEE ALSO *Cancer Sourcebook, 5th Edition, Men's Health Concerns Sourcebook, 3rd Edition*

Rehabilitation Sourcebook

Basic Consumer Health Information about Rehabilitation for People Recovering from Heart Surgery, Spinal Cord Injury, Stroke, Orthopedic Impairments, Amputation, Pulmonary Impairments, Traumatic Injury, and More, Including Physical Therapy, Occupational Therapy, Speech/Language Therapy, Massage Therapy, Dance Therapy, Art Therapy, and Recreational Therapy

Along with Information on Assistive and Adaptive Devices, a Glossary, and Resources for Additional Help and Information

Edited by Dawn D. Matthews. 519 pages. 2000. 978-0-7808-0236-0.

"This is an excellent resource for public library reference and health collections."
—*American Reference Books Annual, 2001*

"Recommended reference source."
—*Booklist, May '00*

Respiratory Disorders Sourcebook, 2nd Edition

Basic Consumer Health Information about Infectious, Inflammatory, and Chronic Conditions Affecting the Lungs and Respiratory System, Including Pneumonia, Bronchitis, Influenza, Tuberculosis, Sarcoidosis, Asthma, Cystic Fibrosis, Chronic Obstructive Pulmonary Disease, Lung Abscesses, Pulmonary Embolism, Occupational Lung Diseases, and Other Bacterial, Viral, and Fungal Infections

Along with Facts about the Structure and Function of the Lungs and Airways, Methods of Diagnosing Respiratory Disorders, and Treatment and Rehabilitation Options, a Glossary of Related Terms, and a Directory of Resources for Additional Help and Information

Edited by Sandra L. Judd. 638 pages. 2008. 978-0-7808-1007-5.

"A great addition for public and school libraries because it provides concise health information . . . readers can start with this reference source and get satisfactory answers before proceeding to other medical reference tools for more in depth information . . . A good guide for health education on lung disorders."
—*ARBAonline, Nov '08*

SEE ALSO *Lung Disorders Sourcebook*

Sexually Transmitted Diseases Sourcebook, 4th Edition

Basic Consumer Health Information about Chlamydial Infections, Gonorrhea, Hepatitis, Herpes, HIV/AIDS, Human Papillomavirus, Pubic Lice, Scabies, Syphilis, Trichomoniasis, Vaginal Infections, and Other Sexually Transmitted Diseases, Including Facts about Risk Factors, Symptoms, Diagnosis, Treatment, and the Prevention of Sexually Transmitted Infections

Along with Updates on Current Research Initiatives, a Glossary of Related Terms, and Resources for Additional Help and Information

Edited by Laura Larsen. 600 pages. 2009. 978-0-7808-1073-0.

SEE ALSO *AIDS Sourcebook, 4th Edition, Contagious Diseases Sourcebook, 2nd Edition, Men's Health Concerns Sourcebook, 3rd Edition, Women's Health Concerns Sourcebook, 3rd Edition*

Sleep Disorders Sourcebook, 2nd Edition

Basic Consumer Health Information about Sleep and Sleep Disorders, Including Insomnia, Sleep Apnea, Restless Legs Syndrome, Narcolepsy, Parasomnias, and Other Health Problems That Affect Sleep, Plus Facts about Diagnostic Procedures, Treatment Strategies,

Sleep Medications, and Tips for Improving Sleep Quality

Along with a Glossary of Related Terms and Resources for Additional Help and Information

Edited by Amy L. Sutton. 567 pages. 2005. 978-0-7808-0743-3.

"This book will be useful for just about everybody, especially the 40 million Americans with sleep disorders."
—*American Reference Books Annual, 2006*

"A welcome addition to public libraries and consumer health libraries."
—*Medical Reference Services Quarterly, Summer '06*

Smoking Concerns Sourcebook

Basic Consumer Health Information about Nicotine Addiction and Smoking Cessation, Featuring Facts about the Health Effects of Tobacco Use, Including Lung and Other Cancers, Heart Disease, Stroke, and Respiratory Disorders, Such as Emphysema and Chronic Bronchitis

Along with Information about Smoking Prevention Programs, Suggestions for Achieving and Maintaining a Smoke-Free Lifestyle, Statistics about Tobacco Use, Reports on Current Research Initiatives, a Glossary of Related Terms, and Directories of Resources for Additional Help and Information

Edited by Karen Bellenir. 595 pages. 2004. 978-0-7808-0323-7.

"Provides everything needed for the student or general reader seeking practical details on the effects of tobacco use."
—*The Bookwatch, Mar '05*

"Public libraries and consumer health care libraries will find this work useful."
—*American Reference Books Annual, 2005*

SEE ALSO *Respiratory Disorders Sourcebook, 2nd Edition*

Sports Injuries Sourcebook, 3rd Edition

Basic Consumer Health Information about Sprains and Strains, Fractures, Growth Plate Injuries, Overtraining Injuries, and Injuries to the Head, Face, Shoulders, Elbows, Hands, Spinal Column, Knees, Ankles, and Feet, and with Facts about Heat-Related Illness, Steroids and Sport Supplements, Protective Equipment, Diagnostic Procedures, Treatment Options, and Rehabilitation

Along with a Glossary of Related Terms and a Directory of Resources for Additional Help and Information

Edited by Sandra J. Judd. 623 pages. 2007. 978-0-7808-0949-9.

SEE ALSO *Fitness and Exercise Sourcebook, 3rd Edition*

Stress-Related Disorders Sourcebook, 2nd Edition

Basic Consumer Health Information about Stress and Stress-Related Disorders, Including Types of Stress, Sources of Acute and Chronic Stress, the Impact of Stress on the Body's Systems, and Mental and Emotional Health Problems Associated with Stress, Such as Depression, Anxiety Disorders, Substance Abuse, Posttraumatic Stress Disorder, and Suicide

Along with Advice about Getting Help for Stress-Related Disorders, Information about Stress Management Techniques, a Glossary of Stress-Related Terms, and a Directory of Resources for Additional Help and Information

Edited by Amy L. Sutton. 608 pages. 2007. 978-0-7808-0996-3.

"Accessible to the lay reader. Highly recommended for medical and psychiatric collections."
—*Library Journal, Mar '08*

"Well-written for a general readership, the 2nd Edition of *Stress-Related Disorders Sourcebook* is a useful addition to the health reference literature."
—*American Reference Books Annual, 2008*

SEE ALSO *Mental Health Disorders Sourcebook, 4th Edition*

Stroke Sourcebook, 2nd Edition

Basic Consumer Health Information about Stroke, Including Ischemic, Hemorrhagic, and Mini Strokes, as Well as Risk Factors, Prevention Guidelines, Diagnostic Tests, Medications and

Surgical Treatments, and Complications of Stroke

Along with Rehabilitation Techniques and Innovations, Tips on Staying Healthy and Maintaining Independence after Stroke, a Glossary of Related Terms, and a Directory of Resources for Stroke Survivors and Their Families

Edited by Amy L. Sutton. 626 pages. 2008. 978-0-7808-1035-8.

"An encyclopedic handbook on stroke that is written in a language the layperson can understand. . . . This is one of the most helpful, readable books on stroke. This volume is highly recommended and should be in every medical, hospital and public library; in addition, every family practitioner should have a copy in his or her office."
— *ARBAonline Dec '08*

SEE ALSO *Hypertension Sourcebook*

▣

Surgery Sourcebook, 2nd Edition

Basic Consumer Health Information about Common Inpatient and Outpatient Surgeries, Including Critical Care and Trauma, Gastrointestinal, Gynecologic and Obstetric, Cardiac and Vascular, Neurologic, Ophthalmologic, Orthopedic, Reconstructive and Cosmetic, and Other Major and Minor Surgeries

Along with Information about Anesthesia and Pain Relief Options, Risks and Complications, Postoperative Recovery Concerns, and Innovative Surgical Techniques and Tools, a Glossary of Related Terms, and a Directory of Additional Resources

Edited by Amy L. Sutton. 645 pages. 2008. 978-0-7808-1004-4.

"Large public libraries and medical libraries would benefit from this material in their reference collections."
— *ARBAonline Aug '08*

SEE ALSO *Cosmetic and Reconstructive Surgery Sourcebook, 2nd Edition*

▣

Thyroid Disorders Sourcebook

Basic Consumer Health Information about Disorders of the Thyroid and Parathyroid Glands, Including Hypothyroidism, Hyperthyroidism,

Graves Disease, Hashimoto Thyroiditis, Thyroid Cancer, and Parathyroid Disorders, Featuring Facts about Symptoms, Risk Factors, Tests, and Treatments

Along with Information about the Effects of Thyroid Imbalance on Other Body Systems, Environmental Factors That Affect the Thyroid Gland, a Glossary, and a Directory of Additional Resources

Edited by Joyce Brennfleck Shannon. 573 pages. 2005. 978-0-7808-0745-7.

"Recommended for consumer health collections."
— *American Reference Books Annual, 2006*

"Highly recommended pick for basic consumer health reference holdings at all levels."
— *The Bookwatch, Aug '05*

SEE ALSO *Endocrine and Metabolic Disorders Sourcebook, 2nd Edition*

▣

Transplantation Sourcebook

Basic Consumer Health Information about Organ and Tissue Transplantation, Including Physical and Financial Preparations, Procedures and Issues Relating to Specific Solid Organ and Tissue Transplants, Rehabilitation, Pediatric Transplant Information, the Future of Transplantation, and Organ and Tissue Donation

Along with a Glossary and Listings of Additional Resources

Edited by Joyce Brennfleck Shannon. 610 pages. 2002. 978-0-7808-0322-0.

"Recommended for libraries with an interest in offering consumer health information."
— *E-Streams, Jul '02*

"This is a unique and valuable resource for patients facing transplantation and their families."
— *Doody's Review Service, Jun '02*

▣

Traveler's Health Sourcebook

Basic Consumer Health Information for Travelers, Including Physical and Medical Preparations, Transportation Health and Safety, Essential Information about Food and Water, Sun Exposure, Insect and Snake Bites, Camping and Wilderness Medicine, and Travel with Physical or Medical Disabilities

Along with International Travel Tips, Vaccination Recommendations, Geographical Health Issues, Disease Risks, a Glossary, and a Listing of Additional Resources

Edited by Joyce Brennfleck Shannon. 619 pages. 2000. 978-0-7808-0384-8.

"Recommended reference source."
—*Booklist, Feb '01*

"This book is recommended for any public library, any travel collection, and especially any collection for the physically disabled."
—*American Reference Books Annual, 2001*

SEE ALSO *Worldwide Health Sourcebook*

Urinary Tract and Kidney Diseases and Disorders Sourcebook, 2nd Edition

Basic Consumer Health Information about the Urinary System, Including the Bladder, Urethra, Ureters, and Kidneys, with Facts about Urinary Tract Infections, Incontinence, Congenital Disorders, Kidney Stones, Cancers of the Urinary Tract and Kidneys, Kidney Failure, Dialysis, and Kidney Transplantation

Along with Statistical and Demographic Information, Reports on Current Research in Kidney and Urologic Health, a Summary of Commonly Used Diagnostic Tests, a Glossary of Related Terms, and a Directory of Resources for Additional Help and Information

Edited by Ivy L. Alexander. 621 pages. 2005. 978-0-7808-0750-1.

"A good choice for a consumer health information library or for a medical library needing information to refer to their patients."
—*American Reference Books Annual, 2006*

SEE ALSO *Prostate and Urological Disorders Sourcebook*

Vegetarian Sourcebook

Basic Consumer Health Information about Vegetarian Diets, Lifestyle, and Philosophy, Including Definitions of Vegetarianism and Veganism, Tips about Adopting Vegetarianism, Creating a Vegetarian Pantry, and Meeting Nutritional Needs of Vegetarians, with Facts Regarding Vegetarianism's Effect on Pregnant and Lactating Women, Children, Athletes, and Senior Citizens

Along with a Glossary of Commonly Used Vegetarian Terms and Resources for Additional Help and Information

Edited by Chad T. Kimball. 337 pages. 2002. 978-0-7808-0439-5.

"Organizes into one concise volume the answers to the most common questions concerning vegetarian diets and lifestyles. This title is recommended for public and secondary school libraries."
—*E-Streams, Apr '03*

"Invaluable reference for public and school library collections alike."
—*Library Bookwatch, Apr '03*

"The articles in this volume are easy to read and come from authoritative sources. The book does not necessarily support the vegetarian diet but instead provides the pros and cons of this important decision. . . . Recommended for public libraries and consumer health libraries."
—*American Reference Books Annual, 2003*

SEE ALSO *Diet and Nutrition Sourcebook, 3rd Edition*

Women's Health Concerns Sourcebook, 3rd Edition

Basic Consumer Health Information about Issues and Trends in Women's Health and Health Conditions of Special Concern to Women, Including Endometriosis, Uterine Fibroids, Menstrual Irregularities, Menopause, Sexual Dysfunction, Infertility, Cancer in Women, and Other Such Chronic Disorders as Lupus, Fibromyalgia, and Thyroid Disease

Along with Statistical Data, Tips for Maintaining Wellness, a Glossary, and a Directory of Resources for Further Help and Information

Edited by Sandra J. Judd. 600 pages. 2009. 978-0-7808-1036-5.

SEE ALSO *Breast Cancer Sourcebook, 3rd Edition, Cancer Sourcebook for Women, 3rd Edition, Healthy Heart Sourcebook for Women, Osteoporosis Sourcebook*

Workplace Health and Safety Sourcebook

Basic Consumer Health Information about Workplace Health and Safety, Including the Effect of Workplace Hazards on the Lungs,

753

Skin, Heart, Ears, Eyes, Brain, Reproductive Organs, Musculoskeletal System, and Other Organs and Body Parts

Along with Information about Occupational Cancer, Personal Protective Equipment, Toxic and Hazardous Chemicals, Child Labor, Stress, and Workplace Violence

Edited by Chad T. Kimball. 610 pages. 2000. 978-0-7808-0231-5.

"As a reference for the general public, this would be useful in any library."
—*E-Streams, Jun '01*

"Provides helpful information for primary care physicians and other caregivers interested in occupational medicine. . . . General readers; professionals."
—*CHOICE, May '01*

Worldwide Health Source-book

Basic Information about Global Health Issues, Including Malnutrition, Reproductive Health, Disease Dispersion and Prevention, Emerging Diseases, Risky Health Behaviors, and the Leading Causes of Death

Along with Global Health Concerns for Children, Women, and the Elderly, Mental Health Issues, Research and Technology Advancements, and Economic, Environmental, and Political Health Implications, a Glossary, and a Resource Listing for Additional Help and Information

Edited by Joyce Brennfleck Shannon. 597 pages. 2001. 978-0-7808-0330-5.

"Named an Outstanding Academic Title."
—*CHOICE, Jan '02*

"Yet another handy but also unique compilation in the extensive *Health Reference Series*, this is a useful work because many of the international publications reprinted or excerpted are not readily available. Highly recommended."
—*CHOICE, Nov '01*

SEE ALSO *Traveler's Health Sourcebook*

Teen Health Series
Complete Catalog
List price $69 per volume. School and library price $62 per volume.

Abuse and Violence Information for Teens

Health Tips about the Causes and Consequences of Abusive and Violent Behavior
Including Facts about the Types of Abuse and Violence, the Warning Signs of Abusive and Violent Behavior, Health Concerns of Victims, and Getting Help and Staying Safe

Edited by Sandra Augustyn Lawton. 411 pages. 2008. 978-0-7808-1008-2.

"A useful resource for schools and organizations providing services to teens and may also be a starting point in research projects."
—*Reference and Research Book News, Aug '08*

"Violence is a serious problem for teens. . . . This resource gives teens the information they need to face potential threats and get help—either for themselves or for their friends."
—*ARBAonline, Aug '08*

Accident and Safety Information for Teens

Health Tips about Medical Emergencies, Traumatic Injuries, and Disaster Preparedness
Including Facts about Motor Vehicle Accidents, Burns, Poisoning, Firearms, Natural Disasters, National Security Threats, and More

Edited by Karen Bellenir. 420 pages. 2008. 978-0-7808-1046-4.

SEE ALSO *Sports Injuries Information for Teens, 2nd Edition*

Alcohol Information for Teens, 2nd Edition

Health Tips about Alcohol and Alcoholism
Including Facts about Alcohol's Effects on the Body, Brain, and Behavior, the Consequences of Underage Drinking, Alcohol Abuse Prevention and Treatment, and Coping with Alcoholic Parents

Edited by Lisa Bakewell. 400 pages. 2009. 978-0-7808-1043-3.

SEE ALSO *Drug Information for Teens, 2nd Edition*

Allergy Information for Teens

Health Tips about Allergic Reactions Such as Anaphylaxis, Respiratory Problems, and Rashes
Including Facts about Identifying and Managing Allergies to Food, Pollen, Mold, Animals, Chemicals, Drugs, and Other Substances

Edited by Karen Bellenir. 410 pages. 2006. 978-0-7808-0799-0.

"This is a comprehensive, readable text on the subject of allergic diseases in teenagers. 5 Stars (out of 5)!"
—*Doody's Review Service, Jun '06*

"This authoritative and useful self-help title is a solid addition to YA collections, whether for personal interest or reports."
—*School Library Journal, Jul '06*

Asthma Information for Teens

Health Tips about Managing Asthma and Related Concerns
Including Facts about Asthma Causes, Triggers, Symptoms, Diagnosis, and Treatment

Edited by Karen Bellenir. 386 pages. 2005. 978-0-7808-0770-9.

"Highly recommended for medical libraries, public school libraries, and public libraries."
—*American Reference Books Annual, 2006*

"Although this volume is nearly 400 pages long, it is so clearly written and well organized that even hesitant readers will be able to find the facts they need, whether for reports or personal information. . . . A succinct but complete resource."
—*School Library Journal, Sep '05*

Body Information for Teens

Health Tips about Maintaining Well-Being for a Lifetime

Including Facts about the Development and Functioning of the Body's Systems, Organs, and Structures and the Health Impact of Lifestyle Choices

Edited by Sandra Augustyn Lawton. 458 pages. 2007. 978-0-7808-0443-2.

Cancer Information for Teens, 2nd Edition

Health Tips about Cancer Awareness, Symptoms, Prevention, Diagnosis, and Treatment

Including Facts about Common Cancers Affecting Teens, Causes, Detection, Coping Strategies, Clinical Trials, Nutrition and Exercise, Cancer in Friends or Family, and More

Edited by Karen Bellenir and Lisa Bakewell. 400 pages. 2009. 978-0-7808-1085-3.

Complementary and Alternative Medicine Information for Teens

Health Tips about Non-Traditional and Non-Western Medical Practices

Including Information about Acupuncture, Chiropractic Medicine, Dietary and Herbal Supplements, Hypnosis, Massage Therapy, Prayer and Spirituality, Reflexology, Yoga, and More

Edited by Sandra Augustyn Lawton. 407 pages. 2007. 978-0-7808-0966-6.

"This volume covers CAM specifically for teenagers but of general use also. It should be a welcome addition to both public and academic libraries."
—*American Reference Books Annual, 2008*

"This volume provides a solid foundation for further investigation of the subject, making it useful for both public and high school libraries."
—*VOYA: Voice of Youth Advocates, Jun '07*

Diabetes Information for Teens

Health Tips about Managing Diabetes and Preventing Related Complications

Including Information about Insulin, Glucose Control, Healthy Eating, Physical Activity, and Learning to Live with Diabetes

Edited by Sandra Augustyn Lawton. 410 pages. 2006. 978-0-7808-0811-9.

"A comprehensive instructional guide for teens. . . . some of the material may also be directed towards parents or teachers. 5 stars (out of 5)!"
—*Doody's Review Service, 2006*

"Students dealing with their own diabetes or that of a friend or family member or those writing reports on the topic will find this a valuable resource."
—*School Library Journal, Aug '06*

"This text is directed to the teen population and would be an excellent library resource for a health class or for the teacher as a reference for class preparation. It can, however, serve a much wider audience. The clinical educator on diabetes may find it valuable to educate the newly diagnosed client regardless of age. It also would be an excellent reference and education tool for a preventive medicine seminar on diabetes."
—*Physical Therapy, Mar '07*

Diet Information for Teens, 2nd Edition

Health Tips about Diet and Nutrition

Including Facts about Dietary Guidelines, Food Groups, Nutrients, Healthy Meals, Snacks, Weight Control, Medical Concerns Related to Diet, and More

Edited by Karen Bellenir. 432 pages. 2006. 978-0-7808-0820-1.

"A very quick and pleasant read in spite of the fact that it is very detailed in the information it gives. . . . A book for anyone concerned about diet and nutrition."
—*American Reference Books Annual, 2007*

SEE ALSO Eating Disorders Information for Teens, 2nd Edition

Drug Information for Teens, 2nd Edition

Health Tips about the Physical and Mental Effects of Substance Abuse

Including Information about Marijuana, Inhalants, Club Drugs, Stimulants, Hallucinogens,

Opiates, Prescription and Over-the-Counter Drugs, Herbal Products, Tobacco, Alcohol, and More

Edited by Sandra Augustyn Lawton. 468 pages. 2006. 978-0-7808-0862-1.

"As with earlier installments in Omnigraphics' Teen Health Series, Drug Information for Teens is designed specifically to meet the needs and interests of middle and high school students. . . . Strongly recommended for both academic and public libraries."
—*American Reference Books Annual, 2007*

"Solid thoughtful advice is given about how to handle peer pressure, drug-related health concerns, and treatment strategies."
—*School Library Journal, Dec '06*

SEE ALSO *Alcohol Information for Teens, 2nd Edition, Tobacco Information for Teens*

Eating Disorders Information for Teens, 2nd Edition
Health Tips about Anorexia, Bulimia, Binge Eating, And Other Eating Disorders
Including Information about Risk Factors, Diagnosis and Treatment, Prevention, Related Health Concerns, and Other Issues

Edited by Sandra Augustyn Lawton. 377 pages. 2009. 978-0-7808-1044-0.

SEE ALSO *Diet Information for Teens, 2nd Edition*

Fitness Information for Teens, 2nd Edition
Health Tips about Exercise, Physical Well-Being, and Health Maintenance
Including Facts about Conditioning, Stretching, Strength Training, Body Shape and Body Image, Sports Nutrition, and Specific Activities for Athletes and Non-Athletes

Edited by Lisa Bakewell. 432 pages. 2009. 978-0-7808-1045-7.

SEE ALSO *Diet Information for Teens, 2nd Edition, Sports Injuries Information for Teens, 2nd Edition*

Learning Disabilities Information for Teens
Health Tips about Academic Skills Disorders and Other Disabilities That Affect Learning
Including Information about Common Signs of Learning Disabilities, School Issues, Learning to Live with a Learning Disability, and Other Related Issues

Edited by Sandra Augustyn Lawton. 400 pages. 2006. 978-0-7808-0796-9.

"This book provides a wealth of information for any reader interested in the signs, causes, and consequences of learning disabilities, as well as related legal rights and educational interventions. . . . Public and academic libraries should want this title for both students and general readers."
—*American Reference Books Annual, 2006*

Mental Health Information for Teens, 2nd Edition
Health Tips about Mental Wellness and Mental Illness
Including Facts about Mental and Emotional Health, Depression and Other Mood Disorders, Anxiety Disorders, Conduct Disorder, Self-Injury, Psychosis, Schizophrenia, and More

Edited by Karen Bellenir. 424 pages. 2006. 978-0-7808-0863-8.

"This excellent overview of the psychological disorders that affect teens provides clear definitions and descriptions, and discusses resources, therapies, coping mechanisms, and medications."
—*School Library Journal Curriculum Connections, Fall '07*

"A well done reference for a specific, often under-represented group."
—*Doody's Review Service, 2006*

SEE ALSO *Stress Information for Teens*

Pregnancy Information for Teens
Health Tips about Teen Pregnancy and Teen Parenting
Including Facts about Prenatal Care, Pregnancy Complications, Labor and Delivery,

Postpartum Care, Pregnancy-Related Lifestyle Concerns, and More

Edited by Sandra Augustyn Lawton. 434 pages. 2007. 978-0-7808-0984-0.

SEE ALSO Sexual Health Information for Teens, 2nd Edition

Sexual Health Information for Teens, 2nd Edition
Health Tips about Sexual Development, Reproduction, Contraception, and Sexually Transmitted Infections
Including Facts about Puberty, Sexuality, Birth Control, Chlamydia, Gonorrhea, Herpes, Human Papillomavirus, Syphilis, and More

Edited by Sandra Augustyn Lawton. 430 pages. 2008. 978-0-7808-1010-5.

"This offering represents the most up-to-date information available on an array of topics including abstinence-only sexual education and pregnancy-prevention methods. . . . The range of coverage—from puberty and anatomy to sexually transmitted diseases—is thorough and extensive. Each chapter includes a bibliographic citation, and the three back sections containing additional resources, further reading, and the index are all first-rate. . . . This volume will be well used by students in need of the facts, whether for educational or personal reasons."
—School Library Journal, Nov '08

SEE ALSO Pregnancy Information for Teens

Skin Health Information for Teens, 2nd Edition
Health Tips about Dermatological Concerns and Skin Cancer Risks
Including Facts about Acne, Warts, Allergies, and Other Conditions and Lifestyle Choices, Such as Tanning, Tattooing, and Piercing, That Affect the Skin, Nails, Scalp, and Hair

Edited by Edited by Kim Wohlenhaus. 400 pages. 2009. 978-0-7808-1042-6.

Sleep Information for Teens
Health Tips about Adolescent Sleep Requirements, Sleep Disorders, and the Effects of Sleep Deprivation

Including Facts about Why People Need Sleep, Sleep Patterns, Circadian Rhythms, Dreaming, Insomnia, Sleep Apnea, Narcolepsy, and More

Edited by Karen Bellenir. 355 pages. 2008. 978-0-7808-1009-9.

SEE ALSO Body Information for Teens

Sports Injuries Information for Teens, 2nd Edition
Health Tips about Acute, Traumatic, and Chronic Injuries in Adolescent Athletes
Including Facts about Sprains, Fractures, and Overuse Injuries, Treatment, Rehabilitation, Sport-Specific Safety Guidelines, Fitness Suggestions, and More

Edited by Karen Bellenir. 429 pages. 2008. 978-0-7808-1011-2.

"An engaging selection of informative articles about the prevention and treatment of sports injuries. . . The value of this book is that the articles have been vetted and are often augmented with inserts of useful facts, definitions of technical terms, and quick tips. Sensitive topics like injuries to genitalia are discussed openly and responsibly. This revised edition contains updated articles and defines sport more broadly than the first edition."
—School Library Journal, Nov '08

"This work will be useful in the young adult collections of public libraries as well as high school libraries. . . . A useful resource for student research."
—ARBAonline, Aug '08

SEE ALSO Accident and Safety Information for Teens

Stress Information for Teens
Health Tips about the Mental and Physical Consequences of Stress
Including Information about the Different Kinds of Stress, Symptoms of Stress, Frequent Causes of Stress, Stress Management Techniques, and More

Edited by Sandra Augustyn Lawton. 392 pages. 2008. 978-0-7808-1012-9.

"Understanding what stress is, what causes it, how the body and the mind are impacted by it, and what teens can do are the general categories addressed here. . . . The chapters are brief but informative, and the list of community-help organizations is exhaustive. Report writers will find information quickly and easily, as will those who have personal concerns. The print is clear and the format is readable, making this an accessible resource for struggling readers and researchers."

—*School Library Journal, Dec '08*

"The articles selected will specifically appeal to young adults and are designed to answer their most common questions."

—*ARBAonline, Aug '08*

SEE ALSO *Mental Health Information for Teens, 2nd Edition*

having to read the entire book. . . . The book is packed full of statistics, with sources to help students look up more."

—*School Library Journal, Sep '07*

"Pulls together a wide variety of authoritative sources to provide a comprehensive overview of tobacco use for this age group. . . . This reasonably priced reference title should be considered a necessary purchase for all public libraries and school media centers, along with academic libraries supporting teacher education."

—*American Reference Books Annual, 2008*

SEE ALSO *Drug Information for Teens, 2nd Edition*

Suicide Information for Teens

Health Tips about Suicide Causes and Prevention
Including Facts about Depression, Risk Factors, Getting Help, Survivor Support, and More

Edited by Joyce Brennfleck Shannon. 368 pages. 2005. 978-0-7808-0737-2.

"Highly Recommended for libraries serving teenagers as well as those who work with them."

—*E-Streams, Apr '06*

SEE ALSO *Mental Health Information for Teens, 2nd Edition*

Tobacco Information for Teens

Health Tips about the Hazards of Using Cigarettes, Smokeless Tobacco, and Other Nicotine Products
Including Facts about Nicotine Addiction, Immediate and Long-Term Health Effects of Tobacco Use, Related Cancers, Smoking Cessation, Tobacco Use Prevention, and Tobacco Use Statistics

Edited by Karen Bellenir. 440 pages. 2007. 978-0-7808-0976-5.

"A comprehensive resource. Each chapter is written to stand alone, so students can dip in and use the information in each section for reports or to answer personal questions without

Adolescent Health Sourcebook, 2nd Edition

Adult Health Concerns Sourcebook

AIDS Sourcebook, 4th Edition

Alcoholism Sourc...

Allergies Sourceb...

Alzheimer Diseas...

Arthritis Sourceb...

Asthma Sourcebook, 2nd Edition

Attention Deficit Disorder Sourcebook

Autism & Pervasive Developmental Disorders
    Sourcebook

Back & Neck Sourcebook, 2nd Edition

Blood & Circulatory Disorders Sourcebook, 2nd
    Edition

Brain Disorders Sourcebook, 2nd Edition

Breast Cancer Sourcebook, 3rd Edition

Breastfeeding Sourcebook

Burns Sourcebook

Cancer Sourcebook, 5th Edition

Cancer Sourcebook for Women, 3rd Edition

Cancer Survivorship Sourcebook

Cardiovascular Diseases & Disorders
    Sourcebook, 3rd Edition

Caregiving Sourcebook

Child Abuse Sourcebook

Childhood Diseases & Disorders Sourcebook,
    2nd Edition

Colds, Flu & Other Common Ailments
    Sourcebook

Communication Disorders Sourcebook

Complementary & Alternative Medicine
    Sourcebook, 3rd Edition

Congenital Disorders Sourcebook, 2nd Edition

Contagious Diseases Sourcebook

Cosmetic & Reconstructive Surgery
    Sourcebook, 2nd Edition

Death & Dying Sourcebook, 2nd Edition

Dental Care & Oral Health Sourcebook, 3rd
    Edition

Depression Sourcebook, 2nd Edition

Dermatological Disorders Sourcebook, 2nd Edition

Diabetes Sourcebook, 4th Edition

Di... Medi... ...k, 3rd Edition

...der Sourcebook

...ebook

Domestic Violence Sourcebook, 3rd Edition

Drug Abuse Sourcebook, 2nd Edition

Ear, Nose & Throat Disorders Sourcebook, 2nd
    Edition

Eating Disorders Sourcebook, 2nd Edition

Emergency Medical Services Sourcebook

Endocrine & Metabolic Disorders Sourcebook,
    2nd Edition

Environmental Health Sourcebook, 2nd Edition

Ethnic Diseases Sourcebook

Eye Care Sourcebook, 3rd Edition

Family Planning Sourcebook

Fitness & Exercise Sourcebook, 3rd Edition

Food Safety Sourcebook

Forensic Medicine Sourcebook

Gastrointestinal Diseases & Disorders
    Sourcebook, 2nd Edition

Genetic Disorders Sourcebook, 3rd Edition

Head Trauma Sourcebook

Headache Sourcebook

Health Insurance Sourcebook

Healthy Aging Sourcebook

Healthy Children Sourcebook

Healthy Heart Sourcebook for Women

Hepatitis Sourcebook

Household Safety Sourcebook

Hypertension Sourcebook

Immune System Disorders Sourcebook, 2nd
    Edition

Infant & Toddler Health Sourcebook

Infectious Diseases Sourcebook

Injury & Trauma Sourcebook